Global Perspectives on ADHD

T0369673

Global Perspectives on ADHD

SOCIAL DIMENSIONS
OF DIAGNOSIS AND TREATMENT
IN SIXTEEN COUNTRIES

Edited by
Meredith R. Bergey
Angela M. Filipe
Peter Conrad
Ilina Singh

Johns Hopkins University Press
Baltimore

Johns Hopkins University Press
2715 North Charles Street
Baltimore, Maryland 21218-4363
www.press.jhu.edu

Library of Congress Cataloging-in-Publication Data

Names: Bergey, Meredith, 1980– editor. | Filipe, Angela, 1983– editor. |
    Conrad, Peter, 1945– editor. | Singh, Ilina, editor.
Title: Global perspectives on ADHD : social dimensions of diagnosis and
    treatment in 16 countries / [edited by] Meredith R. Bergey, Angela M.
    Filipe, Peter Conrad, Ilina Singh.
Description: Baltimore : Johns Hopkins University Press, 2018. |
    Includes bibliographical references and index.
Identifiers: LCCN 2017008832 | ISBN 9781421423791 (paperback : alk. paper) |
    ISBN 9781421423807 (electronic) | ISBN 1421423790 (paperback : alk. paper)
    | ISBN 1421423804 (electronic)
Subjects: | MESH: Attention Deficit Disorder with Hyperactivity | Global
    Health—ethnology | Sociological Factors | Cross-Cultural Comparison |
    Child | Adolescent
Classification: LCC RJ506.H9 | NLM WS 350.8.A8 | DDC 362.196/8589—dc23
    LC record available at https://lccn.loc.gov/2017008832

A catalog record for this book is available from the British Library.

*Special discounts are available for bulk purchases of this book. For more
information, please contact Special Sales at 410-516-6936 or
specialsales@press.jhu.edu.*

Johns Hopkins University Press uses environmentally friendly book
materials, including recycled text paper that is composed of at least
30 percent post-consumer waste, whenever possible.

Contents

List of Contributors   *vii*

Preface   *ix*

1   ADHD in Global Context: An Introduction   1
    Meredith R. Bergey and Angela M. Filipe

2   The Rise and Transformation of ADHD in the United States   9
    Meredith R. Bergey and Peter Conrad

3   In the Elephant's Shadow: The Canadian ADHD Context   34
    Claudia Malacrida and Tiffani Semach

4   Historical, Cultural, and Sociopolitical Influences on Australia's
    Response to ADHD   54
    Brenton J. Prosser and Linda J. Graham

5   The Medicalization of Fidgety Philip: ADHD in Germany   77
    Fabian Karsch

6   ADHD in the United Kingdom: Conduct, Class, and Stigma   97
    Ilina Singh

7   The Emergence and Shaping of ADHD in Portugal:
    Ambiguities of a Diagnosis "in the Making"   118
    Angela M. Filipe

8   Transformations in the Irish ADHD Disorder Regime—
    from a Disorder "You Have to Fight to Get" to One
    "You Have to Wait to Get"   138
    Claire Edwards and Órla O'Donovan

9   The Journey of ADHD in Argentina: From the Increase in
    Methylphenidate Use to Tensions among Health Professionals   162
    Silvia A. Faraone and Eugenia Bianchi

10   Academic and Professional Tensions and Debates around
      ADHD in Brazil   186
      Francisco Ortega, Rafaela Zorzanelli, and Valéria Portugal Gonçalves

11   ADHD in the Italian Context: Children in the Midst of Social
      and Political Debates   208
      Alessandra Frigerio and Lorenzo Montali

12   The French ADHD Landscape: Maintaining and Dealing
      with Multiple Uncertainties   233
      Madeleine Akrich and Vololona Rabeharisoa

13   ADHD in Japan   261
      A Sociological Perspective   261
      Mari J. Armstrong-Hough
      Epidemiology, Treatments, and Cultural Influences   269
      Yasuo Murayama, Hiroyuki Ito, Junko Teruyama, and Masatsugu Tsujii

14   Pharmaceuticalization through Government Funding Activities:
      ADHD in New Zealand   288
      Manuel Vallée

15   From Problematic Children to Problematic Diagnosis:
      The Paradoxical Trajectories of Child and Adolescent
      ADHD in Chile   310
      Sebastián Rojas Navarro, Patricio Rojas, and Mónica Peña Ochoa

16   The Development of Child Psychiatry and the
      Biomedicalization of ADHD in Taiwan   332
      Fan-Tzu Tseng

17   Exploring the ADHD Diagnosis in Ghana: Between
      Disrespect and Lack of Institutionalization   354
      Christian Bröer, Rachel Spronk, and Victor Kraak

18   Reflections on ADHD in a Global Context   376
      Peter Conrad and Ilina Singh

      Index   391

Contributors

Madeleine Akrich, PhD, Director of Research, Mines ParisTech, France

Mari J. Armstrong-Hough, PhD, MPH, Associate Research Scientist in Epidemiology, Yale University, United States

Meredith R. Bergey, PhD, MSc, MPH, Assistant Professor, Villanova University, United States

Eugenia Bianchi, PhD, MSc, Assistant Professor, Universidad de Buenos Aires (UBA), and Researcher, Instituto de Investigaciones Gino Germani (UBA), Argentina. Assistant Researcher, National Scientific and Technical Research Council (CONICET), Argentina

Christian Bröer, PhD, Associate Professor of Sociology, University of Amsterdam, Netherlands

Peter Conrad, PhD, Harry Coplan Professor of Social Sciences, Brandeis University, United States

Claire Edwards, Lecturer, School of Applied Social Studies, University College Cork, Ireland

Silvia A. Faraone, PhD, MPH, Associate Professor, Universidad de Buenos Aires (UBA), and Researcher, Instituto de Investigaciones Gino Germani (UBA), Argentina

Angela M. Filipe, PhD, Research Fellow in Social Science, London School of Hygiene and Tropical Medicine, United Kingdom

Alessandra Frigerio, PhD, Postdoctoral Fellow in Social Psychology, Department of Psychology, University of Milano-Bicocca, Italy

Valéria Portugal Gonçalves, PhD, Postdoctoral Research Fellow, Institute for Social Medicine, State University of Rio de Janeiro, Brazil

Linda J. Graham, PhD, MEd, Associate Professor, Queensland University of Technology, Australia

Hiroyuki Ito, PhD, Assistant Professor, Research Center for Child Mental Development, Hamamatsu University School of Medicine, Japan

Fabian Karsch, PhD, MA, Postdoctoral Lecturer in Sociology and Health Science, Technical University of Munich, Germany

Victor Kraak, MA, Chartered Psychotherapist, NPI, Amsterdam, Netherlands

Claudia Malacrida, PhD, Professor of Sociology and Associate Vice President of Research, University of Lethbridge, Canada

Lorenzo Montali, PhD, Associate Professor of Social Psychology, Department of Psychology, University of Milano-Bicocca, Italy

Yasuo Murayama, PhD, Associate Professor, Faculty of Humanities and Sciences, Kobe Gakuin University, Japan

Órla O'Donovan, Lecturer, School of Applied Social Studies, University College Cork, Ireland

Francisco Ortega, PhD, Associate Professor, Institute for Social Medicine, State University of Rio de Janeiro, Brazil

Mónica Peña Ochoa, PhD, Facultad de Psicología, Universidad Diego Portales, Chile

Brenton J. Prosser, PhD, Senior Research Fellow, Australian National University, Australia

Vololona Rabeharisoa, PhD, Professor of Sociology, Mines ParisTech, France

Patricio Rojas, PhD Candidate, Department of Sociology, Goldsmiths, University of London, United Kingdom

Sebastián Rojas Navarro, Facultad de Psicología, Universidad Diego Portales, Chile and PhD Candidate, Department of Global Health & Social Medicine, King's College London, United Kingdom

Tiffani Semach, MA, University of Lethbridge, Canada

Ilina Singh, PhD, Professor of Neuroscience and Society, University of Oxford, United Kingdom

Rachel Spronk, PhD, Associate Professor of Cultural Anthropology, University of Amsterdam, Netherlands

Junko Teruyama, PhD, Assistant Professor, Faculty of Library, Information, and Media Science, University of Tsukuba, Japan

Masatsugu Tsujii, MA, Professor, School of Contemporary Sociology, Chukyo University, Japan

Fan-Tzu Tseng, PhD, Assistant Professor of Sociology, Fu-Jen Catholic University, Taiwan

Manuel Vallée, PhD, Lecturer in Sociology, University of Auckland, New Zealand

Rafaela Zorzanelli, PhD, Associate Professor, Institute for Social Medicine, State University of Rio de Janeiro, Brazil

Preface

This volume represents the collective effort of the four editors and the range of authors who contributed chapters. The book's origin stems back to a conversation between Peter Conrad and Ilina Singh in 2013. Peter and Ilina each had long-term research interests in ADHD and had conducted research in the United States and the United Kingdom, respectively. That conversation then extended to include two other researchers with interests in ADHD: Meredith Bergey and Angela Filipe. Peter and Meredith had already completed an article on the international migration of ADHD diagnosis and treatment and both Ilina and Angela had explored some comparative aspects of ADHD. Together we knew that there was no extant volume on the social dimensions of ADHD in different countries and we agreed that it would be a worthwhile endeavor to produce such a book. Thus our editorial team was born, with roots extending across both sides of the Atlantic.

The editors decided early on in the project that, with the exception of some general, specific topics that each author would be asked to touch on, chapters should be unique: focusing on case studies of specific countries rather than following formal comparative guidelines for each chapter. Wherever possible we wanted to emphasize the social dimensions of diagnosis and treatment from a social science perspective. Thus we solicited researchers whose work aligned with such a perspective, as opposed to the more clinical discussions that we felt had dominated much of the literature on ADHD. We located these authors through our own networks, contacting scholars who were engaged in ADHD research in a specific country, and asking colleagues about potential contributors. This turned out to be a greater, more time-intensive challenge than we had first anticipated.

In the end, we included authors for 16 countries. These are for the most part a purposive sample of countries, that is, countries where we could locate contributors with appropriate expertise. We were disappointed not to end up with contributions from additional countries, but we could not always locate appropriately involved social researchers or, in several cases, researchers who could provide an article in English. It turned out to be another challenge to edit a book where many of the chapters were contributed by authors for whom English was not their first language. For one country (Japan), we had two different contributors, much by happenstance, as one provided an interesting and important context for the other.

We thank all the contributors who worked with the editors to develop and focus their chapters so they fit the context and goals of the book. In some instances this took several revisions before the chapter met our needs. We appreciate their patience on a project of this size and scope. We are grateful for the assistance of Sharon Hogan, who came on to the project when it was already well on the way and provided her outstanding editorial expertise to improve readability across such a large volume. We also thank Robin W. Coleman, our editor at Johns Hopkins University Press, for his support and enthusiasm for this book. Finally, we are thankful for the electronic technology that facilitated the completion of a project whose editors and authors are scattered around the world.

Global Perspectives on ADHD

1

ADHD in Global Context

An Introduction

Meredith R. Bergey
Angela M. Filipe

A growing body of evidence indicates that attention deficit–hyperactivity disorder (ADHD) is being diagnosed and treated in an increasing number of countries around the world. Recent research suggests that ADHD is now the most common developmental or psychiatric diagnosis among school-age children and adolescents, with worldwide prevalence estimates of 5% and 7.2% (Polanczyk et al. 2014; Thomas et al. 2015). ADHD is being increasingly recognized as a lifespan disorder in many countries (see, e.g., Fayyad et al. 2007; NICE 2009; Nakamura et al. 2013), although far less research has focused on adult ADHD. Data show that the global consumption of psychostimulant medications—the most frequently prescribed treatment for ADHD—is growing as well (Scheffler et al. 2007; INCB 2015).

Findings such as these mark a notable shift in the worldwide picture of ADHD, which until roughly 25 years ago was far less global in scope. Prior to the 1990s, most of the reported diagnosis, treatment, and research related to ADHD occurred in the United States, where the diagnosis was originally devised and institutionalized. The diagnosis of ADHD emerged from the related diagnostic categories of "hyperactivity" and "minimal brain dysfunction." The most recent antecedent of ADHD is the diagnostic category of "attention deficit disorder (ADD: with or without hyperactivity)" from the 1980 American Psychiatric Association's

(APA) *Diagnostic and Statistical Manual of Disorders* (*DSM-III*), which described a disorder characterized by hyperactivity, impulsivity, and inattention (see chapter 2 for details.) The 1987 revision of this manual (*DSM-III-R*) renamed the condition "Attention Deficit / Hyperactivity Disorder," or "ADHD." This term has been used in subsequent revisions and has become the popular designation.

Given this heritage, it is perhaps not surprising that the prevalence of the ADHD diagnosis is highest in the United States, where 11% of school-age children (Visser et al. 2014) and 4% of adults (Kessler et al. 2006) have been diagnosed. The United States is also the country where psychostimulant medication was first widely used to treat symptoms that are associated with ADHD, and it continues to be the largest consumer of the world's supply of methylphenidate (Ritalin; INCB 2015). Until the early 1990s, there were few studies concerning the diagnosis and treatment of ADHD-related behaviors and its antecedents outside the United States, prompting some suggestions that ADHD might be a "culture-bound syndrome" (Canino and Alegria 2008). Given the changes in recent decades and the current dynamics and complexities surrounding ADHD, this is no longer a viable proposition.

A growing body of evidence points to an established and much more international interest in behaviors that constitute ADHD than has often been previously considered. Reports from a few countries outside the United States present historical accounts of troublesome behaviors, restlessness, and inattention that have been deemed not only as problems of childhood but also as objects of medical attention and intervention (e.g., the work of Frederic Still in the United Kingdom and Franz Kramer and Hans Pollnow in Germany). Regardless of whether such manifestations would align exactly with the current ADHD diagnosis, it is evident that increased attention is being paid in various countries to the diagnosis and treatment of what are considered the core symptoms of ADHD in children and adults: inattention, impulsivity, and hyperactivity. In addition, these behaviors have increasingly been diagnosed as ADHD on the basis of the APA's *DSM* criteria (Conrad and Bergey 2014).

Contributing to this increase is a shift in some European countries away from the use of the diagnostic criteria of the World Health Organization's (WHO) *International Classification of Diseases* (*ICD*, now in its tenth edition; WHO 2010). As table 1.1 illustrates, the *ICD* describes a similar diagnostic category called "hyperkinetic disorder." The *ICD* category presents a narrower diagnostic threshold than that described in the *DSM* (Conrad and Bergey 2014), meaning the *DSM* will define a larger number of children and adults as having ADHD.

Table 1.1. Key Differences in Diagnostic Criteria for ADHD and HKD

DSM: ADHD Diagnosis[a]	ICD: HKD Diagnosis
No later than 7 years	No later than 7 years
Symptoms in 1 or more dimension[b]	Symptoms in all dimensions[b]
Some impairment in at least 2 settings	Full criteria met in at least 2 settings
Comorbid conditions permissible (symptoms are not exclusively during comorbid period)	Comorbid conditions are exclusionary for diagnosis (e.g., schizophrenia and anxiety, mood, and pervasive developmental disorders)

[a]*DSM-IV* criteria are presented to align with references to continued usage of the *DSM-IV* in this volume; age of onset in the newly released *DSM-5* is no later than 12 years.
[b]Inattention, hyperactivity/impulsivity.

As is also apparent in table 1.1, the *ICD* and the *DSM* differ when defining the relationship between primary diagnosis and associated comorbidities and with respect to age of onset (with the recent change in the *DSM-5*). While this shift to the use of the *DSM* may be contributing to a redefinition of and an increase in the diagnosis of ADHD worldwide, it is occurring far from evenly and with a remarkable range of responses.

The emerging globalization of ADHD and its diagnostic criteria raises pressing questions and numerous issues for social scientists and clinicians to consider (Singh et al. 2013). For example, are global prevalence estimates homogenizing great differences both across and within various countries (Conrad and Bergey 2014)? How variable and valid are the *DSM*'s diagnostic criteria in various cultural settings (Singh et al. 2013)? How viable are they in different health care systems? Are psychostimulants and related medications considered to be appropriate treatment options, and are they being over- or underprescribed, especially for children (Parens and Johnston 2009)?

It appears that many of these issues manifest differently across countries. Recent reports suggest that the adoption of the *DSM* diagnostic criteria around the world has not been a straightforward affair, particularly if one considers the social dimensions and implications of such adoption or the individual and familial experiences of ADHD. Such factors have been highlighted by the varying reports from countries such as Italy (Frigerio, Montali, and Fine 2013), the Netherlands (Bröer and Heerings 2013), and Portugal (Filipe 2016). Comparative analyses of ADHD in the United States and the United Kingdom (Singh 2011) and in France and Ireland (Edwards et al. 2014) have more formally highlighted variations in the definition of and responses to behaviors that have been associated with ADHD—variations that have salient ethical, sociohistorical, and political aspects. This volume joins this small but growing body of research on the challenges, management, and framing of the diagnosis both across and within various cultural and national contexts.

What strikes us as most interesting is how the ADHD diagnosis is implemented, interpreted, and responded to in different countries. When countries begin to adopt the ADHD diagnosis, they frequently seem to integrate and apply the diagnosis in different and sometimes idiosyncratic ways. For example, some countries appear to adopt a "medications first" treatment strategy, whereas others adopt a "medications last" strategy, with yet others falling somewhere in between. Adoption of ADHD diagnostic criteria appears to have received considerable pushback among professionals and members of the public in some countries, but less so in others, and this adoption has reflected different historical and political circumstances. These are just a few of the heterogeneous circumstances that appear to surround ADHD in various national contexts.

Given this background, it is timely that current global perspectives on ADHD be brought together and considered in a multifaceted discussion that explores factors including the epidemiology, etiology, management, and meaning of ADHD in various contexts from a broad social science perspective. To explore the context and complexities surrounding ADHD in various global settings, we invited authors from around the world to provide case studies of their respective countries. A range of geographically diverse countries with different dominant languages, health care systems, and histories surrounding the adoption of ADHD were purposively sampled. In the end, we included the 16 countries where we could locate scholars who had an interest in and relevant experience with ADHD in their own country (fig. 1.1). Although this volume is not a formal comparative study, the countries it describes represent various historical trajectories, social contingencies, and medical and nonmedical approaches that shape ADHD diagnosis and treatment.

We have organized the chapters roughly in order of when the ADHD diagnosis was adopted in each country, spanning from earlier to more recent "adopters": the United States, Canada, Australia, the United Kingdom, Germany, Portugal, Ireland, Brazil, Argentina, Italy, Chile, France, New Zealand, Japan, Taiwan, and Ghana. We recognize that this list is by no means exhaustive or representative. Only one set of authors is presented for each country and we were unable to locate and include social scientists adequately familiar with ADHD to contribute

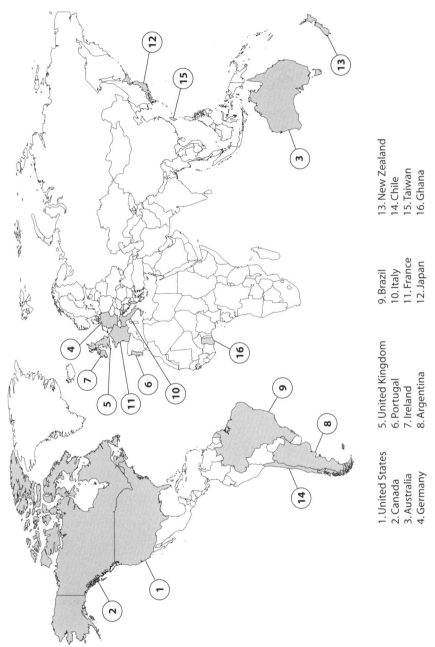

1. United States   5. United Kingdom   9. Brazil   13. New Zealand
2. Canada   6. Portugal   10. Italy   14. Chile
3. Australia   7. Ireland   11. France   15. Taiwan
4. Germany   8. Argentina   12. Japan   16. Ghana

Fig 1.1. Countries included in this volume.

chapters for several large and important parts of the world, including Eastern Europe, India, China, most of Africa, and the Middle East.

What we do have here is a wide range of countries and details regarding how these countries have adopted ADHD as a diagnosis. The chapters contained herein represent a first effort to present a collection of national and local responses to ADHD in a single volume. We see this volume as an initial opportunity to bring together global perspectives in order to better examine the range of adaptations and responses to the diagnosis of ADHD and to cultivate conversations that will broaden our understanding of ADHD in a global context.

Contributors to the volume were asked to provide country-specific analyses of the context surrounding ADHD and to discuss such topics as the emergence and introduction of the diagnosis, its epidemiology, advocacy and resistance groups, and the type and availability of treatments. In addition, authors were asked to discuss any unique country-specific issues that may exist around the diagnosis of ADHD, its treatment, or both. Specific data related to diagnosis and treatment were unreliable or unavailable in some countries, in which case our authors had to use the best estimates available.[1] In this respect, epidemiological and prescription data are presented in the following chapters as they were originally reported in the sources cited by the authors. In several cases, reported ADHD prevalence estimates also relied on different diagnostic criteria and sampling methods. This means that these reported data should be interpreted in the context in which they were generated and cannot be compared in absolute terms (see Singh et al. 2013; Filipe 2016).

This book also explores how behaviors that may be deemed to be consistent with ADHD have been challenged in various medical settings and cultural contexts, albeit in heterogeneous ways that are contingent on specific clinical and professional frameworks (as the chapters on Italy, New Zealand, and France illustrate). A number of authors examine the influence of socioeconomic and political transitions on the adoption of responses to ADHD in countries undergoing substantial changes in recent decades (as the cases of Argentina, Brazil, Ireland, and Portugal show). In addition, authors have considered the impact of various professional and advocacy groups (e.g., HyperSupers in France, the Attention Deficit Disorder Information and Support Service [ADDISS] in the United Kingdom, and Children and Adults with Attention-Deficit/Hyperactivity Disorder [CHADD] in the United States) on the process of adopting diagnostic criteria and treatment.

Both individually and collectively, the chapters in this book lay the foundation for a broader perspective on the social dimensions of the diagnosis and treatment of ADHD in the 16 countries examined. We hope that this volume will encourage a more inclusive conversation around ADHD in a global context, one that is based on a deeper comprehension of the dynamics and complexities of particular contexts. To the extent that we have accomplished this, we will have succeeded in expanding the understandings of the global scope and variations of ADHD.

NOTE

1. We recognize that although a text published in English will facilitate a broad readership, certain meanings may be lost in translation. Wherever possible, original terminology and indications on language variation were included (e.g., for ADHD, for advocacy groups, and for country-specific diagnostic manuals), along with discussion of issues of differentiation and translation in the diagnosis.

REFERENCES

American Psychiatric Association (APA). 1980. *Diagnostic and Statistical Manual of Mental Disorders (DSM-III)*. 3rd ed. Washington, DC: American Psychiatric Association.
———. 1987. *Diagnostic and Statistical Manual of Mental Disorders (DSM-III-R)*. 3rd ed., revised. Washington, DC: American Psychiatric Association.
Bröer, Christian, and Marjolijn Heerings. 2013. "Neurobiology in Public and Private Discourse: The Case of Adults with ADHD." *Sociology of Health & Illness* 35 (1): 49–65. doi:10.1111/j.1467-9566.2012.01477.x.
Canino, G., and M. Alegria. 2008. "Psychiatric Diagnosis—Is It Universal or Relative to Culture?" *Journal of Child Psychology and Psychiatry* 49 (3): 237–50.
Conrad, Peter, and Meredith R. Bergey. 2014. "The Impending Globalization of ADHD: Notes on the Expansion and Growth of a Medicalized Disorder." *Social Science & Medicine* 122: 31–43.
Conrad, Peter, and Deborah Potter. 2002. "From Hyperactive Children to ADHD Adults: Observations on the Expansion of Medical Categories." *Social Problems* 47: 59–82.
Edwards, Claire, Etaoine Howlett, Madeleine Akrich, and Vololona Rabeharisoa. 2014. "Attention Deficit Hyperactivity Disorder in France and Ireland: Parents' Groups' Scientific and Political Framing of an Unsettled Condition." *BioSocieties* 9 (2): 153–72. doi:10.1057/biosoc.2014.3.
Fayyad, J., R. De Graaf, R. Kessler, J. Alonso, M. Angermeyer, K. Demyttenaere, et al. 2007. "Cross-National Prevalence and Correlates of Adult Attention-Deficit Hyperactivity Disorder." *British Journal of Psychiatry* 190: 402–9.

Filipe, Angela M. 2016. "Making ADHD Evident: Data, Practices and Diagnostic Protocols in Portugal." *Medical Anthropology* 35 (5): 390–403. doi:10.1080/01459740.2015.1101102.

Frigerio, Alessandra, Lorenzo Montali, and Michelle Fine. 2013. "Risky and At-Risk Subjects: The Discursive Positioning of the ADHD Child in the Italian Context." *BioSocieties* 8 (3): 245–64. doi:10.1057/biosoc.2013.19.

Hinshaw, Stephan P., and Richard M. Scheffler. 2014. *The ADHD Explosion: Myths, Medication, Money, and Today's Push for Performance.* New York: Oxford University Press.

International Narcotics Control Board (INCB). 2015. "Report of the International Narcotics Control Board for 2014." New York: United Nations.

Kessler, R. C., L. Adler, R. Barkley, J. Biederman, et al. 2006. "The Prevalence and Correlates of Adult ADHD in the United States: Results from the National Comorbidity Survey Replication." *American Journal of Psychiatry* 163: 716–23.

Nakamura, S., M. Ohnishi, and S. Uchiyama. 2013. "Epidemiological Survey of Adult Attention Deficit Hyperactivity Disorder (ADHD) in Japan." *Japanese Journal of Psychiatric Treatment* 28: 155–62.

National Institute for Health and Clinical Excellence (NICE). 2009. *Diagnosis and Management of ADHD in Children, Young People and Adults.* London: The British Psychological Society and the Royal College of Psychiatrists.

Parens, Erik, and Josephine Johnston. 2009. "Facts, Values, and Attention-Deficit Hyperactivity Disorder (ADHD): An Update on the Controversies." *Child and Adolescent Psychiatry and Mental Health* 3 (1). doi:10.1186/1753-2000-3-1.

Polanczyk, G., E. G. Willcutt, G. A. Salum, C. Kieling, and L. A. Rohde. 2014. "ADHD Prevalence Estimates across Three Decades: An Updated Systematic Review and Meta-regression Analysis." *International Journal of Epidemiology* 43 (2): 434–42.

Scheffler, R. M., S. P. Hinshaw, S. Modrek, and P. Levine. 2007. "The Global Market for ADHD Medication." *Health Affairs* 26 (2): 450–57.

Singh, Ilina. 2011. "A Disorder of Anger and Aggression: Children's Perspectives on Attention Deficit/Hyperactivity Disorder in the UK." *Social Science & Medicine* 73 (6): 889–96.

Singh, I., A. M. Filipe, I. Bard, M. Bergey, and L. Baker. 2013. "Globalization and Cognitive Enhancement: Emerging Social and Ethical Challenges for ADHD Clinicians." *Current Psychiatry Reports* 15 (9): 385. doi:10.1007/s11920-013-0385-0.

Thomas, R., S. Sanders, J. Doust, E. Beller, and P. Glasziou. 2015. "Prevalence of Attention-Deficit/Hyperactivity Disorder: A Systematic Review and Meta-analysis." *Pediatrics* 135 (4): 994–1001. doi:10.1542/peds.2014-3482.

Visser, Susanna N., Melissa L. Danielson, Rebecca H. Bitsko, Joseph R. Holbrook, Michael D. Kogan, Reem M. Ghandour, Ruth Perou, and Stephen J. Blumberg. 2014. "Trends in the Parent-Report of Health Care Provider-Diagnosed and Medicated Attention-Deficit/Hyperactivity Disorder: United States, 2003–2011." *Journal of the American Academy of Child and Adolescent Psychiatry* 53 (1): 34–46.

World Health Organization (WHO). 2010. *International Classification of Diseases (ICD-10).* 10th ed. Geneva: World Health Organization.

2

The Rise and Transformation of ADHD in the United States

Meredith R. Bergey
Peter Conrad

The United States has in many ways been the epicenter of attention deficit–hyperactivity disorder (ADHD). The diagnosis of ADHD was developed and institutionalized in the United States in the American Psychiatric Association's (APA) *Diagnostic and Statistical Manual of Mental Disorders (DSM)*, and the United States is where the most frequently used treatments (psychostimulants) were first promoted to treat ADHD and hyperactivity more generally. Until the 1990s, the United States was the country with the highest estimated prevalence of ADHD in the world and this country continues to have some of the highest estimated rates of both diagnosis and treatment (Conrad and Bergey 2014). As of 2011, 11% of American school-age children had been diagnosed with ADHD (6.4 million children and adolescents between the ages of 4 and 17) and 8.8% (5.1 million) currently had ADHD (Visser et al. 2014). Of those children who had a current diagnosis, 69% (3.5 million children) were taking ADHD medications (Visser et al. 2014).

In this chapter we discuss the rise and transformation of ADHD in the United States. We begin by briefly reviewing related historical antecedents of the diagnosis before describing the development of diagnostic and treatment changes in this country. Next we discuss patterns in diagnosis and treatment, along with American ADHD advocacy groups, and some controversies and challenges that have emerged in the United States with respect to ADHD. We close the chapter with some reflections on ADHD in the twenty-first century.

The Emergence of ADHD

Behaviors that might today be consistent with a diagnosis of ADHD—hyperactivity, inattention, and impulsivity—have not always been associated with a medical disorder. There have been claims that evidence of ADHD can be traced back as early as 1845 in the characterization of Zappelphilipp (Fidgety Philip) in Heinrich Hoffmann's popular German children's book *Der Struwwelpeter* (Hoffmann 1845). Others point to Sir George Frederic Still's (1902) Goulstonian Lectures at the Royal College of Physicians of London in which he described conditions related to hyperactivity and impulsivity in children. In yet another example, the German physicians Franz Kramer and Hans Pollnow produced a report in 1932 "Über eine hyperkinetische Erkrankung im Kindesalter" ("On a Hyperkinetic Disease of Infancy"). They described a neurological disorder, called Kramer-Pollnow syndrome, which was characterized by hyperactivity and mental retardation. Examples like these suggest that certain behaviors that are now associated with ADHD have been considered problematic at different points in history (see Lange et al. 2010). None of these cases, however, seemed to prompt widespread diagnosis and/or treatment at the time. That did not occur until the 1960s in the United States.

The Establishment of ADHD in the United States

The medicalization of children's behaviors related to hyperactivity, impulsivity, and inattention (the core symptoms of ADHD) in the United States has historical roots in the early twentieth-century work of the American physician Charles Bradley. Bradley was the medical director of the Bradley Home, a facility in Rhode Island for children with various emotional, behavioral, and neurological impairments. Bradley's neurological evaluations of the children there involved pneumoencephalography, which can lead to intense headaches (Brown 1998). Bradley tried to treat the headaches with the stimulant drug benzedrine and observed something unexpected: although the drug had little effect on the headaches, it appeared to have a positive effect on behavior and school performance (Brown 1998).

Bradley conducted a controlled trial afterward and reported similar effects (Brown 1998). "It appears paradoxical that a drug known to be a stimulant should produce subdued behavior in half of the children," he noted (Bradley

1937: 582). There were a scattering of reports about this effect over the next two decades, mostly by Bradley and his colleagues. Others did not pick up on this finding, however, until roughly 20 years later (Conrad 1975; Lange et al. 2010)— at least in part because it was a treatment without a clear diagnosis. Another contributing factor might have been the wide popularity of psychoanalytical approaches at the time for addressing mental health issues (Brown 1998; Rothenberger and Neumarker 2005).

Two decades later, a group of researchers from the same Bradley Home picked up their predecessor's neglected research on amphetamines (Strohl 2011). Like Bradley, Maurice Laufer, Eric Denhoff, and Gerald Solomons (1957) showed that amphetamines were effective in reducing certain behavioral issues in children. In their 1957 report, they described a condition called hyperkinetic impulse disorder for which hyperactivity was the core symptom. Other characteristics included impulsivity, fidgetiness, and lack of attention. Laufer and his colleagues' (1957) research was influential as it outlined for the first time a specific diagnosis and associated treatment for such behaviors.[1]

The diagnosis of hyperkinetic impulse disorder was only one of several classifications used in the 1960s; others included minimal brain damage, minimal brain dysfunction, hyperkinesis, and hyperactive syndrome. Alongside questions about terminology, questions emerged regarding etiology—specifically around whether certain behavioral problems could occur in the absence of an organic cause (e.g., brain injury or damage). The Oxford International Study Group of Child Neurology held a conference in 1963 on this issue and concluded that the identification of problematic behavioral qualities alone was insufficient evidence from which to infer brain damage (Lange et al. 2010). The group subsequently recommended use of the term "minimal brain dysfunction" as opposed to "minimal brain damage" to emphasize this difference (Rothenberger and Neumarker 2005).

That same year, the National Society for Crippled Children and Adults, Inc., and the Neurological and Sensory Diseases Service Program of the Division of Chronic Diseases (part of the US Public Health Service) organized a symposium and follow-up meetings on the topic of the "child with minimal brain dysfunction" to discuss matters related to terminology, research, identification, and available services (Clements 1966: 3). Minimal brain dysfunction was depicted as a disorder that affects children in the normal range of intelligence; its core symptoms were inattention, impulsivity, and hyperactivity (Clements 1966: 9–10). A report from the meetings described biological causes, suggesting that symptoms "may arise from genetic variations, biochemical irregularities, perinatal brain insults or other illnesses or injuries sustained during the years which are critical for the development and maturation of the central nervous system, or from unknown causes" (Clements 1966: 9–10). Use of the term "minimal brain dysfunction" eventually declined during the 1960s because of concerns that the classification lacked specificity and sufficient empirical evidence (Rothenberger and Neumarker 2005; Barkley 2006).

Diagnostic Changes and Expansions

Emphasis shifted in the latter half of the twentieth century from identifying an organic cause to determining objective observations of deficits in children's behaviors (Barkley 2006: 6). Hyperactivity was the most notable characteristic and remained the central focus for making a diagnosis. A new diagnostic category called "hyperkinetic reaction of childhood" appeared in the 1968 second edition of the APA's *DSM* (*DSM-II*). Symptoms included hyperactivity, restlessness, and a short attention span. Such behaviors were said to typically subside by adolescence (APA 1968).

The *DSM-III* (APA 1980) marked a notable shift in diagnostic criteria by emphasizing inattention, as opposed to hyperactivity, as the primary deficit of concern (Wolraich 2006). The condition was subsequently renamed attention deficit disorder (ADD) and two subtypes were introduced: ADD with hyperactivity and ADD without hyperactivity (APA 1980). Three symptom lists were presented—one for hyperactivity, one for impulsivity, and one for inattention. The greater focus on inattention radically expanded the breadth of the diagnosis. Now not only disruptive and "overactive" children were diagnosed with ADHD but also children (often girls) who were "hypoactive" and "spacey."

The changes appearing in the *DSM-III* instigated debates about whether the new criteria were based in empirical evidence (Barkley 2006); when the revision to the third edition (*DSM-III-R*) was published in 1987, the two subtypes had been eliminated. The symptoms of hyperactivity, impulsivity, and inattention were presented in one list, with one cut-off score (Lange et al. 2010). Hyperactivity was reintroduced into the name and the condition was called attention deficit–hyperactivity disorder (ADHD).

The diagnosis expanded further in the mid-1990s in the fourth edition of the *DSM* (*DSM-IV*) (APA 1994). For most of its history, ADHD has been considered a condition of childhood. This is no longer the case in the United States. The notion that ADHD could extend beyond childhood began to gain acceptance in the

1980s and 1990s as lay, professional, and medical claims emerged to support an expanded diagnosis. Several articles appeared in the medical and psychiatric literature in the mid-1980s suggesting that symptoms of hyperactivity could persist into adulthood (see Conrad and Potter 2000), and a number of books were published in the 1990s that referred specifically to adult ADHD (e.g., Weiss 1992; Kelly and Ramundo 1993; Hallowell and Ratey 1994). The concept of adult ADHD appeared in popular media, including several television programs (e.g., *Good Morning America* and *20/20*) as well as in popular magazine articles (e.g., *Newsweek* and *Ladies' Home Journal*) (Stich 1993; Conrad and Potter 2000). ADHD was being increasingly depicted as a lifespan disorder, rather than just a disorder of childhood and adolescence.

The idea that the ADHD diagnosis could be applicable to adults grew in popularity despite the lack of any strong epidemiological or clinical evidence indicating a population of adults with ADHD (Conrad and Potter 2000). Several factors might have contributed to increased acceptance of the notion of a lifetime disorder. For example, a broad coalition of medical professionals, antipoverty activists, and disability and children's health and welfare advocates lobbied in the 1990s for more generous and expansive interpretations of how individuals qualified for programs designed to aid those with disabilities (Mayes, Bagwell, and Erkulwater 2008). Their efforts contributed to the passage of the Americans with Disabilities Act (ADA) in 1990. This policy "prohibits discrimination and ensures equal opportunity for persons with disabilities in employment, State and local government services, public accommodations, commercial facilities, and transportation" (http://www.ada.gov/2010_regs.htm). ADHD is included under the ADA "as a physical or mental condition, which may rise to the level of disability" (Wolf 2001: 386). This policy helped to further establish adult ADHD as a legitimate condition.

Another policy change occurred in 1991 when Congress included ADHD as a protected disability under the Individuals with Disabilities Education Act (IDEA) (Reid, Maag, and Vasa 1993). This change was due in part to lobbying efforts of parents of children with ADHD. IDEA is a federal funding statute that requires schools to provide a free and appropriate public education (FAPE) to children and adolescents with disabilities (Turnbull 2005). ADHD is included under the following categories: "specific learning disability," "serious emotional disturbance," and "other health impairment" (US Department of Education 2006). A diagnosis of ADHD does not automatically equate with eligibility, however; an individual must have a condition that corresponds with one of the aforementioned disability categories and need special education and associated services because of that disability (US Department of Education 1999). The addition of ADHD as a protected disability under IDEA increased the recognition of the disorder, particularly among educators (Mayes and Erkulwater 2008). As IDEA included adolescents and high school students, this might have contributed to an upward drift in the age bracket of ADHD diagnosis eligibility toward adulthood.

With the ADA and IDEA, the ADHD diagnosis could now position an individual within the broader classification of having a "disability"—a category that can provide an opening for certain accommodations in school (e.g., on homework and tests) as well as in the workplace (Conrad and Potter 2000; Mayes, Bagwell, and Erkulwater 2008). With these policy changes, the medicalization of adult ADHD attained further legal legitimization within the medical profession and with respect to employment and adult education (Conrad and Potter 2000).

The US-based support and advocacy organization Children and Adults with Attention Deficit/Hyperactivity Disorder (CHADD) was also influential in promoting the notion that ADHD can be a lifespan disorder. CHADD worked to bring together professional and lay claims-makers to promote better acceptance, understanding, and treatment of ADHD in general, as well as for adults (Conrad and Potter 2000). The group sponsored a national meeting in 1990 that featured adults with ADD (Jaffe 1995) and in 1993 they added "and Adults" to their name and co-sponsored a national conference called "The Changing World of Adults with ADD." The organization now considers the provision of education and support to adults with ADHD as part of its central mission. CHADD also advocates for legislation that grants certain protections in the workplace for adults with ADHD.

The widely held view that ADHD could persist into adulthood gained medical legitimacy in the *DSM-IV* (APA 1994). The new criteria were more inclusive—for instance, they recognized symptoms that might occur in more adult-specific contexts such as the workplace. Such change further increased the diagnostic reach of ADHD by reconstituting it as a lifespan disorder that was no longer limited to children (Conrad and Potter 2000). In addition to these changes, the *DSM-IV* introduced three subtypes: predominantly hyperactive-impulsive type, predominantly inattentive type, and a combined type (APA 1994). These subtypes reintroduced the possibility of a diagnosis being made for a solely inattentive form (Barkley 2006).

Psychotropic Medication for ADHD

An essential part of the ADHD story in the United States (and more globally) is the increase in the treatment of children with stimulant medications. This is what first brought ADHD to public attention in the 1970s (Conrad 1976), and it remains a topic of much debate in the United States. The main treatment of choice, beginning in the 1960s, was the drug Ritalin (methylphenidate). First synthesized by Leandro Panizzon in 1944, Ritalin was used to treat various conditions including depressive states, lethargy, chronic fatigue, and disturbed senile behavior (Leonard et al. 2004). Although they were not indicated for treating hyperactivity, stimulants had become an accepted treatment approach for behavioral problems in children, and Ritalin was often prescribed "off-label" in pediatric psychiatry (Singh 2006). The drug went through a series of clinical case studies, and was later approved by the US Food and Drug Administration (FDA)[2] for treating certain children's conditions (Chiarello and Cole 1987). Ritalin has since been widely promoted as a treatment for ADHD, and at one point in the 1990s, it was estimated that 90% of the world's Ritalin was sold in the United States—predominantly for ADHD treatment. Ritalin continued to be the main drug of choice until the 1990s (Diller 1998), when other popular drugs (e.g., Adderall, Concerta, and Vyvanse) gained traction in the market.

There is no question that the number of children who are prescribed medication for ADHD in the United States has increased markedly in recent decades. From 1987 to 1996, the annual growth rate in the percentage of children younger than 19 years of age taking stimulants was 17% (Zuvekas and Vitiello 2012).[3] A series of policy changes occurred in the 1990s that might have contributed to such an increase. Managed care practices grew in popularity over the course of that decade in an effort to curb soaring health care costs. The rise in managed care in behavioral health was associated with a growing reliance on prescription therapies to treat psychiatric and life problems (Johnson 1998). Managed behavioral health companies sought less expensive means of treatment with fewer hospitalizations, decreased lengths of hospital stay, decreased use of specialist services, limited psychotherapy, and increased reliance on psychotropic drug treatment (Mayes, Bagwell, and Erkulwater 2008).

Changes to the Supplemental Security Income (SSI) program in the early 1990s contributed to a rise in ADHD diagnosis, which might in turn have influenced the number of children being treated for the condition. The US Supreme

Court ruled in 1990 that the SSI program's provision of financial assistance to individuals with disabilities would include low-income children diagnosed with ADHD (Mayes, Bagwell, and Erkulwater 2008).[4] The number of new children enrolling with an ADHD diagnosis tripled before the expansion was rescinded in 1996 (Mayes, Bagwell, and Erkulwater 2008).

Around the same time that the US Supreme Court made its ruling on the SSI program's expansions, Congress significantly expanded Medicaid eligibility criteria to include a broader number of individuals—particularly children (Kronebusch 2001).[5] Mayes, Bagwell, and Erkulwater (2008) suggest that these expansions contributed to large increases in Medicaid expenditures on psychotropic drugs and stimulants. Medicaid spending on psychotropic drugs grew from $0.6 billion in 1991 to $6.7 billion in 2001; between 1991 and 2001, real (inflation-adjusted) expenditures per child receiving stimulant drugs rose nearly ninefold as the number of prescriptions rose by approximately sixfold (Cuellar and Markowitz 2007).

The use of prescription stimulants continues to rise, with a reported annual growth rate from 1996 to 2008 of 3.4% (Zuvekas and Vitiello 2012). More recent data indicate that the percentage of children 4 to 17 years of age taking ADHD medications increased from 4.8% in 2007 to 6.1% in 2011, a 27% increase in four years (Visser et al. 2014). More drugs for ADHD are prescribed in the United States than in the rest of the world combined (Sharpe 2014). From 1993 to 2003, the United States represented the largest market for ADHD medications, with an 83% to 90% share (Scheffler et al. 2007). Recent International Narcotics Control Board (INCB) (INCB 2015) estimates suggest that the United States continues to account for more than 80% of methylphenidate consumption worldwide.

The pharmaceutical industry has invested deeply in the promotion of the diagnosis and treatment of ADHD in the United States (as well as globally; see, e.g., Conrad and Bergey 2014).[6] Direct-to-consumer advertising (DTCA) in the country increased from $55 million in 1991 to $4.2 billion in 2005 (Conrad and Leiter 2009), and annual spending on DTCA for prescription drugs tripled between 1996 and 2000, reaching $2.5 billion (Rosenthal et al. 2002). Research also suggests that a 330% increase in DTCA occurred between 1996 and 2005 (Conrad and Leiter 2009). The FDA's relaxation of regulations and clarification of rules surrounding DTCA might have contributed to an already apparent increase in such advertising in the 1990s (Rosenthal et al. 2002; Abraham 2010).

DTCA is just one component of money spent on drug promotion. Pharmaceutical companies also market to physicians, psychologists, teachers, and other individuals involved in ADHD diagnosis and treatment (Phillips 2006; Timimi

2008). Companies such as Novartis, Janssen-Cilag, and Shire have helped fund ADHD-related advocacy groups (e.g., CHADD, the ADHD Coaches Organization [ACO], and the Attention Deficit Disorder Association [ADDA]), though it is often difficult to gauge the exact nature and degree of influence related to such investment (Barbarini 2014; Bergey 2015). Such contributions have raised debates about the role pharmaceutical companies should or should not play in supporting advocacy groups—with some criticizing drug-company funding as another mechanism by which pharmaceutical companies promote their goods, and others arguing that drug companies have an obligation to support advocacy groups.

Varied and Increasing Patterns of Diagnosis and Treatment for ADHD

The prevalence of ADHD in the United States continues to be one of the highest in the world. In 2010, the Centers for Disease Control and Prevention (CDC) estimated that 9.5% of US children (4 to 17 years of age) had an ADHD diagnosis. Estimates from the National Survey of Children's Health (NSCH) suggest that in 2011, 11% of school-age children had ever been diagnosed with ADHD—representing approximately 6.4 million children between the ages of 4 and 17 years (Visser et al. 2014). Of those children who had been diagnosed with ADHD, 82% currently had ADHD, for an estimated national prevalence of 8.8% (5.1 million children). These same data indicate a 42% increase between 2003 and 2011 in parent-reported history of ADHD.

Boys continue to be more likely than girls to have been diagnosed with ADHD (15.1% vs. 6.7%, respectively) (http://www.cdc.gov/ncbddd/adhd/data.html). However, the male-to-female ratio in diagnoses appears to have narrowed over time. The male-to-female ratio of ADD with hyperactivity reported in the *DSM-III* was 10:1 (APA 1980). In 1994, the APA suggested somewhere between 4:1 and 9:1, depending on whether the samples were community- or clinic-based (APA 1994; Singh 2008). This change may be due in part to factors such as an increased emphasis on inattention in recent versions of the *DSM*, better representation of females in ADHD studies, and growing awareness that symptoms of ADHD are not male-specific.[7]

There is also growing evidence to suggest that diagnosis is related to such factors as gender, race, ethnicity, household characteristics (e.g., household income, education, and primary language spoken), geographic residence, and health care coverage. Recent reports have raised some concerns about overdiagnosis among white children and underdiagnosis among certain minority groups (Morgan et al. 2013). Morgan et al. (2013) analyzed nationally representative data from the Early Childhood Longitudinal Study and found that blacks had 69% lower odds of being diagnosed with ADHD than whites. Compared to whites, the odds of being diagnosed with ADHD were 50% lower for Hispanics and 46% lower for a combined group of other races/ethnicities. According to aforementioned NSCH data, the prevalence of ADHD (ever-diagnosed) is highest for whites (12.2%), followed by blacks (11.9%) and other racial groups (7.2%) (Visser et al. 2014). These same data suggest that the prevalence of ADHD is roughly twice as high for non-Hispanics (12.3%) as it is for Hispanics (6.9%) (Visser et al. 2014). The CDC's 2013 report (Bloom, Jones, and Freeman 2013) on National Health Interview Survey (NHIS) data from 2012 presents similar findings. Hispanic children were found to be less likely to have an ADHD diagnosis (6%) than non-Hispanic black (9%) and non-Hispanic white (12%) children (Bloom, Jones, and Freeman 2013).

Findings such as these might reflect barriers to receiving a diagnosis; differential awareness of ADHD across segments of the population; biases among physicians who diagnose and treat; cultural differences between patients and providers regarding attitudes toward behavioral issues associated with an ADHD diagnosis; and a lack of culturally appropriate assessments for ADHD (Schmitz and Velez 2003; Stevens, Harman, and Kelleher 2004; Gerdes et al. 2013). Despite such differences, research suggests that from 2001 to 2010, rates of diagnosis for children 5–11 years of age increased among blacks (from 2.6% to 4.1%), Hispanics (from 1.7% to 2.5%), and whites (from 4.7% to 5.6%) (Getahun et al. 2013).

There is evidence that the prevalence of ADHD diagnosis varies according to characteristics of a child's household as well. For instance, children in single-parent families are more likely to have an ADHD diagnosis (12%) than children in families with two parents (8%) (Bloom, Jones, and Freeman 2013). Data from the NSCH indicate that prevalence is higher for children living below 200% of the federal poverty threshold than it is for children from higher-income families (Visser et al. 2014). The prevalence of ADHD is also higher among children living in households with 12 years of education (high school graduate) than it is among children living in households with less or more education (Visser et al. 2014). Children residing in households where English is the first language are more than four times as likely as those living in a household with another primary language to have been diagnosed with ADHD (Visser et al. 2014).

The likelihood of being diagnosed with ADHD also varies according to health insurance status. It is perhaps not surprising that children with health care coverage are more likely to have been diagnosed with ADHD than children without health care coverage (Visser et al. 2014). Comparisons of public versus private health insurance suggest that it is more common for children who have public health insurance to have been diagnosed with ADHD compared to those with private insurance (Visser et al. 2014).

ADHD diagnosis also varies markedly by geographic location. Generally speaking, it is less common to have been diagnosed with ADHD in the western region of the country and more common to have been diagnosed in the South (Visser et al. 2014). State-specific estimates of current ADHD are lowest in Nevada (4.2%) and New Jersey (5.5%) and the highest in Arkansas (14.6%) and Kentucky (14.8%) (Visser et al. 2014). Thus, in the United States, a child's chances of being diagnosed with ADHD appears to vary considerably according to the state she resides in and according to characteristics related to gender, race, ethnicity, household characteristics, and health care coverage. Further research is needed to better understand the social determinants underlying such disparities and whether such figures represent under- or overdiagnosis.

Of the children reported to have ADHD in 2007, 66.3% were taking medication for the condition (representing 4.8% of all children, 4 to 17 years of age, in 2007) (CDC 2010). In 2011, the prevalence of treatment with medication for ADHD was 6.1%—representing approximately 3.5 million children (Visser et al. 2014). Of those with a current diagnosis of ADHD, 69.0% were taking medication for the diagnosis (Visser et al. 2014). Stimulants are the most commonly prescribed medication for ADHD (NIMH 2008). Approximately 1 of every 20 to 25 children in the United States uses a stimulant medication (e.g., Adderall, Concerta, or Ritalin) to treat the condition (Rappley 2005; Zuvekas, Vitiello, and Norquist 2006). Moreover, the use of prescribed stimulants to treat ADHD has risen in recent decades. From 1987 to 1996, the growth rate in the percentage of children younger than 19 years of age using stimulants averaged roughly 17% per year (Zuvekas and Vitiello 2012). Growth in usage continued from 1996 to 2008, with a smaller average yearly increase of 3.4% (Zuvekas and Vitiello 2012). Overall, there is little question that the number of children taking ADHD medications has risen in the United States (Thomas, Mitchell, and Batstra 2013).

Patterns have emerged in medication use as well (Leslie and Wolraich 2007). For example, NSCH data indicate that in 2011 boys were more likely than girls to use medication. Prevalence of medication use was also higher for whites, non-Hispanics, children in households where English was the primary language spoken, children who have public health care, and children residing in the Midwest or the South. The percentage of youth in the 4- to 17-year-old age bracket currently taking medication for ADHD in 2011 was highest in Kentucky (10.1%) and Louisiana (10.4%) and lowest in Hawaii (3.2%) and Nevada (2%) (Visser et al. 2014).

Prescription rates also vary by race and ethnicity (Hoagwood et al. 2000; Stevens, Harman, and Kelleher 2005; Leslie and Wolraich 2007). Stevens, Harman, and Kelleher (2005) examined Medical Expenditure Panel Survey data and found that blacks were less likely both to be diagnosed with ADHD and to start stimulant medication treatment when compared to whites. The analysis of National Ambulatory Medical Care Survey (NAMCS) data from 1995 to 2000 by Hoagwood et al. (2000) suggests that even after controlling for such factors as gender, insurance coverage, length of visit, and age, whites were approximately nine times as likely to obtain a prescription from a clinician for a stimulant medication compared to other groups. Stevens, Harman, and Kelleher (2004) examined the 1995–2000 NAMCS data as well and found that although diagnosis and prescription for stimulant medications were more likely for whites than Hispanics, there were no differences in medication use by ethnicity after a diagnosis had been established.

Far less research pertaining to ADHD has been conducted on adults than on children and adolescents. The research that has emerged suggests that roughly 15% of those diagnosed as children still meet the complete diagnostic criteria as adults, while around half (40% to 60%) are still expected to have some of the ADHD symptoms (Faraone, Biederman, and Mick 2006). The estimated total prevalence of ADHD among adults who are 18 to 44 years of age is 4.4% (Kessler et al. 2006). When adults who are using prescribed stimulants for ADHD are included, the prevalence of pharmacologic treatment has risen by nearly 12% per year since 2000 (Castle et al. 2007). Research also suggests that from March 2002 to June 2005, the number of prescriptions for stimulant medications given to adults increased by 90% (Okie 2006). Further research is necessary to determine patterns of diagnosis and treatment among adults.

Advocacy Groups

Advocacy groups in the United States play an important role in providing ADHD-related information and support for providers, patients, and families around matters such as education, health care, treatment, employment, and public policy. CHADD is the largest support group in the United States and it has a broad reach—with local, national, and even international chapters (e.g., in Canada). CHADD's work and reach are facilitated by the group's large Internet presence. References to the organization and links to its website can be found on various ADHD information sites both in the United States and in other countries.

Although CHADD has largely held center stage, other prominent ADHD-related organizations in the United States include the ADDA and the ACO. The ADDA focuses predominantly on adults, as illustrated in its mission to provide "information, resources and networking opportunities to help adults with Attention Deficit Hyperactivity Disorder lead better lives" (http://www.add.org/). The ADDA also states that it seeks to "provide hope, empowerment and connections worldwide by bringing together science and the human experience for both adults with ADHD and professionals who serve them."

The ACO serves as a professional resource for ADHD coaches and their clients worldwide. ADHD coaching (described in more detail later in this chapter) refers to a nonmedical ADHD management approach with foundations in life coaching and corporate mentoring models (Bergey 2015). One of the ACO's stated aims is to connect potential clients with coaches by providing a repository of contact information for ADHD coaches residing across the United States and in various countries (mainly European) around the world. Like CHADD, both the ADDA and the ACO hold conferences around issues related to ADHD diagnosis, treatment, and advocacy, and the groups have an online presence for information sharing. Participant observation research at these yearly conferences suggests a certain degree of overlap in terms of membership, conference speakers, and leadership across these groups—particularly the latter two (Bergey 2015).

Eye-to-Eye is a national not-for-profit youth-mentoring program for children and young adults with learning disabilities and ADHD. Spread over 50 local chapters in more than 20 states and the District of Columbia, Eye-to-Eye works to build partnerships between a local college or high school and a middle or elementary school. Older students with learning disabilities and/or ADHD mentor younger students with the aim, not of "fixing" the students, but rather of helping them to develop their own unique styles of learning. Eye-to-Eye thus claims to adopt a strength-based approach and considers learning disabilities and ADHD to be "yet another aspect of human individuality to be recognized, embraced, and . . . even celebrated" (eyetoeyenational.org). The organization's stated vision is "to create a world in which people with LD/ADHD are fully accepted, valued, and respected—not just by society, but also by themselves—and that they live free from second thoughts or worry, ready, able, and eager to apply their unique strengths to whatever they encounter in life."

The list of advocacy groups in this section is by no means exhaustive. The groups noted above represent relatively large groups that have an extensive reach across the country, and in some cases more broadly.

Some Challenges to ADHD

ADHD diagnosis and treatment in the United States have not gone uncontested. ADHD has been in the public eye intermittently for decades. For example, a 1970 *Washington Post* article claimed that 10% of the 62,000 elementary school children in Omaha, Nebraska, were being treated with "behavior modification drugs to improve deportment and increase learning potential" (as quoted in Grinspoon and Singer 1973: 546). Although the figures were found later to be somewhat exaggerated, the piece nevertheless spurred a congressional investigation and a government-sponsored conference on treating behaviorally disturbed school children with stimulant drugs (Conrad 1976: 14). This attention did not lead to any restrictions on diagnosis or treatment. It did, however, raise the issue in the public sphere of "hyperactivity" and psychotropic drug treatment of school children. Although the diagnosis and treatment are now well accepted in the educational and medical domains, there are still critiques about "overdiagnosis" or overtreatment of children (see, e.g., Schwarz and Cohen 2013; Schwarz 2014).

In the 1970s, the allergist Ben Feingold (1974) proposed that the causes of hyperactivity were in the artificial food additives and food colors that children ingested as part of their regular diet. Feingold suggested that taking these additives out of children's diets would reduce hyperactive (and inattentive) behavior. As a compelling alternative to drug treatment, the diet received much media publicity. Although there were many personal testimonies about the success of the new diet, scientific studies of the Feingold diet were at best equivocal and most often showed little-to-no positive effect. Despite this, there are still advocates of the Feingold diet (see Smith 2011).

The most extreme and public critics of ADHD and its treatment come from the religious and advocacy organization the Church of Scientology and its offshoot, the Citizens Committee for Human Rights. The Scientologists are an avowedly anti-psychiatry organization, and in the 1980s the organization began a specifically anti-Ritalin campaign (Mieszkowski 2005). Led by media figures such as the Hollywood star Tom Cruise, the Scientologists have engaged in strong and sometimes misleading criticism about ADHD diagnosis and treatment (Neill

2005). Although the impact of this critique on ADHD diagnosis and treatment is probably quite small, it does keep a degree of criticism in the public eye.

There are also numerous professional criticisms of ADHD by psychiatric critics such as Thomas Szasz (2001), Peter Breggin (2001), and others (Timimi and Leo 2009). These perspectives are highly critical of ADHD and its treatment, though they are neither as seemingly animated nor as public as those of the Scientologists. There have been some concerns in the United States with overdiagnosis and treatment of ADHD (Thomas, Mitchell, and Batstra 2013). An article in *Scientific American* recently asked "Are Doctors Diagnosing Too Many Kids with ADHD?" (Lilienfeld and Arkowitz 2013), and a few years ago, the Public Broadcasting Service (PBS) produced a nationally broadcasted documentary entitled *Medicating Kids* that specifically raised the question *Does ADHD Exist?* (http://www.pbs.org/wgbh/pages/frontline/medicatedchild/etc/script.html). These kinds of critiques have led well-regarded ADHD researchers such as the psychologist Russell Barkley to express concern about "periodic inaccurate portrayal of ADHD in media reports" and "non expert doctors" who claim that ADHD does not exist (Barkley et al. 2002). Barkley argues that the scientific evidence overwhelmingly supports consensus that "ADHD is a valid disorder" (Barkley et al. 2002) and advocates for more, rather than less, ADHD treatment.

ADHD in the Twenty-First Century

As we reflect on the growth of ADHD in the twenty-first century in the United States, we can see a few trends that may affect the manifestations of ADHD. We close our chapter with a brief mention of each.

ADHD Medications as Cognitive Enhancement

In recent years, there has been an increasing concern about a "gray market" for stimulant medications where school- and college-age youth are obtaining and taking stimulants without prescription (Outram 2010; Smith and Farah 2011; Ragan, Bard, and Singh 2013). The notion is that these drugs become available when patients with proper prescriptions sell or trade their extra pills, or there is an underground market for drugs such as Ritalin and Adderall. These drugs are then taken as a cognitive enhancement by students who have no ADHD diagnosis, hoping to improve their focus and their academic performance (Singh et al. 2013). In their survey of prescription stimulant use among US undergraduate students across 119 different institutions in 2001, McCabe et al. (2005) found that an estimated 6.9% had used such drugs nonmedically in their lifetime. An estimated 4.1% had used them in the past year (McCabe et al. 2005). Smith and Farah (2011) estimate that the use of drugs for cognitive enhancement among US students ranges somewhere between 5% and 35%. Such diversions of drugs may contribute to public criticism about the rise in stimulant prescriptions. Although the reasons are not entirely clear, in 2012–13 there were actually reported shortages of legitimately prescribed stimulants in pharmacies, making it difficult for those with an ADHD diagnosis to obtain the drugs they were prescribed (Harris 2012).

The Continuing Expansion of the ADHD Diagnosis

As has been evident in this chapter, the threshold of an ADHD diagnosis has changed over the years, casting a wider diagnostic net. This includes the focus on inattention, the expansion of the age range to include adults, and the inclusion of ADHD as a disability. The percentage of the US population diagnosed with ADHD may increase further with the American Academy of Pediatrics' (AAP) newest guidelines, which delineate potential diagnosis and treatment for preschoolers as young as 4 years (AAP 2011; see also Zito et al. 2000). There is also some concern that the criteria for ADHD in the *DSM-5*, published in 2013, has expanded the threshold for diagnosing ADHD further (Thomas, Mitchell, and Batstra 2013). For example, fewer symptoms are required for diagnosis of ADHD in adolescents and adults and the age for the presentation of first symptoms can now be before 12 years rather than before 7 years (APA 2013). Some medical concern with overdiagnosis of ADHD (e.g., Coon et al. 2014) may balance the forces encouraging diagnostic expansion.

Alternative or Adjunct Interventions

Although clinical literature and guidelines have historically recommended medication treatment for ADHD, more recent recommendations often suggest the use of psychosocial interventions (e.g., behavioral therapy) alone or in conjunction with medication (Prince et al. 2006; Kolar et al. 2008; AAP 2011). Medication is increasingly being depicted as a treatment for effectively managing ADHD symptoms; psychosocial approaches, in contrast, are described as a possible adjunctive or alternative approach for addressing any residual symptoms or reducing additional impairments and consequences that may be related to ADHD (Knouse et al. 2008).

The mid-1990s saw the emergence of ADHD coaches as nonmedical advocates for ADHD education and awareness and as proponents of new techniques for managing ADHD. The group has begun to increase in size and national prominence in the past 10–15 years. Related to the wider "coaching" phenomenon (e.g., life coaches, fitness coaches, diabetes coaches), ADHD coaches present an alternative or adjunctive approach to medical or psychological interventions (Bergey 2015). The field is composed mainly of individuals who have ADHD and/ or who have family members with the condition (Wright 2013; Bergey 2015). Research suggests that early pioneers of the field were dissatisfied with what they perceived to be a lack of knowledge and understanding about ADHD among health care professionals. One of the core tenets of the ADHD coach approach is thus to bring awareness and education to individuals with ADHD, health care professionals, and the public at large—both in the United States and internationally (Bergey 2015). Moreover, ADHD coaches have argued that such knowledge should be accessible—not shrouded in scientific, medical jargon—and should be relevant to people's lived experiences with ADHD.

Although they do not deny the medical perspective, ADHD coaches take a more advisory perspective toward managing ADHD. "Pills don't teach skills," they suggest; medicine may be a viable treatment option, but more is needed to manage ADHD in everyday life (Bergey 2015). In contrast to psychological and medical approaches to managing ADHD, ADHD coaches also claim to take a strength-based approach—one that views the individual as creative, resourceful, and whole (Hart, Blattner, and Leipsic 2001; Bergey 2015). With ties to life coaching more broadly, ADHD coaches claim to facilitate one's abilities to clarify goals and devise realistic plans for attaining them (Whitworth et al. 2007). Many ADHD coaches seek to combine their lay expertise and coach training to help clients acquire skills to manage their own individual experiences with ADHD. Initially, ADHD coaching focused primarily on adult ADHD. There is now an increased emphasis on children and specific training programs for ADHD coaches who are interested in working with children as well. A relatively recently emerging, nonmedical approach, it is not yet clear what overall impact the coaching perspective will have on the medicalization of ADHD, or how pervasive the impact of such coaches will be.

GLOBAL MIGRATION OF ADHD

For several decades, the United States has been the center of ADHD diagnosis, research, and treatment along with a few other countries (e.g., Canada and Australia). But since the 1990s, there has been an increasing migration of the ADHD diagnosis and what we have previously referred to as "the impending globalization of ADHD" (Conrad and Bergey 2014). Research emerging from various countries around the globe suggests a diffusion of the ADHD diagnosis well beyond the United States and North America (Conrad and Bergey 2014). Polanczyk et al. (2007), Thomas et al. (2015), and Skounti, Philalithis, and Galanakis (2007) report ADHD prevalence estimates in a large number of countries, and Hinshaw et al. (2011) describe increases in medication usage in Australia, Brazil, Canada, China, Germany, Israel, the Netherlands, Norway, and the United Kingdom. Scheffler et al. (2007) examined IMS Health data from 1993 to 2003 and found that ADHD medication use increased threefold alongside a ninefold rise in global spending. More recent INCB (INCB 2015) data indicate significant increases in per capita consumption of methylphenidate over the past 10 years in Iceland, Norway, Sweden, Australia, Belgium, Germany, and Canada.

We have little doubt that this trend will continue and we have identified previously several vehicles that appear to be driving this migration (see Conrad and Bergey 2014 for details). These include the multinational pharmaceutical industry promoting the ADHD diagnosis and seeking new markets for its medications; the increasing global influence of US psychiatry; the increased adoption of the broader *DSM-IV* (now *DSM-5*) criteria for diagnosis (e.g., as opposed to the criteria from the World Health Organization's [WHO] *International Classification of Diseases [ICD]*); the easy and widespread availability of ADHD information and checklists on the Internet; and the increasing global presence of advocacy groups.

The United States has thus historically been considered to be at the center of much of the history of ADHD diagnosis and treatment. As recent research and the country-specific profiles in this volume will illustrate, this is no longer the case. Both diagnosis and treatment are increasingly being applied internationally. Furthermore, behaviors that may be deemed to be consistent with a diagnosis of ADHD have been discussed, debated, and addressed in heterogeneous ways in various countries. Although it is not yet clear how far ADHD diagnosis and treatment will migrate, it seems evident from our research and the chapters in this book that ADHD is transforming from a primarily North American phenomenon into a broadly global one, with all the medical and social consequences that may entail.

NOTES

1. While their research would have an important impact on the diagnosis and treatment of hyperactivity, reflecting the more dominant psychotherapeutic and Freudian

perspectives in psychiatry at the time, Laufer, Denhoff, and Solomons (1957) subordinated the importance of medication to psychotherapy (Mayes and Rafalovich 2007).

2. The FDA is a federal agency that regulates both prescription and nonprescription drugs, as well as various other types of products (e.g., medical devices, biologics, foods).

3. Analysis was conducted on data from the Medical Expenditures Panel Survey (MEPS), a nationally representative household survey of health care use and costs.

4. The SSI program provides benefits to children and adults with disabilities who lack adequate income and resources. Individuals ≥ 65 years of age who do not have disabilities, but who meet the financial requirements, may also receive benefits (http://www.ssa.gov/disabilityssi/ssi.html).

5. Medicaid is a government health care program, funded through both state and federal government contributions, for low-income and limited-resource families and individuals (http://medicaid.gov).

6. The market research firm Global Industry Analysts reports that "Global ADHD Therapeutics Market Research [Will] Reach $4.2 Billion by 2015" (http://www.strategyr.com/pressMCP-6195.asp).

7. The male-to-female ratios reported in clinic-based samples tend to be higher than those reported from population-based studies (APA 1987; Ramtekkar et al. 2010).

REFERENCES

Abraham, John. 2010. "The Sociological Concomitants of the Pharmaceutical Industry and Medications." In *The Handbook of Medical Sociology*, edited by Chloe E. Bird, Peter Conrad, Allen M. Freemont, and Stefan Timmermans, 290–308. 6th ed. Nashville, TN: Vanderbilt University Press.

American Academy of Pediatrics (AAP). 2011. "ADHD: Clinical Practice Guideline for the Diagnosis, Evaluation, and Treatment of Attention-Deficit/Hyperactivity Disorder in Children and Adolescents." *Pediatrics* 128: 1007–22.

American Psychiatric Association (APA). 1968. *Diagnostic and Statistical Manual of Mental Disorders (DSM-II)*. 2nd ed. Washington, DC: American Psychiatric Association.

———. 1980. *Diagnostic and Statistical Manual of Mental Disorders (DSM-III)*. 3rd ed. Washington, DC: American Psychiatric Association.

———. 1987. *Diagnostic and Statistical Manual of Mental Disorders (DSM-III-R)*. 3rd ed., revised. Washington, DC: American Psychiatric Association.

———. 1994. *Diagnostic and Statistical Manual of Mental Disorders (DSM-IV)*. 4th ed. Washington, DC: American Psychiatric Association.

———. 2013. *Diagnostic and Statistical Manual of Mental Disorders (DSM-5)*. 5th ed. Washington, DC: American Psychiatric Association.

Barbarini, Tatana de Andrade. 2014. "Medicalization through ADHD: Support and Resistance Groups in Brazil." Paper prepared for the meetings of the International Sociological Association.

Barkley, Russell A. 2006. *Attention-Deficit Hyperactivity Disorder: A Handbook for Diagnosis and Treatment*. New York: Guilford.

Barkley, Russell A., et al. 2002. "International Consensus Statement on ADHD." *Clinical Child and Family Psychology Review* 5 (2): 89–111.

Bergey, Meredith R. 2015. "The Rise of Attention Deficit Hyperactivity Disorder (ADHD) Coaching: The Social Meanings and Policy Implications of a New Approach for Managing ADHD." PhD diss., Brandeis University.

Bloom, Barbara, Lindsey I. Jones, and Gulnur Freeman. 2013. "Summary Health Statistics for U.S. Children: National Health Interview Survey, 2012." National Center for Health Statistics. *Vital and Health Statistics* 10 (258): 1–81.

Bradley, Charles. 1937. "The Behavior of Children Receiving Benzedrine." *American Journal of Psychiatry* 94: 577–85.

Breggin, Peter R. 2001. *Talking Back to Ritalin: What Doctors Won't Tell You about Stimulants and ADHD.* Cambridge, MA: Perseus.

Brown, Walter A. 1998. "Charles Bradley, M.D., 1902–1979." *American Journal of Psychiatry* 155: 968.

Castle, Lon, Ronald E. Aubert, Robert R. Verbrugge, Mona Khalid, and Robert S. Epstein. 2007. "Trends in Medication Treatment for ADHD." *Journal of Attention Disorders* 10: 335–42.

Centers for Disease Control and Prevention (CDC). 2010. "Increasing Prevalence of Parent-Reported Attention-Deficit/Hyperactivity Disorder among Children—United States, 2003 and 2007." *MMWR: Morbidity and Morality Weekly Report* 59 (44): 1439–43.

Chiarello, Robert J., and Jonathan O. Cole. 1987. "The Use of Psychostimulants in General Psychiatry: A Reconsideration." *Archives of General Psychiatry* 44: 286–95.

Clements, Sam D. 1966. "Minimal Brain Dysfunction in Children: Terminology and Identification (Phase One of a Three-Phase Project)." Washington, DC: US Department of Health, Education, and Welfare.

Conrad, Peter. 1975. "The Discovery of Hyperkinesis: Notes on the Medicalization of Deviant Behavior." *Social Problems* (October): 12–21.

———. 1976. *Identifying Hyperactive Children: The Medicalization of Deviant Behavior.* Lexington, MA: D. C. Heath.

———. 2007. *The Medicalization of Society: On the Transformation of Human Conditions into Treatable Disorders.* Baltimore: Johns Hopkins University Press.

Conrad, Peter, and Meredith R. Bergey. 2014. "The Impending Globalization of ADHD: Notes on the Expansion and Growth of a Medicalized Disorder." *Social Science & Medicine* 122: 31–43.

Conrad, Peter, and Valerie Leiter. 2009. "From Lydia Pinkham to Queen Levitra: Direct-to-Consumer Advertising and Medicalization." In *Pharmaceuticals and Society: Critical Discourses and Debates*, edited by Simon J. Williams, Jonathon Gabe, and Peter Davis, 12–24. Chichester: Wiley-Blackwell.

Conrad, Peter, and Deborah Potter. 2000. "From Hyperactive Children to ADHD Adults: Observations on the Expansion of Medical Categories." *Social Problems* 47: 59–82.

Coon, Eric R., Ricardo A. Quineoz, Virginia A. Moyer, and Alan R. Schroeder. 2014. "Overdiagnosis: How Our Compulsion for Diagnosis May be Harming Children." *Pediatrics* 134 (5): 1–11.

Cuellar, Alison, and Sara Markowitz. 2007. "Medicaid Policy Changes in Mental Health Care and Their Effect on Mental Health Outcomes." *Health Economics, Policy, and Law* 2: 23–28.

Diller, Lawrence. 1998. *Running on Ritalin: A Physician Reflects on Children, Society and Performance in a Pill.* New York: Bantam.

Faraone, Stephen V., Joseph Biederman, and Eric Mick. 2006. "The Age-Dependent Decline of Attention Deficit Hyperactivity Disorder: A Meta-Analysis of Follow-up Studies." *Psychological Medicine* 36: 159–65.

Feingold, Ben. 1974. *Why Your Child is Hyperactive.* New York: Random House.

Gerdes, Alyson C., Kathryn E. Lawton, Lauren M. Haack, and Gabriela Dieguez Hurtado. 2013. "Assessing ADHD in Latino Families: Evidence for Moving Beyond Symptomatology." *Journal of Attention Disorders* 17 (2): 128–40.

Getahun, Darios, Steven J. Jacobsen, Michael J. Fassett, Wansu Chen, Kitaw Demissie, and George G. Rhoads. 2013. "Recent Trends in Childhood Attention-Deficit/Hyperactivity Disorder." *JAMA Pediatrics* 167 (3): 282–88.

Grinspoon, Lester, and Susan Singer. 1973. "Amphetamines in the Treatment of Hyperactive Children." *Harvard Educational Review* 43: 525–55.

Hallowell, Edward M., and John J. Ratey. 1994. *Driven to Distraction: Recognizing and Coping with Attention Deficit Disorder from Childhood Through Adulthood.* New York: Simon & Schuster.

Harris, Gardner. 2012. "FDA Finds Short Supply of Attention Deficit Drugs." *The New York Times,* January 1, A1.

Hart, Vicki, John Blattner, and Staci Leipsic. 2001. "Coaching versus Therapy: A Perspective." *Consulting Psychology Journal: Practice and Research* 53: 229–37.

Hinshaw, Stephen P., and Richard M. Scheffler. 2014. *The ADHD Explosion: Myths, Medication, Money, and Today's Push for Performance.* Oxford: Oxford University Press.

Hinshaw, Stephen P., Richard M. Scheffler, Brent D. Fulton, Heidi Aase, Tobias Banaschewski, Wenhong Cheng, Paulo Mattos, Arne Holte, Florence Levy, Avi Sadeh, Joseph A. Sergeant, Eric Taylor, and Margaret D. Weiss. 2011. "International Variation in Treatment Procedures for ADHD: Social Context and Recent Trends." *Psychiatric Services* 62: 459–64.

Hoagwood, Kimberly, Peter S. Jensen, Michael Feil, Benedetto Vitiello, and Vinod S. Bhatara. 2000. "Medication Management of Stimulants in Pediatric Practice Settings: A National Perspective." *Journal of Developmental & Behavioral Pediatrics* 21: 322–31.

Hoffmann, Heinrich. 1845. *Der Struwwelpeter.* http://www.struwwelpeter.com.

International Narcotics Control Board (INCB). 2015. "Report of the International Narcotics Control Board for 2014." New York: United Nations.

Jaffe, Paul. 1995. "History and Overview of Adulthood ADD." In *A Comprehensive Guide to Attention Deficit Disorder in Adults: Research, Diagnosis, and Treatment,* edited by Kathleen G. Nadeau, 3–17. New York: Brunner/Mazel.

Johnson, Dale L. 1998. "Are Mental Health Services Losing Out in the U.S. under Managed Care?" *PharmacoEconomics* 14: 597–601.

Kelly, Kate, and Peggy Ramundo. 1993. *You Mean I'm Not Lazy, Stupid, or Crazy?! A Self-Help Book for Adults with Attention Deficit Disorder.* Cincinnati: Tyrell and Jerem.

Kessler, Ronald C., Lenard Adler, Russell Barkley, Joseph Biederman, C. Keith Conners, Olga Demler, Stephen V. Faraone, Laurence L. Greenhill, Mary J. Howes, Kristina Secnik, Thomas Spencer, Bedirhan Ustun, Ellen E. Walters, and Alan M. Zaslavsky. 2006. "The Prevalence and Correlates of Adult ADHD in the United States: Results from the National Comorbidity Survey Replication." *American Journal of Psychiatry* 163: 716–23.

Knouse, Laura E., Christine Cooper-Vince, Susan Sprich, and Steven A. Safren. 2008. "Recent Developments in the Psychosocial Treatment of Adult ADHD." *Expert Review of Neurotherapeutics* 8 (10): 1537–48.

Kolar, Dusan, Amanda Kellar, Maria Golfinopoulos, Lucy Cumyn, Cassidy Syer, and Lily Hechtman. 2008. "Treatment of Adults with Attention-Deficit/Hyperactivity Disorder." *Neuropsychiatric Disease and Treatment* 4: 389–403.

Kramer, Franz, and Hans Pollnow. 1932. "Über eine hyperkinetische Erkrankung im Kindesalter." *European Neurology* 82 (1–2): 1–20.

Kronebusch, Karl. 2001. "Medicaid for Children: Federal Mandates, Welfare Reform, and Policy Backsliding." *Health Affairs* 20: 97–111.

Lange, Klaus W., Susanne Reichl, Katharina M. Lange, Lara Tucha, and Oliver Tucha. 2010. "The History of Attention Deficit Hyperactivity Disorder." *Attention Deficit Hyperactivity Disorders* 2 (4): 241–55.

Laufer, Maurice W., Eric Denhoff, and Gerald Solomons. 1957. "Hyperkinetic Impulse Disorder in Children's Behavior Problems." *Psychosomatic Medicine* 19: 38–49.

Leonard, Brian E., Denise McCartan, John White, and David J. King. 2004. "Methylphenidate: A Review of Its Neuropharmacological, Neuropsychological and Adverse Clinical Effects." *Human Psychopharmacology: Clinical and Experimental* 19: 151–80.

Leslie, Laurel K., and Mark L. Wolraich. 2007. "ADHD Service Use Patterns in Youth." *Ambulatory Pediatrics* 7: 107–20.

Lilienfeld, Scott O., and Hal Arkowitz. 2013. "Are Doctors Diagnosing Too Many Kids with ADHD?" *Scientific American Mind* 24 (2): 72.

Mayes, Rick, Catherine Bagwell, and Jennifer Erkulwater. 2008. "ADHD and the Rise in Stimulant Use Among Children." *Harvard Review of Psychiatry* 16 (3): 151–66.

Mayes, Rick, and Jennifer Erkulwater. 2008. "Medicating Kids: Pediatric Mental Health Policy and the Tipping Point for ADHD and Stimulants." *Journal of Policy History* 20 (3): 309–43.

Mayes, Rick, and Adam Rafalovich. 2007. "Suffer the Restless Children: The Evolution of ADHD and Paediatric Stimulant Use, 1900–80." *History of Psychiatry* 18: 435.

McCabe, Sean Esteban, John R. Knight, Christian J. Teter, and Henry Wechsler. 2005. "Non-Medical Use of Prescription Stimulants among US College Students: Prevalence and Correlates from a National Survey." *Addiction* 100: 96–106.

Mieszkowski, Katharine. 2005. "Scientology's War on Psychiatry." *Salon.* http://www.salon.com/2005/07/01/sci_psy/.

Morgan, Paul L., Jeremy Staff, Marianne M. Hillemeier, George Farkas, and Steven Maczuga. 2013. "Racial and Ethnic Disparities in ADHD Diagnosis from Kindergarten to Eighth Grade." *Pediatrics* 132 (1): 85–93.

National Institute of Mental Health (NIMH). 2008. "Attention Deficit Hyperactivity Disorder." National Institutes of Health Publication No. 08-3572.

Neill, Ushma S. 2005. "Tom Cruise is Dangerous and Irresponsible." *Journal of Clinical Investigation* 115 (8): 1964–65.

Okie, Susan. 2006. "ADHD in Adults." *New England Journal of Medicine* 3254: 2637–41.

Outram, Simon M. 2010. "The Use of Methylphenidate among Students: The Future of Enhancement?" *Journal of Medical Ethics* 36: 198–202.

Phillips, Christine B. 2006. "Medicine Goes to School: Teachers as Sickness Brokers for ADHD." *PLOS Medicine* 3 (4): 182.

Polanczyk, Guilherme, Mauricio Silva de Lima, Bernardo Lessa Horta, Joseph Biederman, and Luis Augusto Rohde. 2007. "The Worldwide Prevalence of ADHD: A Systematic Review and Metaregression Analysis." *American Journal of Psychiatry* 164: 942–48.

Prince, Jefferson B., Timothy E. Wilens, Thomas J. Spencer, and Joseph Biederman. 2006. "Pharmacotherapy of ADHD in Adults." In *Attention Deficit Hyperactivity Disorder: A Handbook for Diagnosis and Treatment*, edited by Russell Barkley, 704–36. 3rd ed. New York: Guilford.

Ragan, C. Ian, Imre Bard, and Ilina Singh. 2013. "What Should We Do about Student Use of Cognitive Enhancers? An Analysis of Current Evidence." *Neuropharmacology* 64: 588–95.

Ramtekkar, Ujjwal P., Angela M. Reiersen, Alexandre A. Todorov, and Richard D. Todd. 2010. "Sex and Age Differences in Attention-Deficit/Hyperactivity Disorder Symptoms and Diagnoses: Implications for DSM-5 and ICD-11." *Journal of the American Academy of Child and Adolescent Psychiatry* 49 (3): 217–28.

Rappley, Marsha D. 2005. "Attention-Deficit Hyperactivity Disorder." *New England Journal of Medicine* 352: 165–73.

Reid, Robert, John W. Maag, and Stanley F. Vasa. 1993. "Attention Deficit Hyperactivity Disorder as a Disability Category: A Critique." *Exceptional Child* 60: 198–214.

Rosenthal, Meredith B., Ernst R. Berndt, Julie M. Donohue, Richard G. Frank, and Arnold M. Epstein. 2002. "Promotion of Prescription Drugs to Consumers." *New England Journal of Medicine* 346 (7): 498–505.

Ross, Dorothea M., and Sheila A. Ross. 1976. *Hyperactivity: Research, Theory and Action.* New York: Wiley.

Rothenberger, Aribert, and Klaus-Jurgen Neumarker. 2005. *Wissenschaftsgeschichte der ADHS. Kramer-Pollnow im Spiegel der Zeit.* Darmstadt: Steinkopff.

Scheffler, Richard M., Stephen P. Hinshaw, Sepideh Modrek, and Peter Levine. 2007. "The Global Market for ADHD Medication." *Health Affairs* 26 (2): 450–57.

Schmitz, Mark F., and Maricruz Velez. 2003. "Latino Cultural Differences in Maternal Assessments of Attention Deficit/Hyperactivity Symptoms in Children." *Hispanic Journal of Behavioral Sciences* 25 (1): 110–22.

Schwarz, Alan. 2014. "Thousands of Toddlers are Medicated for ADHD Report Finds, Raising Worries." *The New York Times*, May 16, A1.

Schwarz, Alan, and Sarah Cohen. 2013. "A.D.H.D. Seen in 11% of U.S. Children as Diagnoses Rise." *The New York Times*, March 31.

Sharpe, Katherine. 2014. "Evidence is Mounting that Medication for ADHD Doesn't Make a Lasting Difference to Schoolwork or Achievement." *Nature* 506: 146–48.

Singh, Ilina. 2008. "Beyond Polemics: Science and Ethics of ADHD." *Nature Reviews Neuroscience* 9: 657–64.

———. 2006. "A Framework for Understanding Trends in ADHD Diagnoses and Stimulant Drug Treatment: Schools and Schooling as a Case Study." *BioSocieties* 1 (4): 439–52.

Singh, Ilina, Angela M. Filipe, Imre Bard, Meredith Bergey, and Lauren Baker. 2013. "Globalization and Cognitive Enhancement: Emerging Social and Ethical Challenges for ADHD Clinicians." *Current Psychiatry Reports* 15: 385–93.

Skounti, Maria, Anastas Philalithis, and Emmanouil Galanakis. 2007. "Variations in Prevalence of Attention Deficit Hyperactivity Disorder Worldwide." *European Journal of Pediatrics* 166 (2): 117–23.

Smith, M. Elizabeth, and Martha J. Farah. 2011. "Are Prescription Stimulants 'Smart Pills'? The Epidemiology and Cognitive Neuroscience of Prescription Stimulant Use by Normal Health Individuals." *Psychological Bulletin* 137 (5): 717–41.

Smith, Matthew. 2011. *An Alternative History of Hyperactivity: Food Additives and the Feingold Diet.* New Brunswick, NJ: Rutgers University Press.

Stevens, Jack, Jeffrey S. Harman, and Kelly J. Kelleher. 2004. "Ethnic and Regional Differences in Primary Care Visits for Attention-Deficit Hyperactivity Disorder." *Journal of Developmental and Behavioral Pediatrics* 25: 318–25.

———. 2005. "Race/Ethnicity and Insurance Status as Factors Associated with ADHD Treatment Patterns." *Journal of Child and Adolescent Psychopharmacology* 15: 88–96.

Stich, Sally. 1993. "Why Can't Your Husband Sit Still?" *Ladies Home Journal* (September): 74–77.

Still, George Frederic. 1902. "Some Abnormal Psychical Conditions in Children: The Goulstonian Lectures." *The Lancet* 1: 1008–12.

Strauss, Alfred A., and Laura E. Lehtinen. 1947. *Psychopathology and Education of the Brain-Injured Child.* Vol. 1. New York: Grune and Stratton.

Strohl, Madeleine P. 2011. "Bradley's Benzedrine Studies on Children with Behavioral Disorders." *Yale Journal of Biology and Medicine* 84: 27–33.

Szasz, Thomas. 2001. *Pharmacracy: Medicine and Politics in America.* New York: Praeger.

Thomas, Rae, Geoffrey K. Mitchell, and Laura Batstra. 2013. "Attention-Deficit Hyperactivity Disorder: Are We Helping or Harming?" *British Medical Journal* 347: f6172.

Thomas, Rae, Sharon Sanders, Jenny Doust, Elaine Beller, and Paul Glasziou. 2015. "Prevalence of Attention-Deficit/Hyperactivity Disorder: A Systematic Review and Meta-analysis." *Pediatrics* 135 (4): 994–1001.

Timimi, Sami. 2008. "Child Psychiatry and Its Relationship with the Pharmaceutical Industry: Theoretical and Practical Issues." *Advances in Psychiatric Treatment* 14: 3–9.

Timimi, Sami, and Jonathan Leo. 2009. *Rethinking ADHD: From Brain to Culture.* New York: Palgrave Macmillan.

Turnbull, H. Rutherford. 2005. "Individuals with Disabilities Education Act Reauthorization: Accountability and Personal Responsibility." *Remedial and Special Education* 26 (6): 320–26.

US Department of Education. 2006. 34 CFR Parts 300 and 301. Assistance to States for the Education of Children With Disabilities and Preschool Grants for Children With Disabilities; Final Rule.

———. 1999. "Children with ADD/ADHD—Topic Brief." http://www2.ed.gov/policy/spe ced/leg/idea/brief6.html.

Visser, Susanna N., Melissa L. Danielson, Rebecca H. Bitsko, Joseph R. Holbrook, Michael D. Kogan, Reem M. Ghandour, Ruth Perou, and Stephen J. Blumberg. 2014. "Trends in the Parent-Report of Health Care Provider-Diagnosed and Medicated Attention-Deficit/Hyperactivity Disorder: United States, 2003–2011." *Journal of the American Academy of Child and Adolescent Psychiatry* 53 (1): 34–46.

Weiss, Lynn. 1992. *Attention Deficit Disorder in Adults: Practical Help for Sufferers and Their Spouses.* Dallas: Taylor.

Whitworth, Laura, Karen Kimsey-House, Henry Kimsey-House, and Phillip Sandahl. 2007. *Co-active Coaching: New Skills for Coaching People toward Success in Work and Life.* Mountain View, CA: Davies-Black.

Wolf, Lorraine E. 2001. "College Students with ADHD and Other Hidden Disabilities: Outcomes and Interventions." *Annals of the New York Academy of Sciences* 931: 385–95.

Wolraich, Mark L. 2006. "Attention-Deficit/Hyperactivity Disorder." *Infants and Young Children* 19 (2): 86–93.

Wright, Sarah D. 2013. *ADHD Coaching Matters: The Definitive Guide.* College Station, TX: ACO Books.

Zito, Julie Magno, Daniel J. Safer, Susan dosReis, James F. Gardner, Myde Boles, and Frances Lynch. 2000. "Trends in the Prescribing of Psychotropic Medications to Preschoolers." *JAMA* 283 (8): 1025–30.

Zuvekas, Samuel H., and Benedetto Vitiello. 2012. "Stimulant Medication Use in Children: A 12-year Perspective." *American Journal of Psychiatry* 169 (2): 160–66.

Zuvekas, Samuel H., Benedetto Vitiello, and Grayson S. Norquist. 2006. "Recent Trends in Stimulant Medication Use among U.S. Children." *American Journal of Psychiatry* 163: 579–85.

3

In the Elephant's Shadow

The Canadian ADHD Context

Claudia Malacrida
Tiffani Semach

The trajectory of the emergence and solidification of attention deficit–hyperactivity disorder (ADHD) in Canada is, as former Canadian Prime Minister Pierre Trudeau once famously said about Canada-US relations in general, reflective of sleeping with an elephant, in that "no matter how friendly and even-tempered is the beast . . . one is affected by every twitch and grunt" (O'Malley and Thompson 2003: vii). The introduction of ADHD as a legitimate diagnosis and of psychopharmaceutical medication as its primary treatment, the populist reactions to those developments, and the grassroots activism and regulatory policies that have arisen in Canada to manage ADHD and its treatment have all unfolded within the context of American influence by way of a highly permeable US-Canadian border. As will be discussed more fully below, suspicions have been expressed in the popular media and among the general public and some professionals that the emergence of ADHD in Canada has not only been influenced by, but also echoes, the United States in terms of diagnosis and treatment. That said, more recent developments in advocacy and professional practice relating to ADHD indicate that there have been efforts to move away from American models to carve out a more specifically Canadian approach.

The Perceived Legitimacy of ADHD and US-Canadian Border Permeability

Part of the shared context centers on the criteria used in diagnosing ADHD in Canada and the United States. Canada has long accepted the American Psychiatric Association (APA) guidelines outlined in its *Diagnostic and Statistical Manual of Mental Disorders* (*DSM*), which includes much broader symptoms and earlier acceptable ages of identification than those outlined by the World Health Organization's (WHO) *International Classification of Diseases* (*ICD*) (Malacrida 2003). In addition, the contexts of public discourse relating to both favorable and critical arguments about ADHD and its treatment are similar in Canada and the United States. Of course, mommy blogs, psychological and medical information sites, and virtual support groups have the capacity to transcend all national borders in terms of transferring information and support, but in Canada both the blogosphere and more traditional media are heavily influenced by US content. In terms of lay literature on health, "problem" children, education, and ADHD, most of the parenting magazines available on Canadian newsstands are American; Canadian bookstores carry books about self-help, health, psychology, and parenting that are primarily published in the United States; and American television programming dominates Canadian airwaves (Clarke 2011).

Finally, up until recently, the US-based Children and Adults with Attention Deficit/Hyperactivity Disorder (CHADD), which describes itself as a recognized authority on ADHD and which has sustained a strong lobbying effort toward legitimating the disorder (Conrad and Schneider 1980; Conrad 2006), has operated as many as 40 chapters in Canada (Malacrida 2003).[1] Among the activities sponsored through the Canadian CHADD groups have been a number of regular "ADD fairs" that offered workshops for professionals, a place for service providers to market their wares, and information for parents about both mainstream and alternative treatments for ADHD. At these venues, much of the information (including US-based keynote speakers) and most of the products, ranging from biofeedback techniques and behavior modification protocols to "nutraceuticals" (dietary supplements and super-vitamins), came from US sources (Malacrida 2002, 2003). Given the pervasive presence of American media, products, and services available to concerned parents and educators, it is fair to state that the US-based normalization of ADHD as a common childhood disorder (Mayes, Bagwell, and Erkulwater 2009) has deeply influenced how Canadian parents, medical professionals, and educators respond to ADHD.

Although much of the information and knowledge that crosses the US-Canadian border is positive in tone, it also includes a significant amount of negative coverage about ADHD as a diagnosis and, most pressingly, about the aggressive and inappropriate use of medication in young children, producing an ambivalent context in which educators and parents must operate (Clarke 2011). Much of this discourse draws on strong anti-Ritalin activism originating from the United States, in particular through Peter Breggin, a prominent anti-psychiatry figure who has conducted speaking tours in Canada and whose books and website are part of the populist Canadian landscape concerning ADHD. During the late 1990s, several series of articles in local and national newspapers and related television media engendered and reflected a general backlash against what was seen as an alarming propensity to label children's behavioral problems as psychiatric diagnoses and a new willingness to medicate children with psychopharmaceuticals (see, e.g., Palmer and Bongers 1997; Rees and Dawson 1998; Rees 1998a, 1998b; Schatsky and Yaroshevsky 1997). While much of this critique does reference or reflect US-based critiques, there is also an ironic anti-American slant to the criticisms, in which the United States is frequently portrayed as a looming and negative influence because of its purported pill-popping culture, skyrocketing ADHD rates, and for-profit medical complex. Much of this criticism has rested on the claim that Canada's own diagnostic and medication rates echoed similar trends occurring south of the border in the United States (Chisholm 1996; Bongers 1997; Mate 2000), which has not in fact necessarily been the case.

The American effect on Canadian medical and psychological professionals' thoughts and practices is hard to trace, although it is fair to speculate that professionals encounter influences similar to those of any other Canadian in terms of exposure to American popular media on health and education. Further, although professional research on ADHD is international in scope, the United States remains a leader in the field, with some of the literature and research on ADHD going so far as to conflate Canada with the United States, characterizing the two as North America as though the two countries are synonymous in their handling of ADHD (Buitelar et al. 2006). American professional associations for doctors, psychiatrists, psychologists, and educators are much larger than their Canadian counterparts, and they actively recruit and include Canadian membership and attendance at their conferences and annual meetings. Similarly, the American pharmaceutical industry disseminates its research and markets its products through Canadian doctors' offices and through professional events such as sponsored conferences and marketing/informational retreats (Malacrida 2003). In sum, the professional and research context in which Canadian physicians, educators, and psychologists operate is strongly embedded within American discourse and practice.

Rates of Diagnosis and Treatment in Canada

As noted above, in populist Canadian critiques and in some of the more critical professional and academic literature, it is often claimed that ADHD rates in Canada have echoed those of the United States. In addition, much of the available research on ADHD in Canada uncritically reports statistics that actually come out of the United States as though they were Canadian data. For example, Statistics Canada, the national government bureau that collects and analyzes Canadian population, educational, and medical information, issued a major report on mental health in Canada, using US sources and US data to explain the status of ADHD in Canada (Langlois et al. 2011). That report repeated the American research—that ADHD is one of the most common of childhood conditions, with 1 in 20 children being so labeled, that boys are three times more likely than girls to "develop" it, and that symptoms persist into adulthood in 75% of all cases—as though these claims apply universally to the Canadian context (Langlois et al. 2011). The rate of 1 in 20 directly reflects figures presented in the APA's *DSM-5*, which estimates a worldwide childhood ADHD diagnostic rate of 5% (APA 2013).

In actuality, it is difficult to know whether the permeable border relating to the legitimation and acceptance of ADHD has actually resulted in similar rates of diagnosis or in similar treatment options in the two countries. In Canada, medical coverage and public education, although funded primarily through federal taxation, is administered and regulated at provincial levels. As a result, published research on medication rates (rather than diagnostic rates) has been predominantly based on medical record-keeping at the provincial level, and none of these data have been reported in a systemic way.

In Ontario, where almost one-third of Canada's 35 million people live, one fairly early study found that 9.6% of all boys and 3.3% of all girls under the age of 18 years had been diagnosed, which is in keeping with some reported US diagnostic rates (Szatmari, Offord, and Boyle 1989). More recent provincial studies on diagnostic rates in Ontario and Quebec suggest that the reported national statistics of less than 3% of children—which we discuss more fully below—may actually under-report Canadian diagnostic rates; in the early 2000s, the Ontario Child Health Study reported diagnostic rates of 6.1% among children and youth between 4 and 16 years of age, and the Quebec Child Mental Health Survey reported a diagnostic rate of 5.4% across the same ages (Charach, Lin, and To 2010). A notable difference between the Ontario and Quebec provincial studies and the National Longitudinal Survey of Children and Youth (NLSCY) is the inclusion of teacher-reported symptoms in the provincial studies, supporting the proposition that parent-reported surveys may underestimate the rates of affected youth (Charach, Lin, and To 2010).

Another concern about inter-provincial ADHD rates in Canada is raised in a study in British Columbia that examined the effect of age-of-entry to school and likelihood of diagnosis. In this study, questions arise about the influence of school entry age on the likelihood of increasing ADHD diagnoses. In most provinces, including British Columbia, the cut-off date for admission to first grade occurs when a child turns 6 prior to December 31, so that children born in January must wait considerably longer to enter school than children born before year-end. Researchers conducted a cohort study of 937,943 children between the ages of 6 and 12 years and compared birth dates and diagnostic rates, finding that boys born in December were 30% more likely than boys born in January to receive an ADHD diagnosis, while for girls that difference skyrocketed, with December-born girls 70% more likely than January-born girls to be diagnosed (Morrow et al. 2012). The increases are even higher in terms of the likelihood of being medicated; December-born boys are 41% more likely and December-born girls are 77% more likely to be taking psychoactive medication for the ADHD diagnosis (Morrow et al. 2012).

Education (like health care) is a provincial rather than a federal matter in Canada; however, not all provinces use the same cut-off dates. Ontario, Canada's most populous province, holds March 31 as its cut-off, as does Alberta; however, in response to concerns about school-readiness, the Alberta Catholic School Board and numerous local public boards have opted for dates that would make their entering students older than in other jurisdictions (CBC 2013). Over and above how problematic it is that the age of a child being admitted to school seems to have an undue effect on his likelihood of being diagnosed with a mental disorder, these variances also mean that there is probably significant variation in overall diagnostic rates among Canadian provinces.

Nationally aggregated data about ADHD diagnoses and the use of various medical treatments have only been collected in Canada since 1994 through the biannual NLSCY, and even this instrument has not consistently included questions about ADHD, nor has it regularly included children in all age groups even when ADHD rates have been measured (Brault and Lacourse 2012). Because the NLSCY survey is primarily parent-reported, researchers have suggested actual rates of affected children may be underestimated since some parents may not accept an "ADHD" label for their children (Charach, Lin, and To 2010; Brault and Lacourse 2012). Further problems with this instrument arise from the fact that it has excluded children from the Northwest Territories, Yukon, and Nunavut (with predominantly indigenous populations); First Nation reserves; institutional facilities; and children with an immediate family member in the army (Brault and Lacourse 2012). The exclusion of children from indigenous groups and those living in correctional, mental health, and child welfare facilities may mean that ADHD rates are significantly underreported in the NLSCY, given the high rates of disability and social, learning, and behavioral challenges among children in these categories (Fuchs et al. 2010; Chapman 2012; Lindblom 2014).

The NLSCY does not include children who have been labeled informally by parents or teachers (rather than by a physician or psychologist), or who are being treated through nonmedical interventions at school (such as decreased classroom size, in-class supports, breaking up daily routines, and behavioral feedback techniques) and at home (such as diet, fish oil supplements, nutraceuticals, biofeedback, and behavioral programs). Rather, reports on formally labeled children, based on prescription rates for Ritalin, Strattera, Dexedrine, Adderall XR, and Vyvanse, are used to measure ADHD levels across the country (Brault and Lacourse 2012). Finally, none of these data include diagnoses or treatment of adults identified with ADHD, a sector that has burgeoned since changes were made in the *DSM* to include adult-onset and adult-identified symptoms (Conrad 2007; Loe 2008), although it has been estimated that between 2% and 6% of adults may have the diagnosis (Weiss and Murray 2003). The dearth of data on adults identified and treated means that the overall figures on ADHD diagnosis and treatment for all Canadians remains something of a black box.

Given the above caveats, a hallmark paper on the diagnostic rates among preschool and school-age children in Canada drew on the NLSCY data to outline the prevalence and trajectory of ADHD, using three cross-sectional samples from 1994 to 2007. The authors concluded that "the estimated prevalence of prescribed medications and ADHD diagnosis in Canada was . . . less than 3%" (Brault and Lacourse 2012: 93) and that while the prevalence among boys was higher than that among girls, the prevalence among girls was increasing more rapidly than that among boys. The authors also noted that between 1994 and 2007, the use of prescribed ADHD medications had significantly increased by 1.6-fold for all children. The increase was most marked among school-age children, at 1.9-fold (i.e., almost double), which they attributed to the introduction of new long-acting medications and to the publication, beginning in the year 2006, of national guidelines through the Canadian ADHD Resource Alliance (CADDRA), which have contributed to parents' and professionals' awareness of symptoms and bolstered trust in the use of pharmaceuticals in treating ADHD (Brault and Lacourse 2012).[2]

Bearing in mind the gaps produced by excluding adults; individuals in the child welfare, mental health, and justice systems; non-medicated children; and many indigenous people, the 2006–7 round of the NLSCY provides the most recent Canadian data on childhood diagnostic rates for ADHD. According to NLSCY data, the reported percentage of preschool and school-age boys and girls who are diagnosed is now 3.7% and 1.5%, respectively—figures that are significantly below the 1 in 20 estimate anticipated in the *DSM-5* (Charach, Lin, and To 2010).

Canadian Regulations and Clinical Guidelines

Until 2006, there were no national guidelines for practice concerning the diagnosis or treatment of ADHD in Canada. To illuminate how diagnosis operated prior to these guidelines, Malacrida's research examining assessment and treatment in the province of Alberta found that there were really no consistent guidelines in operation (Malacrida 2001, 2003, 2004). Rather, children could be referred for assessment through their family physician, a pediatrician or psychiatrist, several private-fee assessment centers, or a medical setting such as the Alberta Children's Hospital. Each of these sites offered widely divergent assessment protocols. For example, parents described processes with general practitioners and pediatricians that involved extremely brief consultations in response to educator or parental self-referrals. These then resulted in a seemingly pro forma process of diagnosis by administering medication trials—sometimes coupled with paper-and-pencil behavioral checklists and sometimes just medication alone. In these reports, it seems that if the medication changed the child's behavior, this was taken as proof that ADHD was the correct diagnosis for the original referral. Other, more affluent parents described using private clinics of specialist psychologists and related child development experts, whose approach was to recommend an assessment process that involved multidisciplinary professionals observing and assessing the child in multiple sites, including at home and in school

(Calgary Learning Centre 1997). Other parents described how the impetus for assessment originated and remained in the child's school. Such assessments were guided in principle by municipal and district school boards, sometimes drawing on provincial Ministries of Education policies on special education guidelines to inform the accommodations.

In Alberta, one such board suggested at the time that a multimodal and multisite assessment process that would involve parents, school-based psychologists, educators, and resource specialists was the ideal standard for diagnosis (Calgary Board of Education 1999). However, public funding for these specialists was limited and children experienced lengthy wait-lists due to high demand (Malacrida 2003). Because parents either experienced pressure from educators to have their children tested, or were themselves impatient to obtain help for their struggling children, a number of them sought private services offering the recommended multimodal, multisite psychological assessments. However, those private assessments were not paid for through public health care coverage in Canada, and the costs for many parents were prohibitive. As a result, it remained typical that parents and children used the quicker, if perhaps less reassuring, route of government-funded, medically driven physician assessments rather than the recommended multimodal process (Malacrida 2003).

Relying on family physicians to provide reassuring and well-managed assessments may not always be optimal. A survey of more than 800 family physicians in the province of British Columbia indicated that many of them preferred to refer their patients to a pediatrician because of their lack of comfort in dealing with ADHD, which one can reasonably anticipate would be a common psychosocial problem facing patients of family physicians (Miller et al. 2005). Surprisingly, these family physicians expressed more comfort and confidence in taking on primary care responsibility for children's mood disorders such as depression or bipolar disorder than ADHD, admitting a lack of confidence about dealing with behavior problems among their charges (Miller et al. 2005). Similarly, researchers in the province of Manitoba conducted a study that drew on the medical records of almost 5,000 ADHD-identified children, controlling for variables such as age, sex, region, neighborhood income level, and physician specialty. They found that while a relatively low 1.9% of children were diagnosed and an even lower 0.89% received stimulant medication, children in urban areas were four times more likely than rural children to be identified with ADHD, and they were eight times more likely to be prescribed stimulant medication, regardless of physician specialty or socioeconomic factors (Brownell and Yogendran 2001).

The authors conclude that these extreme variations in diagnosis and treatment were strongly influenced by the individual practice styles of the physicians, calling for better training of medical practitioners in managing this childhood disorder.

In an attempt to improve diagnosis and treatment in Canada, in the early 2000s, CADDRA, a national nonprofit group of professionals, was formed and in 2006 it published its first set of guidelines in the hopes that they would be taken up as standardized practice in Canada (CADDRA 2011). The makeup of CADDRA is decidedly and narrowly medical; the editorial board for the 2011 guidelines was composed of seven psychiatrists, five medical doctors (mostly pediatricians), and one psychologist. All the editors, with the exception of the psychologist, indicate working as advisory board members, speakers, or grant-holders for major pharmaceutical companies involved in producing ADHD medications. In addition, the actual membership of the organization operates hierarchically along medical and nonmedical lines: "full membership" with voting privileges is only open to "practising physicians or specialists with Canadian certification to practice medicine in Canada," whereas non-voting "associate membership" is offered to "certified and practising health care professionals such as psychologists, social workers . . . and nurses who have an interest in the field of ADHD" (CADDRA 2014: n.p.).

The guidelines committee reviewed policies and guidelines from the United States (including the *DSM* and the American Academy of Pediatrics [AAP] guidelines) and from the United Kingdom (including the National Institute for Health and Care Excellence [NICE] guidelines and the British Association for Psychopharmacology guidelines), noting that the difference between American and British approaches is almost contradictory. The US guidelines suggest medicine first and the addition of other treatments second, whereas the UK guidelines suggest medication only for extreme cases. CADDRA notes that its guidelines are intended to enhance and standardize Canadian practices, which the authors argue are characterized by "holistic-based care, individualized to the patients" (CADDRA 2011: v). According to the authors, this kind of holistic-based care is characterized as something of a third way between the British and American models. The idealized holistic model includes educating "patients" and their families, behavioral strategies, psychological treatment, educational accommodations, and, finally, "medical management (as a way to facilitate the other interventions)" (CADDRA 2011:vii). This latter characterization of medical management as a mere facilitator is perhaps overly optimistic, as we will see in this chapter's section on treatment. Further, despite these stated goals of medicine as just one plank in the platform of standard treatment for Canadians identified with ADHD, it has been suggested that this publication of a set of comprehensive Canadian guidelines has coincided with a fairly steep rise in medication rates. Indeed, some authors speculate that this rise has occurred because of increased physician confidence in ADHD as a diagnosis and enhanced trust in the use of psychopharmaceuticals engendered by these guidelines (Brault and Lacourse 2012).

Although CADDRA recommends its guidelines for all Canadian physicians and "other professionals" in diagnosing ADHD, neither the government nor the Canadian Medical Association requires physicians to follow the CADDRA guidelines. As such, the choice of diagnostic guidelines and manuals remains at the discretion of individual doctors, and in practice, doctors may follow American-based resources because they are more readily accessible and recognized by physicians across North America. Even Canadian advocacy groups direct parents of children affected by ADHD to American-based resources; for example, the Centre for ADHD Awareness Canada (CADDAC), a national group endorsed by CADDRA, directs individuals to several US websites for information on assessment and treatment protocols (CADDAC 2014b).

That said, there are commonalities between the CADDRA guidelines and those indicated in the APA's *DSM-IV* (APA 1994) and, more recently, the *DSM-5* (APA 2013). All three guidelines are highly medical in their approach, with a medical examination recommended as the first order of an assessment, and with medication highlighted as, at the very least, a core rather than last-option treatment. Each recommends that the behavior of children and adolescents across all social settings should be a significant factor considered during the diagnostic process; in addition, they all recommend that assessments include input from parents and other adults such as teachers, daycare providers, and coaches who are in substantial daily contact with the children. It is thus difficult to say how truly different the CADDRA guidelines actually are from US models. Nevertheless, the ideals proposed in all guidelines—whether Canadian or American—do not necessarily get spooled out in Canadian children's actual assessments, where a need for expediency and a lack of funding and resources for these ideal assessments often mean that children are diagnosed without multisite observations or input from multiple adults in the child's life.

Canadian Approaches to Nonmedical Treatment

In terms of treatment options in Canada, CADDRA's national guidelines recommend medication as a facilitating part of a holistic treatment protocol that should include behavioral strategies; psychological treatment; classroom and workplace accommodation; counseling and supports for time management, social and organizational skills; and support for individuals, families, and professionals as they advocate for these accommodations at home, in the school, and in the workplace (CADDRA 2011: vii, 6.1–6.10). That said, it is difficult to know how well these goals are being met for Canadians who have been identified with ADHD. Canada enjoys a generous federally funded but provincially administered system of public health care, so that the services of doctors and psychiatrists—but *not* those of social workers, educational specialists, or psychologists—are covered through public health funding. This may mean that children and adults with ADHD have differential access to nonmedical treatment; in effect, poorer individuals may be more bound to stay within the medical-model coverage provided by the government, whereas wealthier individuals may have increased scope to seek nonmedical interventions. It also means that the scope of nonmedical services being provided in Canada remains hidden. Although physicians and psychiatrists are required to submit information on prescriptions for most ADHD-related drugs for reporting through their provincial medical associations, nonmedical professionals do not have such reporting requirements. There are undoubtedly large profits derived from both medical and nonmedical treatments of ADHD in Canada as elsewhere (as evidenced in the listing of professional services and supports on the CADDAC resource pages). That said, because services such as biofeedback, nutraceuticals, dietary supplements, individual and group counseling, specialty camps, specialist schools, self-esteem workshops, tutoring and supplemental classes, and behavioral programs are not tracked in any methodical way, it is difficult to know exactly the extent of those profits or how many people with ADHD are being treated in nonmedical ways either alone or in tandem with medication.

Schools are, or should be, key players in providing support and accommodation for children identified with ADHD, and there have been suspicions that (over)medicating children occurs simply because schools fail to provide adequate educational accommodations for children with ADHD (Kean 2004; Malacrida 2004). Unfortunately, as with other nonmedical interventions, it is difficult to trace the exact extent of the demand for educational accommodations or to assess Canadian educators' responses to that demand—although it is often stated that most Canadian classrooms, because of a general ethos of classroom inclusion, will house at least two or three children who are either formally or informally diagnosed with ADHD (Martinussen et al. 2006). At present, ADHD diagnosis and treatment in Canada are managed through medical professionals without significant input from or collaboration with educators; although teachers frequently initiate the referral, once the actual diagnostic process is initiated it is handled almost exclusively by medical personnel (Edmunds and Martsch-Litt 2008). Thus, although the CADDRA guidelines indicate that medication should simply be used to reduce the core symptoms of ADHD, and thus permit a more effective response to behavioral and educational interventions, in practice it is unlikely that such interventions will be implemented as part of a sustained, collaborative treatment approach. It is also unlikely that the medical personnel involved in diagnosing and medicating a child would have any involvement in, information about, or perhaps even interest in nonmedical treatments for their patients. This disconnect can have profound implications for the successful treatment of Canadian children diagnosed with ADHD, leading to poor case management of a child's problems at best, and an over-reliance on medication at worst.

In addition to the negative impact of a system of diagnosis and treatment that separates medical from nonmedical personnel, funding arrangements and teacher training can also contribute to gaps in the Canadian treatment context. Education is a provincial matter in Canada, and local school boards are granted significant autonomy within the confines of federal and provincial educational jurisdictions. In practice, this means that in some provinces, funding for a child identified with ADHD may result in some form of individualized funding that would provide that specific child with personalized supports. In some jurisdictions, however, funding for children who are identified as requiring special accommodations for ADHD will not find its way to the individual child, but will instead be folded into the broader educational budget of a classroom or sometimes even a school (Malacrida 2003). Finally, in many cases, funding specific to ADHD is not really an option; rather, it is only available for individuals identified with ADHD if they also have disorders such as learning disabilities, or severe behavioral challenges, so that children whose ADHD is not coupled with other disorders that are disruptive to the general classroom will not be eligible for classroom supports beyond that of any other child in the classroom (Martinussen et al. 2006). Formal supports for a child with ADHD in Canada are thus contingent on a number of things, including funding arrangements, the kind of diagnosis the child receives, and the policies of inclusion and support that are specific to the educational jurisdiction of the child's school.

In terms of informal supports, although there is broad evidence that teacher attitudes and knowledge can have a significant effect on the likelihood of a child being diagnosed, and further, that teachers have the capacity to meaningfully support children with ADHD by providing them with educational and social accommodation in classes, there is little research in the educational, psychological, or disability studies literature that specifically speaks to the availability or efficacy of classroom or workplace accommodation for children and adults with ADHD in Canada. It is clear, however, that even though classrooms in Canada ostensibly operate under an ethos of inclusion, teachers are not always trained in providing special accommodations for children with ADHD. Because ADHD is not formally recognized (as evidenced by the funding situation described above) in most Canadian educational systems, and because educators are so marginalized within the assessment and treatment approaches in Canada, there is little collaboration or knowledge transfer between medical and educational systems. Further, this marginalization has meant that education systems express little motivation for training teachers about how to address or treat ADHD. Indeed, most teacher training programs at Canadian universities do not have a requirement that "special" education be included as part of teachers' coursework, and there is significant evidence that post-graduation professional development is an ineffective corrective to these gaps (Chaban 2010).[3] As a result, it is fair to assume that despite CADDRA guidelines to the contrary, many ADHD-identified children in Canadian classrooms are being treated solely through medication since teachers lack the training or institutional supports needed to implement meaningful classroom accommodations.

Canadian Support and Advocacy

In light of these significant gaps between medical and educational funding, and between teacher and medical professional engagement with children's ADHD assessments and treatment, it is important to examine the kinds of community support and advocacy available to individuals with ADHD that might help bridge those gaps. As noted earlier, in the late 1990s there were as many as 40 branches of the US-based CHADD offering support meetings, conferences, workshops, and information fairs in Canada (Malacrida 2003), but currently only the Calgary and Vancouver branches appear to continue with an active local program. The Calgary chapter—which simultaneously represents itself online as CHADD-Canada—appears to have been inactive since 2012 (CHADD Canada 2014). According to the CHADD-Canada site, CHADD first developed in Ontario through the work of a social worker and a psychologist working in ADHD parent support groups. These two, along with a handful of interested parents, began the first Canadian branch of CHADD in Ottawa, Ontario, in 1991. By 1993, the organization had obtained charitable status and had branches across Canada (CHADD Canada 2014). The subsequent attrition of CHADD chapters may simply reflect that Canadian parents seeking information are still doing so through CHADD, but they are doing so online using the American site, which offers a wide range of information and services.

Another possibility may be the establishment of CADDAC, a national, not-for-profit network of educators and professionals offering both face-to-face and online education, awareness, and advocacy about ADHD-related issues in Canada for the past five years (CADDAC 2014b). CADDAC is a remarkably well-structured and well-connected organization: the group's president and executive director also served as the executive director of CADDRA (the group that produces Canada's national ADHD guidelines); the board includes high-profile philanthropists and fundraisers; and the advisory board includes well-placed academics and researchers in education, pediatrics, and psychiatry across the country (CADDAC 2014a). CADDAC's activities are extensive, including offering public speakers and workshops through local clinics and schools, and providing advice on setting up and obtaining funding for local support groups. CADDAC also moves beyond the local setting by posting polished public service announcements and conference presentations on YouTube (including a number of talks by the renowned American ADHD proponent Russell Barkley); offering an online research clearing-house about parenting, adult-identified ADHD, stress management, and workplace/school challenges; providing an extensive listing of local support groups across the country and information about available funding, scholarships, and bursaries for individuals diagnosed with ADHD; operating a blog and a Facebook page about ADHD and its related problems; posting lists of specialized schools and helping professionals serving learning and attentionally challenged children; providing detailed information about the kinds of classroom accommodations that parents should expect and lobby for; organizing fundraisers and distributing its promotional and information materials to local branches as part of a national ADHD Awareness Month; and providing interviews to local and national media outlets about ADHD awareness (CADDAC 2014b). In sum, this group offers a cornucopia of information and supports to parents, professionals, and adults interested in ADHD.

In keeping with this mandate, one of CADDAC's more recent foci is on increasing awareness of ADHD in adulthood, arguing that "this is worth repeating since it's one of the key reasons why we must up the awareness towards government and physicians . . . It is estimated that 90 per cent of adults living with ADHD are untreated, mainly due to lack of diagnosis and access to knowledgeable physicians. BTW, the vast majority of ADHD kids grow up to be ADHD adults!" (CADDAC 2014c).[4] Thus, like CHADD in its early years in America, CADDAC is working not only to serve existing ADHD needs, but it is also actively seeking to broaden acceptance of the ADHD diagnosis and its intervention (Conrad 2006). Unlike CHADD, however, CADDAC's funding is not tied to the pharmaceutical industry. The organization relies instead on donations, membership fees, and conference fees. A key and apparently effective means of obtaining funding operates through its membership mechanisms, in that organizations that join are also given a place on the site's resource listings; thus, in return for a relatively inexpensive $100 annual membership fee, support groups, service providers, and related organizations are then listed on CADDAC's information clearinghouse service. This arrangement undoubtedly provides a significant income since the resource lists hundreds of services, including private assessment clinics; private schools; ADHD coaches; psychologists; camps; clubs, tutors, and online tutoring; and support groups. In sum, CADDAC is a powerhouse of information and dissemination that seeks not only to support and empower people with ADHD but also to enhance the scope and legitimacy of that disorder in Canada.

A clear indication that the legitimation of ADHD is virtually complete in Canada is evidenced by the fact that for the past several years, ADHD has been recognized as a disability at both provincial and federal levels, meaning some diagnosed individuals may be eligible for a disability tax credit. A tax credit is not a straight reimbursement of fees, but instead offers the individual a reduced level of taxation to compensate for costs incurred related to the disability. Thus, individuals who hire consultants, counselors, or lifestyle/behavioral coaches; who attend specialist private schools; who participate in camps and workshops; or whose medications and assessments are not covered through other means may receive part of those costs back as a tax refund if the impairment is deemed to warrant such support.

In the case of a child or adolescent under the age of 18 years affected by ADHD, the parent or guardian may be eligible to receive the credit on the child's behalf. In order to qualify for the disability tax credit, an individual must be documented as severely physically or mentally affected for a prolonged period by her ADHD diagnosis, or be significantly affected by what are considered to be typical comorbid disorders such as autism spectrum disorder, oppositional defiance disorder, depression, or certain learning disabilities (Government of Canada 2013). In order to access this funding, a health care practitioner capable of diagnosing and treating ADHD—in Canada this would typically be a family physician, pediatrician, psychologist, or psychiatrist—must assess the individual and fill out the tax form for either the individual or the parent/guardian who is filing for credit. The application is then further reviewed by the Canadian Revenue Agency in order to determine whether the credit will be received. Combined, provincial and federal tax credits may total up to $15,000; however, typical payouts are much lower, and obtaining the tax credit is challenging (Blackwell 2011). Recently, the Canadian Revenue Agency, along with several ADHD specialists, has expressed concern that some individuals may be taking advantage of this credit or falsifying information in an attempt to qualify, and some professionals and advocates worry that inappropriate applications may flood the system and ultimately result in the government ending the credit for individuals legitimately affected by the disorder to the degree that they require assistance (Blackwell 2011).

Conclusion

At the beginning of this chapter, we argued that the Canadian context has developed in the shadow of American ways of understanding and managing ADHD. Much of this has changed in recent years, and there have been efforts among medical professionals and parent support groups to engender a more tailored Canadian set of resources, knowledge, and practice relating to ADHD. Despite the creation of national guidelines for professional practice and a national knowledge network for consumer support, however, significant gaps remain in the Canadian landscape. Much remains unknown about the situation of ADHD in Canada, ranging from the lack of consistent and comprehensive statistics concerning prevalence and treatment rates, to the almost inexplicable lack of communication and collaboration between medical and educational professionals. Further, little is known about the effect of those gaps on the lives of individuals identified with ADHD and their families and supporters. What does seem clear, however, is that despite guidelines that at least superficially seem geared toward containing medication rates and producing a holistic and comprehensive set of supports for people with ADHD, the actual conditions on the ground mean that nonmedical interventions remain a poor second, while ADHD's medicalization in Canada continues as the first—and often—the only option.

NOTES

1. As discussed later in this chapter, the activities of CHADD in Canada have declined in the past decade, with currently only a couple of community chapters remaining.

2. The CADDRA organization and its guidelines are discussed more fully below.

3. Canadian schools are closed to students for 10 to 11 school days each year so that teachers can obtain specialized training in recent pedagogical advances. This professional development is a requirement of continued teacher certification (Alberta Teachers' Association 2015).

4. The original source for this quote was not cited on the CADDAC pages.

REFERENCES

Alberta Teachers' Association. 2015. *Professional Development.* http://www.teachers.ab.ca
  /For%20Members/Professional%20Development/Pages/Index.aspx.
American Psychiatric Association (APA). 1994. *Diagnostic and Statistical Manual of Mental
  Disorders (DSM-IV).* 4th ed. Washington, DC: American Psychiatric Association.
———. 2013. *Diagnostic and Statistical Manual of Mental Disorders (DSM-5).* 5th ed. Washing-
  ton, DC: American Psychiatric Association.
Blackwell, Tom. 2011. "Disability Tax Credit Program Being Abused, Psychiatrist Says."
  National Post, July 19.
Bongers, Agnes. 1997. "At Attention: Critics Worry Ritalin Is Being Used as 'Sit Down
  and Shut Up Drug' in Classrooms." *Calgary Herald,* June 30.
Brault, Marie-Christine, and Eric Lacourse. 2012. "Prevalence of Prescribed Attention-
  Deficit Hyperactivity Disorder Medications and Diagnosis among Canadian Preschool-
  ers and School-Age Children: 1994–2007." *Canadian Journal of Psychiatry* 57 (2): 83–101.
Brownell, Marni D., and Marina S. Yogendran. 2001. "Attention-Deficit Hyperactivity
  Disorder in Manitoba Children: Medical Diagnosis and Psychostimulant Treatment
  Rates." *Canadian Journal of Psychiatry* 46 (3): 264–72.
Buitelar, Jan K., Joanne Barton, Marina Damckaerts, Edgar Friedrichs, Christopher Gill-
  bert, Philip L. Hazell, Hans Hellmans, Mats Johnson, Luuk J. Klverdijk, Gabriele Masi,
  David Michelson, Alivier Revol, Javier San Sebastian, Shuyu Zhang, and Alessandro
  Zuddas. 2006. "A Comparison of North American versus Non-North American
  ADHD Study Populations." *Euopean Child and Adolescent Psychiatry* 15: 177–81.

Calgary Board of Education (CBE). 1999. *Chief Superintendent's Operating Policy: Policy 3003—Special Education*. Calgary, AB: Calgary Board of Education.

Calgary Learning Centre. 1997. *Calgary Learning Centre News*. Calgary, AB: Calgary Learning Centre.

Canadian ADHD Resource Alliance (CADDRA). 2011. "Canadian ADHD Practice Guidelines (CAP-Guidelines), Third Edition."

———. 2014. "Membership Types & Fees." October 10.

Canadian Broadcasting Company (CBC). 2013. "Elk Island Schools to Change Kindergarten Admission Age." http://www.cbc.ca/news/canada/edmonton/elk-island-schools -to-change-kindergarten-admission-age-1.1858310.

Centre for ADHD Awareness Canada (CADDAC). 2014a. "About Us." Markham, ON: Centre for ADHD Awareness Canada.. http://www.caddac.ca/cms/page.php?63.

———. 2014b. "Centre for ADHD Awareness Canada." https://www.facebook.com /CADDAC/timeline.

———. 2014c. "Centre for Awareness of ADHD in Canada." https://www.facebook.com /CADDAC/timeline.

Chaban, Peter. 2010. "ADHD: From Intervention to Implementation." *Education Canada* 50 (2): 32–35.

CHADD Canada. 2014. "Welcome to C.H.A.D.D. Canada Inc." http://www.chaddcanada .com/.

Chapman, Chris. 2012. "Colonialism, Disability, and Possible Lives: The Residential Treatment of Children Whose Parents Survived Indian Residential Schools." *Journal of Progressive Human Services* 23 (2): 127–58.

Charach, Alice, Lizabeth Lin, and Teresa To. 2010. "Evaluating the Hyperactivity/Inattention Subscale of the National Lngitudinal Survey of Children and Youth." Statistics Canada. http://www.statcan.gc.ca/pub/82-003-x/2010002/articles/11234-3ng.htm.

Chisholm, Patricia. 1996. "The ADD Dilemma: Is Ritalin the Best Way to Treat Attention Deficit Disorder?" *MacLean's Magazine*, March 11, 46–48.

Clarke, Juanne N. 2011. "Magazine Portrayals of Attention Deficit/Hyperactivity Disorder (ADD/ADHD): A Post-Modern Epidemic in a Post-Trust Society." *Health, Risk & Society* 13 (7): 632–46.

Conrad, Peter. 2006. *Identifying Hyperactive Children: The Medicalization of Deviant Children*. 2nd ed. Ashgate Classics in Sociology. Aldershot, UK: Ashgate.

———. 2007. *The Medicalization of Society: On the Transformation of Human Conditions into Treatable Disorders*. Baltimore: Johns Hopkins University Press.

Conrad, Peter, and Joseph W. Schneider. 1980. *Deviance and Medicalization: From Badness to Sickness*. St. Louis: C. V. Mosby.

Edmunds, Alan, and Shelley Martsch-Litt. 2008. "ADHD Assessment and Diagnosis in Canada: An Inconsistent but Fixable Process." *Exceptionality Education Canada* 18 (2): 3–23.

Fuchs, Don, Linda Burnside, Sheila Marchenski, and Andria Mudry. 2010. "Children with FASD-Related Disabilities Receiving Services from Child Welfare Agencies in Manitoba." *International Journal of Mental Health & Addiction* 8 (2): 232–44.

Government of Canada. 2013. "Disability Tax Credit." Canada Revenue Agency. http:// www.cra-arc.gc.ca/E/pbg/tf/t2201/t2201-12e.pdf.

Kean, Brian. 2004. "What the Multimodal Treatment Study Really Discovered about Intervention for Children Diagnosed with ADHD: Implications for Early Childhood." *Ethical Human Psychology and Psychiatry* 6 (3): 193–200.

Langlois, Kelly, Andriy V. Samokhvalov, Jürgen Rehm, Selene T. Spence, and Sarah Connor Gorber. 2011. "Health State Descriptions for Canadians: Mental Illnesses." Health Analysis Division, Statistics Canada, Ottawa, Canada.

Lindblom, Anne. 2014. "Under-Detection of Autism among First Nations Children in British Columbia, Canada." *Disability & Society* 29 (8): 1248–59.

Loe, Meika. 2008. "Grappling with the Medicated Self: The Case of ADHD Collge Students." *Symbolic Interaction* 31 (3): 303–23.

Malacrida, Claudia. 2002. "Alternative Therapies and Attention Deficit Disorder: Discourses of Motherhood, Science and Risk." *Gender & Society* 16 (3): 366–85.

———. 2003. *Cold Comfort: Mothers, Professionals and ADD.* Toronto: University of Toronto Press.

———. 2004. "Medicalization, Collaboration and Social Control: Educators and ADD/ADHD." *Health: An Interdisciplinary Journal for the Social Study of Health, Illness and Medicine* 8 (1): 61–80.

———. 2001. "Motherhood, Resistance and Attention Deficit Disorder." *Canadian Review of Sociology and Anthropology* 38 (2): 141–65.

Martinussen, Rhonda L., Rosemary Tannock, Peter Chaban, Alison McInnes, and Bruce Ferguson. 2006. "Increasing Awareness and Understanding of Attention Deficit Hyperactivity Disorder (ADHD) in Education to Promote Better Academic Outcomes for Students with ADHD." *Exceptionality Education Canada* 16 (2–3): 107–28.

Mate, Gabor. 2000. "Attention Please: Doctors Must Stop Thinking of ADD as a Disease That Can Only Be Controlled with Drugs." *Globe and Mail*, May 4, 15.

Mayes, Rick, Catherine Bagwell, and Jennifer Erkulwater. 2009. *Medicating Children: ADHD and Pediatric Mental Health.* Cambridge, MA: Harvard University Press.

Miller, Anton, Charlotte Johnston, Anne Klassen, Stuart Fine, and Michael Papsdorf. 2005. "Family Physicians' Involvement and Self-reported Comfort and Skill in Care of Children with Behavioral and Emotional Problems: A Population-based Survey." *BMC Family Practice* 6 (1): 10–12.

Morrow, Richard I., E. Jane Garland, James M. Wright, Malcolm Maclure, Suzanne Taylor, and Colin R. Dormuth. 2012. "Influence of Relative Age on Diagnosis and Treatment of Attention-Deficit/Hyperactivity Disorder in Children." *Canadian Medical Association Journal* 184 (7): 755–61.

O'Malley, Martin, and Justin Thompson. 2003. "Prime Ministers and Presidents." Canadian Broadcasting Corporation, November 22. http://www.cbc.ca/canadaus/pms_presidents1.html.

Palmer, David, and Agnes Bongers. 1997. "Ritalin Use in Canada Up 35%—and Climbing." *Calgary Herald*, June 30.

Rees, Ann. 1998a. "Drug's Success Fuels Misdiagnosis." *Calgary Herald*, March 13.

———. 1998b. "Rise in ADHD Cases Worrying—Expert." *Calgary Herald*, March 11.

Rees, Ann, and Chris Dawson. 1998. "Use of Ritalin under Attack: Some Parents Too Quick to Seek Medication for Behavioral Disorders, says Calgary Doctor." *Calgary Herald*, March 9.

Schatsky, David, and Felix Yaroshevsky. 1997. "Ritalin, Ritalin, Who's Got the Ritalin?" *Globe and Mail*, September 3, 15.

Szatmari, Peter, David Offord, and Michael Boyle. 1989. "Ontario Child Health Study: Prevalence of Attention Deficit Disorder with Hyperactivity." *Journal of Child Psychology & Psychiatry* 30 (2): 219–30.

Weiss, Margaret, and Candice Murray. 2003. "Assessment and Management of Attention-Deficit Hyperactivity Disorder in Adults." *Canadian Medical Association Journal* 168 (6): 715–22.

4

Historical, Cultural, and Sociopolitical Influences on Australia's Response to ADHD

Brenton J. Prosser
Linda J. Graham

The Emergence of ADHD in Australia

By Western standards, Australia has a relatively short official history. Originally inhabited by a diverse array of more than 500 Indigenous groups, the "Australia" that is widely recognized today first came into being as a British penal colony in the late 1700s. Over the period of the next 150 years, the Anglo-Australian population grew and diversified through several waves of European immigration, but retained its deep cultural, political, and economic ties with Britain. The Second World War became a turning point in this relationship. Disquiet over the rising death toll of Australians fighting to protect British interests in Europe, Indo-China, the Middle East, and North Africa, along with fear from the threat from Japan in the Pacific, led to a change in Australia's economic and defense posture, resulting in a growing alliance with the United States (Lee 1992). From the 1950s, Australia increasingly identified with the United States—first strategically and then culturally. This shift also had material effects, particularly in the areas of medicine and health (Graham 2010). Since the 1970s, Australia has tended to follow the United States in mental health directions, especially in relation to a cultural preference for pharmacological treatment within a medical model of care.

An example of this tendency can be found in the case of the diagnostic category of hyperactivity (a precursor to ADHD). The 1970s were a turning point for public and professional opinion in relation to mental disabilities in Australia (AIHW 2004), with greater recognition of their existence (through the adoption of the American Psychiatric Association's [APA's] *Diagnostic and Statistical Manual of Mental Disorders [DSM]* and the impact of the deinstitutionalization movement) and the responsibility of governments to provide support for greater social participation for affected individuals. Hyperactivity became well known during this period, with a number of advocacy groups (including independent state-based hyperactivity support associations such as the Hyperactivity Association of South Australia and the Hyperactive Children's Association of Victoria) emerging across Australia. These groups facilitated conferences and educational seminars (most of which focused on medical and educational interventions for individuals), whereas the public debate focused on a range of questions that are still commonly raised with ADHD more than three decades later (such as its "reality" and the appropriateness of treatment with psychostimulants). In the Australian context, "hyperactivity" was the launch point for a diagnostic category that evolved into other nomenclatures (e.g., "ADD" and "ADHD") that were identified within the *DSM* (Smith 2008) and were to come to the attention of Australian practitioners, professionals, and the public in the early 1980s.

GROWTH AND PREVALENCE IN AUSTRALIA

Since the 1970s, Australian medical practitioners have drawn primarily on the *DSM*, which is now in its fifth edition (APA 2013). Although this manual covers an ever-growing array of disorders, ADHD and its precursors have held a consistent place within it. Due to the historical and cultural influences identified above, there has been relatively little use of the World Health Organization's (WHO's) *International Classification of Diseases (ICD-10)* (1992), which has been preferred in Europe. Whereas the *ICD-10* refers to hyperkinetic disorder—and requires symptoms relating to the full triad of impairments (impulsivity, hyperactivity, and inattention) to be present for a diagnosis to be made—the *DSM*, in contrast, categorizes these symptoms into three subtypes (predominantly inattentive, predominantly hyperactive, and combined type). This allows a diagnosis to be made when only some symptoms are present (Thomas, Mitchell, and Batstra 2013). The use of the *ICD-10* is frequently associated with lower rates of diagnosis (Amaral 2007); consequentially, the standardization of diagnostic protocols around the *DSM* in Australia has been identified as one factor in the dramatic increase in ADHD diagnosis and psychostimulant treatment (Prosser and Reid 1999), paralleling trends in the United States (Conrad 2007).

Like the United States, Australia experienced a fivefold increase in medication use for ADHD during the 1990s (Hazell, McDowell, and Walton 1996). Rates and growth of prescription varied among Australian states, possibly because of differing recording procedures, but growth did occur in all states (Valentine, Zubrick, and Sly 1996). New prescriptions for ADHD grew 26% per year between 1984 and 2000 (Berbatis, Sunderland, and Bulsara 2002) and by almost 73% between 2000 and 2011 (Paterson 2013). Meanwhile, the average growth rate of children being medicated for ADHD in Australia was 4.7% per year between 2002 and 2009, as compared with 2% per year in the United States over the same period (Stephenson, Karanges, and McGregor 2013). Notably, this growth in ADHD medication occurred during a period when the level of dispensation of other psychotropic drugs remained relatively constant (Stephenson, Karanges, and McGregor 2013). Increases in the use of atypical antipsychotic drugs and antidepressants were identified as well, though no data are kept on the specific use of antidepressants for ADHD. Australia now ranks second highest in the world behind Iceland in the prescription of antidepressants (Carter 2013) and third highest in the world behind the United States and Canada in the prescription of stimulants (Graham 2010).

Estimates of the prevalence of ADHD among Australian children and adolescents (i.e., younger than 18 years) have ranged from 1.6% (Valentine, Zubrick, and Sly 1996) to 11% (Sawyer et al. 2002). The most widely accepted estimates of ADHD prevalence place it between 6% and 9% (Al-Yagon et al. 2013), including a recent estimate of 6.8% based on a community sample of Australian children (RACP 2009). Rates of psychostimulant prescription for ADHD grew dramatically from the early 1990s, but they appear to have plateaued in Australia since the mid-2000s (Prosser and Reid 2009). However, psychostimulants are the only ADHD medications about which official records are kept and there might have been some transfer to other medical treatments. That said, it was the explosion in ADHD diagnosis and treatment with dexamphetamine in the 1990s that captured the popular consciousness and catalyzed the formation of the first national guidelines for ADHD.

Australia's First National Guidelines for ADHD

Public and professional concern about the dramatic increase in the diagnosis of ADHD and the associated growth in stimulant drug prescription prompted health authorities to approach the Australian National Health and Medical Research Council (NHMRC) for advice on assessment and management. The resultant NHMRC (1997) national guidelines were the first of their kind in Australia. The terms of reference for these guidelines were to draw on scientific literature to determine appropriate diagnostic methods and use of stimulant medication, ascertain the safety of long-term treatment, and formulate advice about the best methods of management for ADHD. They were also intended to formulate advice for researchers, health professionals, educators, parents, and consumers. The major contribution of these early guidelines was to establish the *DSM-IV* (APA 1994) as the preferred mechanism in Australia by setting its criteria as the minimum on which a diagnosis should be made. These guidelines were therefore overwhelmingly medical in their focus on interventions for individuals. Although the content of this document noted the importance of multimodal approaches, it was largely dismissive of treatments other than stimulant medication and gave only cursory attention to sociocultural, economic, and policy considerations. In practice, the NHMRC guidelines formalized a medical "best practice" approach to ADHD in Australia and consolidated an alignment with similar emphases in the United States. The result was an increase in the prescription of medication as a "first-line" approach, leading to a growing number of critiques of both education and social support systems (Graham 2007), as well as questions within the field of pediatrics itself as to whether comprehensive assessments were indeed being made, and which or whose needs the medical model was serving (Issacs 2006).

That said, the concerns about appropriate medication use that served as a catalyst for the creation of these guidelines have not been ignored, with a range of state and territory government measures being introduced to provide safeguards against factors that might contribute to overdiagnosis and overprescription. As a result, the Australian context has a number of additional "checks and balances" that are not present in the United States. These include national bans on the advertisement of all prescription medications (not just those used in the treatment of ADHD), jurisdictional restrictions on who has the authority to prescribe medication for ADHD, and the centralization of control over the authority to prescribe at the state and territory levels. However, these measures have not quelled concerns about a potential over-reliance on medication as a first-line response (Prosser 2006), the reported overrepresentation of disadvantaged children in ADHD prescription rates (Prosser and Reid 2009), and evidence of doctor-shopping and polypharmacy (which can result in some individuals taking multiple medications prescribed by more than one specialist and the selling of stimulant medications on the black market) (Whitely 2012b; Graham 2015b). These concerns continue to be expressed publicly by a number of academic, practitioner, professional, and community advocates who claim that psychostimulant treatment is too often the first (or only) Australian response to the behaviors that have come to be associated with ADHD.

Diagnosis and Treatment of ADHD in Australia

As indicated above, there are clear restrictions on who can participate in the diagnosis and prescription of medication for treatment of ADHD in Australia. This is managed independently by jurisdictions (which can result in slight variations between each). A number of broad features, however, can be identified. First, unlike the United States, where primary care physicians (or general practitioners) are the dominant actors (AAP 2011; Thomas, Mitchell, and Batstra 2013), ADHD diagnosis and treatment in Australia is limited to pediatricians and psychiatrists (Starling 2013). Second, although medical, health, and educational professionals are strongly encouraged to refer their clients to these specialists, there is limited evidence of these groups being involved in the provision of information to support diagnostic assessment (Prosser and Reid 2013). Third, there is not a widespread presence of psychologists within Australian schools, which further establishes the dominance of medical specialists in child and family care. In fact, in some jurisdictions, long-standing government policies state that educational professionals are not to suggest assessments, anticipate the potential outcome of assessments, or question a doctor's diagnosis (e.g., DETE 1999), although research has found that this does indeed happen (Skellern, Schluter, and McDowall 2005; Graham, Sweller, and Van Bergen 2010; Graham 2015a). Together, these features perpetuate a situation in which the medical model is central to the diagnosis, treatment, and management of the behaviors that have come to be associated with ADHD in Australia, while the availability of other multimodal treatments can be inconsistent and more costly than prescription medication, which is subsidized through the Pharmaceutical Benefits Scheme (PBS) (Graham 2010).

To be clear, the provision of health care in Australia is a joint federal and jurisdictional responsibility. The basic delineation is that states provide hospital services through their health departments, whereas the federal government supports the states with health funding grants, as well as subsidizes private medical services through the publicly funded Medicare Benefits Scheme (MBS). Under Medicare, citizens purchase approved services from authorized medical practitioners and are then paid a rebate as a subsidy. Whether this subsidy meets the full cost of providing a service may depend on additional fees charged by the provider, although a service user with a welfare status will usually receive a "free" consultation. In practice, this system provides universal access to medical services within Australia. What this means in relation to ADHD diagnosis and treatment is that the MBS provides a cheap and effective mechanism for referrals from medical practitioners to specialists, as well as a number of "free" or subsidized consultations with those specialists. Further, the PBS provides subsidies for the purchase of medications (including psychostimulants for ADHD) to all Australians who hold a Medicare Benefits Card. The context noted above creates a situation in which psychostimulants are potentially the most accessible and affordable treatment response to the behaviors that have come to be associated with ADHD. When considered in relation to the relative costs of accessing a range of health and other professional supports (which are not usually subsidized), concerns have been raised about the accessibility (or potential for sustained use) of nonmedical and multimodal treatments among poorer Australian families (Prosser, Shute, and Atkinson 2002; Prosser 2014).

Conditions for Diagnosis and Treatment

A number of principles guide the practices of approved Australian prescribing specialists. Again, these vary between state and territory jurisdictions but, by way of example, we provide a brief overview of the arrangements in New South Wales (NSW) (Australia's most populated state), which are indicative of arrangements more broadly.

In this context, diagnosis must align with criteria set by the NSW Ministry of Health (MoH 2014). These diagnostic criteria are identical to the previously noted national guidelines (NHMRC 1997) and stress the use of the *DSM* as the minimum grounds for ADHD diagnosis. These guidelines also clarify that a pharmacist cannot dispense a prescription for ADHD medication unless it bears an authority number from the MoH (regardless of in which state or territory jurisdiction the prescription was issued). Within NSW, data on authorizations for psychostimulant prescription are recorded in the Pharmaceutical Drugs of Addiction System, which is maintained and monitored by the MoH. Since psychostimulants are classified as "drugs of addiction," eligible specialists in NSW are required to access either a general or individual authorization from the MoH. General approvals are available to consultant pediatricians and consultant child psychiatrists who are members of the Royal Australian and New Zealand College of Psychiatrists. These medical practitioners do not need to gain individual approval for each prescription as long as they follow the set of routine prescribing criteria in the guidelines. The maximum duration for a prescription under general approval is six months, after which a renewal is required. Other medical practitioners who wish to prescribe or specialists who wish to vary from the set criteria for prescriptions for individuals younger than 4 years of age require individual approval. Similar arrangements apply in all Australian jurisdictions and comprise a relatively regulated diagnostic and treatment environment.

The above conditions also result in a context that is highly reliant on the provisions of the *DSM*, with any revisions of the *DSM* having direct implications for practice. For instance, the potential growth in referrals for ADHD diagnosis under the expanded diagnostic criteria in the new *DSM-5* (APA 2013) risks creating tensions in a context of medical workforce shortages, where the number of child and adolescent psychiatric specialists is in the low hundreds (Prosser and Reid 2013). This could result in less rigorously examined assessments or longer delays before specialists can be seen. These new diagnostic arrangements (particularly the inclusion of later onset of ADHD) may also result in new responsibilities and new resource demands, such as testing for alternative causes of ADHD-like behaviors as part of assessment and greater sensitivity to the temporal evolution of behaviors through adolescence (Sibley et al. 2013). Further, a renewed emphasis on the inclusion of teacher reports in the new *DSM* will have implications when applied in the Australian school context. In the elementary school years (kindergarten through year 6), students spend most of their time in a class with one teacher, which makes reporting to clinicians easier. However, in the secondary years (year 7 through year 12), any given teacher may see more than 150 students each week, which raises practical considerations about the accuracy and accessibility of teacher reports to clinicians. Together, these factors will add to ongoing questions about the appropriateness of medical assessments that include educational assessments.

Although the changes in the *DSM* are expected to result in a shift in practices and increased demands on medical specialists, it is anticipated that there will be minimal influence on the health and education systems (Al-Yagon et al. 2013), mainly because there is little alignment between ADHD diagnosis and access to additional government health, education, and social services.

"Falling through the Cracks" of Australian Public Policy

As has been indicated above, the respective Australian jurisdictions play a pivotal role in the clinical diagnosis, treatment, and management of ADHD. However, they are also crucial in providing potential access to health and education supports. This is due primarily to the conditions of federation within Australia.

As noted at the start of this chapter, the modern independent nation of Australia was formed in 1901 when the British Parliament passed legislation allowing the six Australian colonies to govern in their own right within the Commonwealth of Australia. As part of the establishment of these arrangements, clear principles were laid down to delineate between central federal and former colony (now state) responsibilities. The federal government was granted responsibility for areas of national interest (such as taxation, defense, communications, and foreign affairs), while the states retained legislative powers over matters within their borders (such as police, education, hospitals, and transport). However, this division also resulted in areas of overlap; this is most pertinent in the case of health (and mental health) and has important implications in the context of ADHD.

One of the difficulties for children diagnosed with ADHD in Australia is that in practical terms the condition "falls through the cracks" between state and federal policy (Prosser et al. 2002) and between policy areas, such as health and education policy. ADHD is recognized as a neurological disorder under the Federal Disability Discrimination Act, and as a result, private and public bodies are expected to make "reasonable adjustments" so that persons diagnosed with ADHD are not disadvantaged. However, in most cases, state health or education services do not recognize "ADHD" as a disability category; nor does the diagnosis alone qualify someone for additional support. The latter is because a diagnosis of disability does not necessarily translate into additional support for learning, and the emphasis within Australian education systems is increasingly on functional assessment, rather than diagnosis. That said, long-term policy incoherence between medical and educational models has led to considerable confusion as to what "support" means and who should provide it, particularly at the level of school practice. Since primary and secondary school student support policies are broadly similar across the states and because NSW enjoys considerable influence in educational debates and policy development (Graham 2015a), we will again take the state of NSW as our example.

The NSW Department of Education and Communities (DEC) student support policy maintains that all children are eligible for additional support for learning but not all are eligible for individual targeted funding. Additional support for learning is provided via two programs in NSW government schools: (1) Every Student, Every School (ESES), and (2) Integration Funding Support (IFS). ESES provides a global resource allocation—including access to school-based specialist learning support teachers—to all schools via a census-based funding approach. Conceptualized as the "first line of defense" in supporting students with any type of learning or behavioral difficulty, ESES requires adjustments and accommodations by the classroom teacher with support from the Learning Support Team and other specialist staff (including the school counselor). However, the requirement that teachers and school staff act as the first line of defense through adjustments and accommodations to curriculum and practice—and that all schools receive a funding allocation to support this—is not well understood on the ground in schools, even by specialist learning support teachers (Graham 2015a). This is where children with learning and attentional difficulties typically slip through the cracks as teachers may continue to teach in ways that do not serve individual student needs in the belief that adjustments and modifications are required only for students with a confirmed diagnosis from one of the six categories of disability that are eligible for support through the IFS program (see below). This is a fundamental misunderstanding of inclusive practice but one that is still common (Graham 2015a).

In the NSW government school system, students with disabilities and high-support needs who are enrolled in a regular class in a mainstream school, but who require significantly more support than is available through ESES, can access individual targeted funding through the IFS program. Entry requires a confirmed diagnosis of disability within one of DEC's six eligibility categories—physical disability, moderate-to-severe intellectual disability, hearing impairment, vision impairment, autism spectrum disorders, and mental health problems. A diagnosis of ADHD is not sufficient to attract individual targeted funding. However, many children and young people who receive additional support under the categories of "emotional disturbance" or "behavior disorder" will have a primary diagnosis of ADHD (Van Bergen et al. 2015).

IFS is also the program that has registered the most significant growth in recent years, despite numerous attempts by successive NSW governments to limit eligibility through funding caps and changes to eligibility (see Graham and Jahnukainen 2011). For example, the proportion of students receiving IFS rose from 0.58% to 3.5% of total enrollments in the 13 years between 1993 and 2006, with some extraordinary jumps year to year, including a 41% increase between 2001–2 and 2002–3, equating to 6,183 new children in the space of 12 months (Graham and Sweller 2011).

Research has revealed that significant pressure is placed on health professionals to provide a diagnosis that will secure individual support funding in Australian schools, with some erring "on the side of positive diagnosis of autism and ASD [autism spectrum disorders] when they are less than certain . . . as a strategy to facilitate a child's access to funding sources which demand categorical diagnoses despite the complex spectrum of clinical reality" (Skellern, Schluter, and McDowall 2005: 412). Senior policy officers and public servants have confirmed these reports (Graham 2015a), noting that a high proportion of students now receiving individual targeted funding under the category of ASD were originally diagnosed with ADHD and/or oppositional defiance disorder and had received a diagnosis of ASD much later (and typically in the high-functioning range). Since a diagnosis of ADHD is not enough to trigger eligibility for individual targeted funding in the NSW government school system, students end up with multiple diagnoses because their parents are forced to return to pediatricians or child psychiatrists for reassessment (Graham 2015a). Diagnostic substitution—particularly between ADHD and ASD—is not uncommon in NSW and occurs in order to secure funding support eligibility or placement in a separate special educational setting (Graham 2015a).

The provision of special education support services is one area in which there is a key difference between Australia and the United States. In recognition of the perverse incentives created by categorical support allocation methods, Australia is increasingly moving toward tiered support mechanisms based on functional assessment and demonstrated need (such as ESES), and away from a costly and retrospective medical model that drives diagnosis within "fundable" disability categories (Graham and Jahnukainen 2011). The challenge for Australian systems of education, however, is that teachers have become skilled at identifying students with additional support needs, but have yet to become proficient at making adjustments and accommodations to curriculum and practice (Graham 2015a). The result for many children with learning and behavioral difficulties is a prescription for psychoactive medication and little else despite how ineffective some young people consider such responses to be (Graham 2015b).

ADHD, Medicalization, and Resistance

A common perspective among Australian social scientists has been to see ADHD as another example of the medicalization of society, with psychostimulants being a technology of social control for youth from lower socioeconomic backgrounds who are deemed to be unruly (Prosser 2014). This view varies significantly from commonly held views in the United States (where ADHD is identified more widely across socioeconomic groups). Such a view draws on the central premise of the medicalization perspective, namely, that once a medical means of social control exists, then it is only a matter of time before a label emerges to justify its treatment of a social problem, after which these labels may expand beyond their original domain to claim other social conditions (Conrad 1976: 2007). Initially, in the 1970s, medicalization theory focused on medical technologies of social control, with hyperactivity as a prime example. However, as part of the evolution to ADHD, the theoretical trajectory has taken a post-structuralist turn (Tait 2005). Internationally, scholars have come to focus on a psycho-medical discourse to see how it shapes diagnostic criteria (Singh 2004; Bailey 2010) and responses through pathologization (Timmi 2005) or pharmaceuticalization (Abraham 2010), as well as acts as a dominant discourse that manages blame for professionals, parents, and teachers (Graham 2007). These insights have been influential and have helped Australian scholars to explore how expert knowledge and authoritative discourses act to regulate behavior in that context.

However, such perspectives have been less helpful in identifying what should be done for children and families in a situation in which Australian policy sees clinical interventions as the most likely "real-world" response. This is because classical medicalization theory focuses on the responsibility of medical practitioners (or pharmaceutical companies), whereas the poststructural is more concerned with critiquing the status quo than proposing solutions to it. In response, as we will explore later in this chapter, we propose a less structuralist approach to the medicalization perspective than has been taken previously by Australian (and many international) social scientists in relation to ADHD.

Although not conceptualized exactly in terms of medicalization as first proposed by Conrad (1976), public debate around ADHD in Australia has shown an awareness of the potential for the medical profession to label social ailments as medical conditions. Within Australian popular culture, there remain echoes from 1960s advertising campaigns that added "take a Bex and lie down" to the

national lexicon as it encouraged stay-at-home mothers to consume these cura-
tive powders daily. They were dissolved in a cup of tea and were recommended as
a "fix all" for everything from headaches, colds, and flu, to nerve pains, rheuma-
tism, and stress. However, during the 1970s, it was recognized that these
substances were addictive and large doses resulted in kidney disease and other
health conditions (*News Australia* 2014; School of Medicine: UNSW 2015). The
public outcry and subsequent government regulation of this uniquely Australian
"mother's little helper" has left an indelible mark and contributes to strong antimedication views in the community.

More recently, there have been expressions of concern about the growing
levels in use of over-the-counter pain medications from Australian pharmacies
(*Sydney Morning Herald* 2015). Medical professionals identify dangers associated
with excess painkiller use (in the form of codeine), including nausea, constipation,
memory problems, and, in rare cases, cardiac and respiratory arrest (Iedema
2011). Also likely is the occurrence of ulcers, dysfunctional bowels or liver, and
pancreas and kidney damage. The growing dependence on pain killers has been
located in what is seen as an Australian addiction to medical quick fixes and part
of a national normalization of taking a "pill to cure every ill."

It is in the echoes of these debates that considerations of the psychostimulant
treatment for ADHD are given voice. With unfaltering regularity, Australian
media present stories on the "reality" of ADHD and the controversy around
prescribing "addictive" drugs to young people and their potential for unin-
tended recreational and performance enhancement purposes (e.g., Snow 2010).
Although important questions remain to be considered, the sensational nature of
these reports contributes to "black or white" responses (Prosser 2014) that are
ultimately unhelpful and can result in an emphasis on allocating blame or responsibility. Such simplistic representations of ADHD neither better inform
families nor challenge misconceptions about ADHD in the community (Singh
2004; Lloyd, Stead, and Cohen 2006). Further, these popular representations
present children out of control, fears about drug use, allegations of poor parenting, and links with crime, which may be highly influential on parental and
community views. Such powerful everyday discourses are evident in Australian
talkback radio, current affairs, news, and newspapers. In Australia, the "ADHD"
label is now also referred to regularly in television and popular music, and has a
prominent presence in other entertainment media (see Prosser 2006: 2014).
Such media representations have contributed to a situation in which ADHD and
its controversial treatment with psychostimulants are very much a part of the

Australian popular consciousness. The label "ADHD" has come to be associated with any "bad behavior" and no longer needs to have been diagnosed or treated with drugs for the label to be used by parents, teachers, and health professionals (Slee 2010; Prosser 2014).

Feeding into this are key sites of critique and resistance to the medical model of ADHD. These include significant opposition from within health professional and lobby groups, in addition to ongoing controversy and robust debate about ADHD and its treatment within Australian medical and psychiatric journals (Whitely 2012b; Paterson 2013). This has been seen most recently in responses to the revised national guidelines for ADHD in Australia.

A CASE OF RESISTANCE: THE REVISED NATIONAL GUIDELINES FOR ADHD

As a result of concerted lobbying by a wide range of politicians and professional and health advocates (some of whom originally supported the initial national guidelines for ADHD), Australia's first national guidelines were rescinded in December 2005. These critics (e.g., see Whitely 2012) described the guidelines as deeply flawed and unduly influenced by multinational pharmaceutical companies. In response, the NHMRC requested the Royal Australian College of Physicians (RACP) to develop a new set of national guidelines. Almost immediately after their completion (RACP 2009), they were dogged by public and professional criticism (Starling 2013).

The draft's validity was at the center of the controversy after it was revealed that a well-known medical researcher whose published research had significantly influenced the development of the draft guidelines had not acknowledged a potential conflict of interest over payments from drug companies (Sikora 2009). Further, there were allegations that members of the group responsible for preparing the guidelines had links to pharmaceutical companies and advocated primarily for drug interventions for ADHD (Whitely 2012a). The NHMRC responded by distancing itself from the draft, and by November 2009, it had been withdrawn.

However, in 2011, the NHMRC released a set of draft clinical practice points for consultation. The NHMRC (2011) described these practice points as a profound and almost fundamental shift in outlook on the role of medication treatment for ADHD. This shift meant looking beyond the symptoms of ADHD to recognize children's behavior as it exists in a wider context. It also meant the exclusion of more than a half dozen other conditions before a formal ADHD diagnosis is made, and it renewed the potential for diagnosis based on *ICD-10* criteria in Australia.

These new practice points have been accepted broadly by critics and the community, with state and territory governments and professional bodies endorsing them. However, not all are convinced on the fundamental nature of any shift. Prominent Australian critics (Whitely 2012a) have argued that they are contradictory since they are based on a convenient compromise between pro-medical and anti-pharmaceutical views (rather than evidence-based consensus) and that they are the product of a committee that included a cross section of medication advocates and skeptics. The practice points are also quite brief and focus specifically on practical interventions to be used by psychiatrists and neuropsychologists. There is only scant reference to educational or other supports, and no consideration of sociocultural influences on behavior or its interpretation. Such matters could be appropriately addressed within a new set of guidelines (which were set for 2014). However, to date, there has been no public indication that they have been prepared or released. At this time, because of a stalemate between the above medical advocacy and resistance advocates, Australia has no active formal guidelines for ADHD.

ADHD, Disadvantage, and Social Control

Meanwhile, geographic variations in psychostimulant treatment for ADHD have continued to be identified within Australia (Prosser and Reid 2009; Whitely 2012b). This has contributed to the ongoing public controversy around the primacy of medical responses to ADHD in Australia. Underlying such controversy is an association between psychostimulant treatment for ADHD and lower socioeconomic status (SES) that has been identified in Australia for more than a decade. Two studies from the early 2000s relied on parent surveys and found more psychostimulant use for ADHD according to low SES and social adversity (Graetz et al. 2001; Sawyer 2002). Since that time, six Australian studies have been conducted (all based on federal or state government drug-approval records), with the majority finding an association between psychostimulant treatment and low SES. Of these studies, two have considered a state with relatively high levels of prescription and found geographical, with possible SES, associations (Valentine et al. 1996; Calver et al. 2007). Another two were decade-long studies from the same state and have identified an association between prescription drug use and low SES regions (Reid, Hakendorf, and Prosser 2002; Prosser and Reid 2009). Furthermore, a study of 20 years of archival data in NSW found higher drug use in lower socioeconomic areas (Prosser, Lambert, and Reid 2013, 2014) and that the average duration of psychostimulant use for ADHD was declining to less than two years across all groups (Lambert et al. 2015). One nationwide assessment of drug data according to the political electorate identified an association with low SES (Harwood 2010).

By way of comparison, diagnosis and drug treatment of ADHD in the United States has been identified as being more prevalent among the middle classes. Some have framed this in policy terms, such that reduced levels of Medicaid use and private insurance among lower socioeconomic groups may result in lower levels of access to diagnosis and treatment of ADHD (Pastor and Reuben 2008). Associated with this may be lower levels of diagnosis and treatment among African American and Latino groups, who make up a large part of low SES communities and whose negative associations with psychostimulants may contribute to resistant parental attitudes toward medication (McLeod et al. 2007; Pham, Carlson, and Kosciulek 2009; Eiraldi and Diaz 2010). Whatever the cause, the findings in the Australian context are an important point of difference with the stated situation in the United States.

Another distinction emerges around powerful images of cultural and national identity in Australia. For instance, the active, earthy, rebellious, and exuberant qualities of First World War Australian soldiers form the origins of the Australian and New Zealand Army Corps (ANZAC) legend, which remains influential on social constructions of Australian national identity (McKenna 2014). And yet, these same behaviors are open to being associated with ADHD diagnosis and medical treatment (Prosser 2006). Further, there would appear to be much lower levels of acceptance of diagnosis and medication treatment of ADHD among Indigenous Australian and Asian Australian families (Prosser 2006). This may be due to different cultural attitudes in relation to behavior or parenting, or alternative institutional explanations for the behaviors associated with ADHD. These examples point to how cultural identity can interact with attitudes toward ADHD and how it may result in different levels of acceptance of diagnosis and medical treatment. Hence, a consideration of differing influences on ADHD in Australia illustrates the need for social scientists to conduct more detailed examination of the role of socioeconomic and cultural factors in the experience of ADHD.

These examples also highlight the importance of the inclusion of the perspective of human agents in understanding differing experiences of ADHD. For instance, research has indicated that Australian parents and children (irrespective of SES) are not passive receptors of medical labels (as is sometimes implied by overly structuralist renditions of medicalization perspectives; Prosser 2014). Some Australian studies have explored the effect of the "ADHD" label on adolescent identity development (Prosser 2008), which speaks to the ways that youth and families come to adopt, refine and use, or even reject "ADHD" labels (Taylor, O'Donoghue, and Houghton 2006; Graham 2015b).

A common theme in work with adolescents in Australian schools (who had been labeled with ADHD) was their description of themselves as having "mild ADHD" (Prosser 2006). From a biomedical or structuralist medicalization perspective, such a claim makes no sense—either one has (or has been labeled with) ADHD or one has not. Moreover, there are no criteria within either the *DSM-IV* (APA 1994) or *DSM-5* (APA 2013) to differentiate mild, moderate, and severe ADHD (Thomas, Mitchell, and Batstra 2013). While these young people voiced strong opposition to what they saw as highly influential (mis)representations of ADHD and stereotypes in Australian media, they also maintained that they encountered difficulties at school for which they needed support. They were not willing to incorporate the "ADHD" label into their identity in the form it was provided to them; neither were they in a position in which they were able to reject completely a label that was endorsed by their family and was seen to assist them in practical ways to manage relationships at home and succeed academically at school. Hence, "mild ADHD" can be seen as an identity that has been created by actors to negotiate contradictory demands of structure and agency. Such insights warn against assumptions that a particular attitude toward the ADHD diagnosis and medical treatment is held uniformly within a particular social class group or enforced through medical dominance.

In recent years, the concept of "medical dominance" has come under increased scrutiny within Australian scholarship. "Medical dominance" is a term used to describe the power of the medical profession to control its work, to shape health policy, and to reify the knowledge that it creates about individuals (Willis 2006). This concept was highly influential around the time when ADHD was first used as an example of medicalization in the 1970s (Conrad 1976). However, in recent years, some scholars have argued that traditional medical roles and authority are being challenged by other health professionals and by greater patient autonomy (Germov 2009), that medicine and psychiatry never had complete control over patients and resources (Roach-Anleu 2009), and that the medical profession is not a unified force in society (Willis 2006). Conrad (2007) recognized such critiques in his revision of the medicalization thesis, which factors in market forces and notes the role of pharmaceutical companies.

However, in the United States (where the medicalization perspective was developed), there have historically been stronger links between the pharmaceutical industry and ADHD support groups (Conrad 2007). Although support groups exist in Australia, they are small, survive on the voluntary contributions of parents, and occasionally benefit from government grants to underpin basic support and information services. In Australia, pharmaceutical companies have been restricted in the direct marketing of information and products for the treatment of ADHD. Parents thus rely on sources of information that are not dependent on pharmaceutical industry research and medical professional advice (such as popular health and parenting websites), which can further challenge the authority of the medical profession (Broom 2005). All these factors suggest that assumptions that the emergence of ADHD as an explanatory narrative for particular behaviors in Australia is the product of global medicalization, medical discourses, and all-powerful pharmaceutical companies bear further examination (Prosser 2014). However, this raises a new question for research: in the absence of many of the conditions for medicalization, how do we develop new ways to understand the factors that shape ADHD in the Australian context?

Conclusion

ADHD, as a mental "disorder," is just as much a social as it is a clinical phenomenon (Wakefield 1992). Yet, within the social sciences there has been an emphasis on ADHD as an example of the medicalization of Western society, which has brought with it the risks that it is seen solely as an extension of North American trends and that it overlooks ADHD as a topic of social and cultural study in its own right (Rafalovich 2001; Prosser 2014). This leaves unexplored the particular social and policy conditions that have contributed to Australian trends in ADHD diagnosis and medical treatment broadly mirroring the United States, while obscuring the important differences that exist within Australia. Although the medicalization perspective remains a vital theoretical tool to help understand ADHD nationally and internationally, it is also open to revision because of emerging evidence in the Australian context of the potential decline of medical dominance, the lesser influence of markets, and a recognition of the important role of human agents in "real-world" ADHD experiences. In our view, an important way forward will be efforts to rework the overtly structuralist focus within the medicalization perspective with one that better accommodates agency and resistance to (and around) the label on the part of individuals and their families. Although some work has been done to explore a greater role for agency within medicalization perspectives previously, this was within gender studies (e.g., Gunson 2010), and has not been thoroughly explored in relation to mental disorders generally (or for ADHD specifically). Such new approaches will, we believe, not only offer a better understanding of the epidemiological, historical, and social contexts that have shaped ADHD diagnosis and treatment internationally, but they will also support more rigorous national comparisons and a growing body of work that examines a unique Australian experience of ADHD.

REFERENCES

Abraham, John. 2010. "Pharmaceuticalization of Society in Context: Theoretical, Empirical and Health Dimensions." *Sociology* 44 (4): 603–22.

Al-Yagon, Michal, Wendy Cavendish, Casare Cornoldi, Angela J. Fawcett, Matthias Grunke, Li-Yu Hung, Juan E. Jimenez, Sunil Karande, Christina E. van Kraayenoord, Daniela Lucangeli, Malka Margalit, Marjorie Montague, Rukhshana Sholapurwala, Georgios Sideridis, Patrizio E. Tressoldi, and Claudio Vio. 2013. "The Proposed Changes for *DSM-5* for SLD and ADHD: International Perspectives—Australia, Germany, Greece, India, Israel, Italy, Spain, Taiwan, United Kingdom, and United States." *Journal of Learning Disabilities* 46 (1): 58–72.

Amaral, Olavo. 2007. "Psychiatric Disorder as Social Constructs: ADHD as a Case in Point." *American Journal of Psychiatry* 164 (10): 1612.

American Academy of Pediatrics (AAP). 2011. "ADHD: Clinical Practice Guideline for the Diagnosis, Evaluation and Treatment of Attention-Deficit/Hyperactivity Disorder in Children and Adolescents." *Pediatrics* 128: 1007–22.

American Psychiatric Association (APA). 1994. *Diagnostic and Statistical Manual of Mental Disorders (DSM-IV)*. 4th ed. Washington, DC: American Psychiatric Association.

———. 2013. *Diagnostic and Statistical Manual of Mental Disorders (DSM-5)*. 5th ed. Washington, DC: American Psychiatric Association.

Australian Institute of Health and Welfare (AIHW). 2004. *Children with Disabilities in Australia*. Cat. no. DIS 38. Canberra: Australian Institute of Health and Welfare.

Bailey, Simon. 2010. "The DSM and the Dangerous School Child." *International Journal of Inclusive Education* 14 (6): 581–92.

Berbatis, Constantine G., V. Bruce Sunderland, and Max Bulsara. 2002. "Licit Psychostimulant Consumption in Australia, 1984–2000: International and Jurisdictional Comparisons." *Medical Journal of Australia* 177 (10): 539–43.

Broom, Alex. 2005. "Medical Specialists' Accounts of the Impact of the Internet on the Doctor/Patient Relationship." *Health* 9 (3): 319–38.

Calver, Janine, David B. Preen, Max Bulsara, Frank M. Sanfilippo, and C. D'Arcy J. Holman. 2007. "Prescribing for the Treatment of ADHD in Western Australia: Socioeconomic and Remoteness Difference." *Medical Journal of Australia* 186 (6): 124–27.

Carter, Lucy. 2013. "OECD Snapshot Ranks Australia Second in World in Anti-depressant Prescriptions." November 22. http://www.abc.net.au/news/2013-11-22/australia-second -in-world-in-anti-depressant-prescriptions/5110084.

Conrad, Peter. 1976. *Identifying Hyperactive Children: The Medicalization of Deviant Behavior.* Lexington, MA: D. C. Heath.

———. 2007. "From Hyperactive Children to Adult ADHD." In *The Medicalization of Society*, 46–69. Baltimore: Johns Hopkins University Press.

Department of Education, Training and Employment (DETE). 1999. *Attention Difficulties, Poor Impulse Control, Overactivity or ADHD (Attention Deficit/Hyperactivity Disorder).* Adelaide, South Australia: Department of Education, Training and Employment.

Eiraldi, Ricardo, and Yamalis Diaz. 2010. "Use of Treatment Services for Attention-Deficit/ Hyperactivity Disorder in Latino Children." *Current Psychiatry Reports* 12 (5): 403–8.

Germov, John. 2009. "Challenges to Medical Dominance." In *Second Opinion: An Introduction to Health Sociology*, edited by John Germov, 392–415. 4th ed. South Melbourne: Oxford University Press.

Graetz, Brian W., Michael G. Sawyer, Philip L. Hazell, Fiona Arney, and Peter Baghurst. 2001. "Validity of DSM-IV ADHD Subtypes in a Nationally Representative Sample of Australian Children and Adolescents." *Journal of the American Academy of Child & Adolescent Psychiatry* 40 (12): 1410–17.

Graham, Linda J. 2007. "From ABCs to ADHD: The Role of Schooling in the Construction of Behaviour Disorder and Production of Disorderly Subjects." *International Journal of Inclusive Education* 12 (1): 7–33.

———. 2010. "Teaching ADHD?" In *(De)constructing ADHD: Critical Guidance for Teachers and Teacher Educators*, edited by Linda J. Graham, chapter 1. Vol. 9. New York: Peter Lang.

———. 2015a. "A Little Learning Is a Dangerous Thing: Factors Influencing the Increase in Diagnosis of Special Educational Needs from the Perspective of Educational Policymakers and School Practitioners." *International Journal of Disability, Development and Education* 62 (1): 116–32.

———. 2015b. "To be Well Is to Be Not Unwell: The New Battleground inside Our Children's Heads." In *Rethinking Youth Wellbeing: Critical Perspectives*, edited by Katie Wright and Julie McLeod, 11–33. Dordrecht: Springer.

Graham, Linda J., and Markku Jahnukainen. 2011. "Wherefore Art Thou, Inclusion? Analysing the Development of Inclusive Education in New South Wales, Alberta and Finland." *Journal of Education Policy* 26 (2): 263–88.

Graham, Linda J., and Naomi Sweller. 2011. "The Inclusion Lottery: Who's In and Who's Out? Tracking Inclusion and Exclusion in New South Wales Government Schools." *International Journal of Inclusive Education* 15 (9): 941–53.

Graham, Linda J., Naomi Sweller, and Penny Van Bergen. 2010. "Detaining the Usual Suspects: Charting the Use of Segregated Settings in New South Wales Government Schools, Australia." *Contemporary Issues in Early Childhood* 11 (3): 234–48.

Gunson, Jessica S. 2010. "'More Natural but Less Normal': Reconsidering Medicalisation and Agency through Women's Accounts of Menstrual Suppression." *Social Science & Medicine* 71 (7): 1324–31.

Harwood, Valerie. 2010. "The New Outsiders: ADHD and Disadvantage." In *(De)constructing ADHD: Critical Guidance for Teachers and Teacher Educators*, edited by Linda J. Graham, 119–42. Vol. 9. New York: Peter Lang.

Hazell, Phillip L., M. J. McDowell, and J. M. Walton. 1996. "Management of Children Prescribed Psychostimulant Medication for Attention Deficit Hyperactivity Disorder in the Hunter Region of NSW." *Medical Journal of Australia* 165 (9): 477–80.

Iedema, Joel. 2011. "Cautions with Codeine." *Australian Prescriber* 34 (5). http://www.australianprescriber.com/magazine/34/5/133/5.

Isaacs, D. 2006. "Attention-Deficit/Hyperactivity Disorder: Are We Medicating for Social Disadvantage?" *Journal of Paediatrics and Child Health* 42 (9): 544–47.

Lambert, Matthew C., Robert Reid, Brenton Prosser, and Regina Bussing. 2015. "Psychostimulant Prescription in New South Wales from 1990 to 2010: A Survival Analysis." *Journal of Child and Adolescent Psychopharmocology* 25 (6): 475–81.

Lee, David. 1992. "Australia, the British Commonwealth, and the United States, 1950–1953." *The Journal of Imperial and Commonwealth History* 20 (3): 445–69.

Lloyd, Gwynned, Joan Stead, and David Cohen. 2006. *Critical New Perspectives on ADHD*. London: Routledge.

McKenna, Mark. 2014. "Keeping in Step: The Anzac Resurgence and Military Heritage in Australia and New Zealand." In *Nation, Memory and Great War Commemoration*, edited by Shanti Sumartojo and Ben Wellings, 151–68. Oxford: Peter Lang.

McLeod, Jane D., Danielle L. Fettes, Peter S. Jensen, Bernice A. Pescosoldio, and Jack K. Martin. 2007. "Public Knowledge, Beliefs, and Treatment Preferences concerning Attention Deficit Hyperactivity Disorder." *Psychiatric Services* 58 (5): 626–31.

National Health and Medical Research Council (NHMRC). 1997. *Attention Deficit Hyperactivity Disorder*. Canberra: Australian Government Publishing Service.

———. 2011. *Clinical Practice Points on the Diagnosis, Assessment and Management of ADHD in Children and Adolescents*. May 22. https://www.nhmrc.gov.au/guidelines/publications/mh26.

News Australia. 2014. "Cancer Council NSW: Bex Powder Killed More Than Pain." July 29. http://www.news.com.au/national/cancer-council-nsw-bex-powder-killed-more-than-pain/story-fncynjr2-1227041736061.

New South Wales Ministry of Health (MoH). 2014. *Prescribe a Psychostimulant*. May 22. http://www.health.nsw.gov.au/pharmaceutical/doctors/Pages/prescribe-psychostimulant.aspx.

Pastor, Patricia N., and Cynthia A. Reuben. 2008. "Diagnosed Attention Deficit Hyperactivity Disorder and Learning Disability: United States, 2004–2006." *Vital Health Statistics* 10 (206): 237.

Paterson, Roger. 2013. "The ADHD Debate: To Bury National Guidelines or to Praise Them." *Australian New Zealand Journal of Psychiatry* 47 (10): 959–60.

Pham, Andy V., John S. Carlson, and John F. Kosciulek. 2009. "Ethnic Difference in Parental Beliefs of Attention-Deficit/Hyperactivity Disorder and Treatment." *Journal of Attention Disorders* 13 (6): 584–91.

Prosser, Brenton. 2006. *ADHD: Who's Failing Who?* Lane Cove: Finch.

———. 2008. "Beyond ADHD: A Consideration of Attention Deficit Hyperactivity Disorder and Pedagogy in Australian Schools." *International Journal of Inclusive Education* 12 (1): 81–97.

———. 2014. "Attention Deficit Hyperactivity Disorder in Australia: Perspectives from the Sociology of Deviance." *Journal of Sociology* 50. doi:10.1177/1440783313514643.

Prosser, Brenton, Matthew C. Lambert, and Robert Reid.. 2013. "Psychostimulant Use for ADHD across Two Australian Jurisdictions." Paper presented at the 4th International Conference on Behavioral, Cognitive and Psychological Sciences, London, November 19.

———. 2014. "Psychostimulant Prescription in New South Wales: A Longitudinal Perspective." *Journal of Attention Disorders.* doi:10.1177/1087054714553053.

Prosser, Brenton, and Robert Reid. 1999. "Psychostimulant Use for Children with Attention Deficit Hyperactivity Disorder in Australia." *Journal of Emotional and Behavioral Disorders* 7 (2): 110–17.

———. 2009. "Changes in Use of Psychostimulant Medication for ADHD in South Australia (1990–2006)." *Australian and New Zealand Journal of Psychiatry* 43 (4): 340–47.

———. 2013. "The DSM-5 Changes and ADHD: More Than a Tweak of Terms." *Australian and New Zealand Journal of Psychiatry* 46 (12): 1196–97.

Prosser, Brenton, Robert Reid, Rosaline H. Shute, and Ivan J. Atkinson. 2002. "Attention Deficit Hyperactivity Disorder: Special Education Policy and Practice in Australia." *Australian Journal of Education* 46 (1): 65–78.

Rafalovich, Adam. 2001. "The Conceptual History of Attention Deficit Hyperactivity Disorder: Idiocy, Imbecility, Encephalitis and the Child Deviant, 1877–1929." *Deviant Behavior* 22 (1): 93–115.

Reid, Robert, Paul Hakendorf, and Brenton Prosser. 2002. "Use of Psychostimulant Medication for ADHD in South Australia." *Journal of the American Academy of Child and Adolescent Psychiatry* 41 (8): 1–8.

Roach-Anleu, Sharyn. 2009. "The Medicalisation of Deviance." In *Second Opinion: An Introduction to Health Sociology,* edited by John Germov, 242–68. 4th ed. South Melbourne: Oxford University Press.

Royal Australian College of Physicians (RACP). 2009. *Draft Australian Guidelines on Attention Deficit Hyperactivity Disorder.* May 22. https://www.racp.edu.au/index.cfm?objectid=393DD54A-04C5-85AC-B35FE82BA4849595.

Sawyer, Michael G., Joseph M. Rey, Brian W. Graetz, Jennifer J. Clark, and Peter A. Baghurst. 2002. "Use of Medication by Young People with Attention Deficit/Hyperactivity Disorder." *Medical Journal of Australia* 177 (1): 21–25.

School of Medicine: UNSW. 2015. "Bex Powders." July 29. https://medicalsciences.med.unsw.edu.au/node/302500715.

Sibley, Margaret H., James G. Waxmonsky, Jessica A. Robb, and William E. Pelham. 2013. "Implications of Changes for the Field: ADHD." *Journal of Learning Disabilities* 46: 34–42.

Sikora, Kate. 2009. "ADHD Guidelines Pulled after Payment Scandal." September 2. http://www.news.com.au/national-news/adhd-guidelines-pulled-after-payment-scandal/story-e6frfkvr-1225801902002.

Singh, Ilina. 2004. "Doing Their Jobs: Mothering with Ritalin in a Culture of Mother-Blame." *Social Science & Medicine* 59 (6): 1193–1205.

Skellern, Catherine, Philip Schluter, and Michael McDowell. 2005. "From Complexity to Category: Responding to Diagnostic Uncertainties of Autistic Spectrum Disorders." *Journal of Paediatrics and Child Health* 41 (8): 407–12.

Slee, Roger. 2010. "Bad Behaviour." In *(De)Constructing ADHD: Critical Guidance for Teachers and Teacher Educators*, edited by Linda Graham, 41–62 . Vol. 9. New York: Peter Lang.

Smith, M. 2008. "Psychiatry Limited: Hyperactivity and the Evolution of American Psychiatry, 1957–1980." *Social History of Medicine* 21 (3): 541–59.

Snow, Deborah. 2010. "Ritalin the New Drug of Choice for Parties and Studying." *Sydney Morning Herald*, February 27. http://www.smh.com.au/national/ritalin-is-students -new-drug-of-choice-for-parties-and-studying-20100226-p953.html.

Starling, Jean. 2013. "Commentary on Levy (2012) Politics vs. Practice: Withdrawal of the Draft NHMRC ADHD Guidelines." *Australian and New Zealand Journal of Psychiatry* 47 (1): 91–92.

Stephenson, Chris P., Emily Karanges, and Iain S. McGregor. 2013. "Trends in the Utilization of Psychotropic Medications in Australia from 2000 to 2011." *Australian and New Zealand Journal of Psychiatry* 47 (1): 74–87.

Sydney Morning Herald. 2015. "Over-the-Counter Sale of Codeine Pain Killers Such as Nurofen Plus and Panadeine May End," July 29. http://www.smh.com.au/national /health/overthecounter-sale-of-codeine-pain-killers-such-as-nurofen-plus-and -panadeine-may-end-20150425-1mt2fl.html.

Tait, Greg. 2005. "The ADHD Debate and the Philosophy of Truth." *International Journal of Inclusive Education* 9 (1): 17–38.

Taylor, Myra, Tom O'Donoghue, and Stephen Houghton. 2006. "To Medicate or Not to Medicate? The Decision Making Process of Western Australian Parents Following Their Child's Diagnosis with Attention Deficit Hyperactivity Disorder." *International Journal of Disability, Development and Education* 53 (1): 111–28.

Thomas, R., G. K. Mitchell, and L. Batstra. 2013. "Attention-Deficit/Hyperactivity Disorder: Are We Helping or Harming?" *British Medical Journal* 347. doi:https://doi.org/10 .1136/bmj.f6172.

Timmi, Sammi. 2005. *Naughty Boys: Anti-social Behaviour, ADHD and the Role of Culture.* New York: Palgrave Macmillan.

Valentine, Jane, Stanley Zubrick, and Peter Sly. 1996. "National Trends in the Use of Stimulant Medication for Attention Deficit Hyperactivity Disorder." *Journal of Pediatric Child Health* 32 (3): 223–27.

Van Bergen, Penny, Linda Graham, Naomi Sweller, and Helen Dodd. 2015. "The Psychology of Containment: (Mis)representing Emotional and Behavioural Difficulties in Australian Schools." *Emotional and Behavioural Difficulties* 15 (1).

Wakefield, James. 1992. "The Concept of Mental Disorder: On the Boundary between Biological Facts and Social Values." *American Psychologist* 47 (3): 373–88.

Whitely, Martin. 2012a. "New Australian ADHD Clinical Practice Points—after 6 Years of Frustrated Advocacy at Last a Small Victory over Big Pharma." October 2. http://speed

upsitstill.com/australian-adhd-clinical-practice-points-6-years-frustrated-advocacy
-small-step-direction.

———. 2012b. "The Rise and Fall of ADHD Child Prescribing in Western Australia: Issues and Implications." *Australian and New Zealand Journal of Psychiatry* 46 (5):
400–403.

Willis, Evan. 2006. "Introduction: Taking Stock of Medical Dominance." *Health Sociology Review* 15 (5): 421–31.

World Health Organization (WHO). 1992. *The ICD-10 Classification of Mental and Behavioural Disorders: Clinical Descriptions and Diagnostic Guidelines.* Geneva: World Health
Organization.

5

The Medicalization of Fidgety Philip

ADHD in Germany

Fabian Karsch

E ven though attention deficit–hyperactivity disorder (ADHD) is relatively successfully medicalized in Germany, it remains contested. One could even go so far as to say that it is the controversial nature of ADHD itself that helped to promote the success story of the syndrome. The history of ADHD in Germany is often traced back to the children's story "Zappelphilipp" ("Fidgety Philip") by the German author and psychiatrist Heinrich Hoffmann, dating back to 1845. Fidgety Philip is described as a little boy who will not sit still at the dinner table. To some, this story includes an early description of a boy with ADHD symptoms. Yet the story of Fidgety Philip is largely understood as a pedagogical parable that points out a moral misbehavior rather than a disease-related inability. Thus, the question is raised regarding when (and how) the moral framework of interpretation was replaced by a medical interpretation. If Philip really was a "sick" child, then the evaluation of his behavior would not be a matter of why he would not sit still—he simply wasn't able to control himself. Interestingly enough, Hoffmann published another story in the same book, entitled "Hans Guck-in-die-Luft" ("Johnny Head-in-Air"), about a daydreamer whose behavior could nowadays be understood as that of a child with ADD symptoms, the predominantly inattentive type without hyperactivity.

What we can learn from the stories of Fidgety Philip and Johnny is that the violation of certain social norms can today be understood as being a result of an impaired cognitive performance rather than just morally inadequate behavior. The stories can also be interpreted as an indicator that ADHD is not merely a recent conception of teachers, doctors, patients, or the media, but that it might have been there all along as a certain variation of the norm that is now framed in medical terms. Yet the medical frame of interpretation, the "medicalization" of this phenomenon, has significantly changed the way in which societies, predominantly Western, deal with that type of deviant behavior. Not only has medicalization opened up new ways of social control, but accepting socially deviant behavior as a consequence of a biological status shifts responsibilities and may ease the burden of both the parents and the deviator. With further medicalization and decreasing stigmatization, the acceptance of the disease category grows and benefits emerge; access to medication and the legitimization of deviant behavior seem to be the main factors in this development. The pointed striving toward the sick role can thus be observed especially in adult ADHD patients, who are often very aware of those benefits.[1] Consequently, psychiatrists as well as nonprofessional stakeholders (e.g., individuals affected by ADHD, including patient organizations) have been seen to promote the disease category. These groups are a strong driving force in establishing and continuously stabilizing the medicalization of ADHD. This chapter traces the emergence of ADHD in Germany, its dissemination, and how ADHD is now processed, medically, politically, and socially. Included are the description of ADHD's current epidemiology, developments in the governance of ADHD, and different forms of stakeholder activism. Finally, I discuss living and performing with ADHD in daily life. In that context, the question is raised as to whether the practice of using pharmaceutical neurostimulants is best understood as a form of treatment or if the medicalization of certain behaviors is leading toward the establishment of cognitive-enhancing drugs in everyday life.

Emergence and Expansion of a Disease Category

In the late nineteenth century, children in Germany who would not comply with the moral system characterized by Protestant-Calvinist ethics and the then valid set of rules—emphasizing self-control and obedience—entered the realm of modern medicine. In 1845, the German psychiatrist Wilhelm Griesinger described children suffering from a "nervous constitution" and "showing no attention" (Rothenberger and Neumärker 2005a: 14). In 1890, the German

psychologist Ludwig Strümpell described in his treatise "Pädagogische Patholo-
gie oder die Lehre von den Fehlern der Kinder" ("Pedagogical Pathology or the
Theory of Children's Defects") "restlessness" and "inattention" as moral deficits
and flaws of character (Seidler 2004: 241). The assessment of deviant behavior in
moral categories was common, and even severe mental illnesses were framed as
loss of self-control and "relapse into immorality" (Fangerau 2006: 369).

Historic retrospectives of ADHD show that the British physician George
Frederic Still was among the first who suspected that the observed behavioral
shortcomings in children could have a somatic etiology (Doyle 2004). This hypothesis was supported by the finding that many of the children he examined
had suffered from actual verifiable brain damage and showed symptoms similar
to those of hyperactivity. Still speculated further that the children without a
known history of brain damage might have genetically inherited a malfunction-
ing of the brain (Doyle 2004: 2). Whatever the cause, it is remarkable that Still
associated brain malfunction with an impairment of moral control. Thus, what
was understood as the moral constitution of a person might, in his view, be biologically determined.

Another important yet often overlooked contribution in the history of ADHD
is the work by the German psychiatrists Franz Kramer and Hans Pollnow (1932).
In the study "Über eine hyperkinetische Erkrankung im Kindesalter" ("On a Hyperkinetic Condition in Childhood"), Kramer and Pollnow described a syndrome
that was characterized by restlessness and distractibility (Kramer and Pollnow
1932 in Rothenberger and Neumärker 2005a) and termed it "hyperkinetic condition." According to Neumärker (2005: 438), it appears that Kramer and Pollnow
(1932) proposed a remarkably contemporary description of ADHD:

In all patients the symptoms were observed for the first time when the children
were between three and four years of age, the "climax seeming to be at the age
of approximately six." Kramer and Pollnow maintained that "the uniformity of
symptoms and the manifold affinities in the course of the illness in the individual cases suggest that pathogenetically we do indeed have a homogenous
syndrome." As examples of these uniform symptoms, the authors listed an
elementary movement disorder together with a "chaotic character," lack of
concentration, insufficient goal orientation, increased distractibility, walking
around aimlessly, touching of chairs, boards, etc.—of everything "that comes
their way." Furthermore, patients showed no persistence (being affected "by
momentary external stimuli only"), occasional increased irritability, mood

lability, and inclination towards fits of rage or aggression. At school, children "affected" by hyperkinetic disease often caused extreme educational difficulties. (Neumärker 2005: 438)

Kramer and Pollnow's work can accordingly be understood as an important benchmark leading toward the notion of an organic etiology. They linked the symptoms to encephalitis or so-called minimal brain damage, later termed "minimal brain dysfunction" (MBD). In 1954, the East German psychiatrist Gerhard Göllnitz connected the hyperkinetic syndrome further to brain damage experienced during early childhood (Göllnitz 1954). A consensus was reached in the United States in 1966 when a task force formulated an official definition for the term "minimal brain dysfunction," which "refers to children of near average, average, or above average general intelligence with certain learning or behavioral disabilities ranging from mild to severe, which are associated with deviations of function of the central nervous system. These deviations may manifest themselves by various combinations of impairment in perception, conceptualization, language, memory, and control of attention, impulse, or motor function" (Clements 1966: 9). Substantial adaptations to the concept of MBD in Germany and Austria can be found in the works of Göllnitz (1970), Lempp (1973), and Corboz (1977).

In the 1970s, attention deficit was brought to the fore, finally resulting in the concept of "attention deficit disorder" (ADD) that was introduced in the American Psychiatric Association's (APA) third edition of the *Diagnostic and Statistical Manual of Mental Disorders (DSM-III)* in 1980, thereby abandoning the concept of "MBD." ADD was understood as a neuropsychiatric disorder with strong hereditary factors (Enseroth 2011: 22). The symptoms were considered strongly related to accompanying impairments in social sectors such as at school or at home, and whereas MDB was in its definition mono-causally linked to an organic brain lesion, ADD was defined by three different behavioral categories, thus focusing on the symptoms as opposed to the cause (Enseroth 2011: 22). With the integration of the diagnosis into the *DSM-III* in 1980, ADD was further legitimized as a valid diagnosis (Stiehler 2007: 47).

The criteria for "hyperkinetic disorder" (HKD) in the World Health Organization's (WHO) *International Classification of Diseases (ICD-10)* (WHO 1992), used mainly in Europe, are similar to the criteria in the *DSM-IV* (APA 2000), but they do not recognize the differentiation between the predominantly inattentive and the predominantly hyperactive subtypes. In the *ICD-10*, six of nine typical symptoms of attention deficit, three of five symptoms of hyperactivity, and one of four symptoms of impulsivity have to be present for a diagnosis. This may be the reason why diagnostics following *DSM-IV* criteria show a lower prevalence than those following *ICD-10* criteria (Krause and Krause 2014: 9). In contrast to the *ICD-9*, the *DSM* acknowledged the possibility of the persistence of the disorder into adulthood in the revised version (*DSM-III-R*), and facilitated a specific type of adult ADHD in the fourth edition (*DSM-IV*). In the German version of the *ICD-10* (GM [German Modification]),[2] ADHD is subsumed under the category of "disorders with onset in childhood or adolescence," thus also recognizing a possible chronicity of the disorder. As of the latest iteration of the *DSM*, the *DSM-5* (APA 2013), ADHD is no longer listed as a disruptive disorder but instead is classified as a neurodevelopmental disorder.

The medicalization of ADHD in Germany, understood as the widespread discursive and institutional establishment of the categories "HKD" and "ADHD," is strongly linked to the global spread and worldwide cultural impact of the label "ADHD." In Germany the condition is mostly referred to as "ADHS" (Aufmerksamkeitsdefizit-/Hyperaktivitätsstörung), mirroring the English label "ADHD." The globalization of disease categories (see Watters 2010) and maybe also the absence of a specialized handbook for the codification of mental illness in Germany contributed to the popularity of the *DSM* term of "ADHD" over the term "HKD" that is used in the *ICD* system, even though officially German physicians are required to use the *ICD-10* GM in communication with health insurance providers.[3] The effectiveness of treatment with methylphenidate since the 1960s, the lack of nonmedical means of social control, and the ever-growing acceptance of the condition within the realm of medicine itself led to a sustained and successful medicalization of ADHD in Germany as well as other countries. Thus, the 1990s showed a constant rise in the prescribed amount of daily doses of methylphenidate in Germany. Schubert et al. (2003) even suggest a 34-fold increase from 1991 to 2000, showing a drastic doubling of the amount between 1995 and 1996 as well as a sharp increase between 1999 and 2000. This resulted in an increase from around 400,000 daily doses in 1991 to 13.5 million daily doses in 2000 in Germany (Schubert et al. 2003: 4).

Medical Care and Epidemiology

The official clinical guidelines for ADHD are compiled and published by the Deutsche Gesellschaft für Kinder- und Jugendpsychiatrie (DGKJP) and are marked as outdated. The DGKJP is currently working on a revised guideline for adult and youth ADHD in cooperation with the Deutsche Gesellschaft für Psychiatrie und Psychotherapie, Psychomatik und Nervenheilkunde (DGPPN). The still available outdated guidelines use both *ICD-10* and *DSM-IV* criteria, but as the range of ADHD variants are subsumed as "hyperkinetic disorders," its wording distinctly tends toward the *ICD-10*. However, referring to the *DSM-IV*, the guidelines identify hyperactivity, impulsivity, and inattention as the core symptoms and differentiate the following subtypes: the predominantly inattentive type, the predominantly hyperactive-impulsive type, and the combined type. The authors of the guidelines add that there has not been any consensus regarding the classification of subtypes (DGKJP 2007: 239). They also explain which comorbid disorders might be encountered and how multimodal treatment should be carried out. There is a wide range of available treatments for ADHD in Germany (ranging from physical therapy to counseling, and more recently, neurofeedback), but a multimodal approach, mostly combining cognitive-behavioral therapy and medication, is proclaimed as the gold standard (DGKJP 2007: 245).

Adult patients with ADHD seeking medication have long been suffering from the restrictions of Germany's drug-regulation laws, which have prevented or at least complicated access to methylphenidate treatment. Since the Bundesinstitut für Arzneimittel und Medizinprodukte (BfArM) only recently approved methylphenidate for the treatment of adult patients in 2011 (BfArM 2011), off-label use was the only way to proceed. This meant not only that patients had poor prescription coverage through their health insurance for ADHD medication, but also that prescribing physicians took a bigger liability risk. Despite the recent approval of adult treatment (BfArM 2011), there has not been a rise in the usage of methylphenidate. In 2014, the BfArM even stated that according to the most recent statistics, there has not been a rise in the prescription of methylphenidate for the first time in 20 years. With 1,839 kilograms in 2012 and 1,803 kilograms in 2013, it might be too early to discern a downward trend, but the development certainly points toward the stagnation of a so-far ongoing rise in methylphenidate usage. This might be the result of a more critical handling of the drug, as BfArM President Walter Schwerdtfeger suggests (BfArM 2014).

There might be another reason for the seeming stagnation of the usage of methylphenidate in Germany. The Gemeinsamer Bundesausschuss (G-BA), being the highest decision-making body of the joint self-government of physicians, hospitals, and health insurance funds in Germany, announced in 2010 a further restriction on the prescription of methylphenidate-based stimulants. Due to the "risk potential" of the stimulants, the diagnosis must follow diagnostic criteria, "for example, the *DSM-IV*," more strictly, implying a shortcoming in previous ways of diagnosing that were presumably conducted without using any formal guidelines. Furthermore, stimulants can only be prescribed by specialized medical practitioners (ideally psychiatrists) as part of an "overall diagnostic strategy" (G-BA 2010).[4] This restriction can be understood as a reaction to the ongoing dispute about the substantial number of methylphenidate prescriptions over the past few years.

Germany operates with a so-called universal health care system, which is based on a compulsory state-governed health insurance system with coexisting private insurance groups. Eighty-five percent of German citizens take part in the compulsory public health insurance scheme, which is financed by contributions that are calculated as a percentage of gross salary. There has been an ongoing debate about an exponential increase in the cost of the German health care system and related reforms (see Porter and Guth 2012). An ever-rising number of diagnosed ADHD patients means more expenses for treatment, and the expansion of diagnostic criteria to include adult ADHD further intensifies that problem. Schlander, Trott, and Schwarz (2010: 297) estimate the cost of ADHD to the public health care system to be 260 million euros per year and warn of further overdiagnosis.

So what is the actual prevalence of ADHD in Germany? The Studie zur Gesundheit von Kindern und Jugendlichen in Deutschland (KiGGs), conducted between 2003 and 2006 (Schlack et al. 2007), presents nationally representative data for the age range of 3 to 17 years and shows a parent-reported lifetime prevalence of 4.8% based on diagnosis made by medical professionals or psychologists. Parents of 7,569 boys and 7,267 girls 3 to 17 years of age took part in the study. Participants whose parents reported that they had received an ADHD diagnosis by a doctor or psychologist were classified as ADHD cases. ADHD had been diagnosed in 7.7% of the boys and 1.8% of the girls. Another 4.9% of the participants can be considered as suspected cases (showing significant signs of ADHD deduced by parental judgment, but without having received an official diagnosis). Among primary school-age children (7 to 10 years old) the frequency of diagnosis was 5.3% and even higher for the age group 11 to 13 years (7.1%). At ages 11 to 17 years, ADHD had been diagnosed in 1 in 10 boys and 1 in 43 girls. Furthermore, ADHD was diagnosed significantly more frequently among participants of low socioeconomic status (SES) than among participants of high SES. A diagnosis of ADHD in Germany was reported less often for migrants, who rank more frequently among the suspected cases. The discrepancy between confirmed and suspected cases of ADHD among migrants may point to lower rates of diagnosis or lower utilization of medical services (Schlack et al. 2007). So what is the latest development of the epidemiology in Germany? Lange et al. (2014) come to the conclusion that there were no significant changes in the frequency of ADHD diagnosis between the years 2003 and 2012. A follow-up to the nationally representative KiGGs study based on the years 2009–12 showed a prevalence of 5.0% among children and adolescents between 3 and 17 years of age (compared to 4.8% in the baseline study). Another report, based on a sample of health insurance data between 2006 and 2011, shows a marginally lower prevalence of 4.1% of hyperkinetic disorder diagnoses following *ICD-10* criteria (Grobe, Bitzer, and Schwartz 2013).

Different studies show different persistence rates of ADHD depending on their methods, the demographic structure of the sample, and the diagnostic criteria used. The persistence of ADHD diagnosis can thus vary between 10% and 78% (Krause and Krause 2014: 12). Fayyad et al. (2007) conducted a survey in 10 different countries (Belgium, Colombia, France, Germany, Italy, Lebanon, Mexico, the Netherlands, Spain, and the United States) and found an average prevalence of 3.4% among adults (4.1% male and 2.7% female), with Germany showing a prevalence of 3.1%. A more recent survey that was based on a self-report questionnaire found a higher prevalence of 4.7% among adults in Germany (de Zwaan et al. 2012). The quality of health care for ADHD appears to change drastically with the patient's 18th birthday. A study conducted by the German health insurance provider Barmer GEK (Lehmkuhl and Schubert 2013) queried 3,728 diagnosed ADHD patients between the ages of 18 and 21. The survey showed that 49% of the participants reported that their pharmaceutical treatment was terminated when they turned 18, with only 12% reporting that their attending physician was arranging a follow-up treatment with another professional (Lehmkuhl and Schubert 2013: 6). A total of 18% found it difficult to receive ongoing therapy, and 14% reported a transition to another physician. All these factors indicate challenges in the trajectory of ADHD, when diagnosed children and adolescents transition into adulthood. This is most likely due to the fact that ADHD in Germany is often still framed and perceived as a childhood disorder. Although the BfArM approved the prescription of methylphenidate for adult patients in 2011, the study indicates that adult ADHD has not been fully established yet.

Discourses on ADHD

Public discourses on ADHD in Germany have mainly been critical in nature for a long time. In Germany, like in many other countries, ADHD has become a synonym for medicalization, or even disease mongering. Imprecise and interpretable diagnostic criteria (such as "has difficulty organizing tasks"; see *DSM-IV*) led to the impression that anyone could be suffering from ADHD symptoms—more or less. The core issue, however, has always been pharmaceutical treatment. Over the course of the ongoing debate on ADHD, methylphenidate (Ritalin) has become one of the most well-known but also notorious and contested pharmaceuticals. In retrospect, the main pattern of interpretation in the German public discourse is that of a medicalization critique, which either sees ADHD as a case of disease mongering or dismisses a biological etiology and with it the need for pharmaceutical treatment. The headline "Koks für Kinder" ("Cocaine for Kids") in the popular German magazine *FOCUS* (Bartholomäus 2002) is indicative of the critical media coverage.[5] Public discourse has not been the sole source of criticism around ADHD. Social scientists picked up the perception of ADHD as a social problem early on and contributed to the understanding of "ADHD" as a label mainly used as a mechanism of control. As early as 1983, a publication with the controversial title *Pillen für den Störenfried* (*Pills for the Troublemaker*; Voss 1983) critically discussed hyperkinetic syndrome and the associated medication of children. The book includes a contribution by the renowned sociologist Peter Conrad, and presents the only translation of Conrad's work into German (Conrad 1983). In the context of this critical anthology, Conrad's balanced description of ADHD as an example of the medicalization of deviant behavior was perceived as a much more normative (and thus critical) standpoint. But gradually another frame of interpretation entered the discourse on ADHD in Germany.

Groups of concerned persons, including parents, relatives, and adult patients began actively promoting ADHD in Germany and united in self-help groups and other associations. The first self-help groups formed as early as the 1990s, but grew larger and gained greater recognition over the course of the following decades. In 2007, two larger associations, the Bundesverband Aufmerksamkeitsstörung/Hyperaktivität e.V. (BV-AH e.V.) and the Bundesverband Arbeitskreis Überaktives Kind e.V. (BV AÜK e.V.) fused to form ADHS Deutschland e.V., the largest German ADHD self-help organization to date. Such organizations can exert substantial influence on health care politics and discourses. In

2002, the German Bundestag issued a statement (Bundesdrucksache 2002) entitled "Methylphenidat bei ADHS verantwortungsbewusst einsetzen" ("Toward a Responsible Use of Methylphenidate"), proclaiming new legal parameters to include "abuse of medications": "[Methylphenidate] is an underestimated medicinal drug, used to achieve what parents cannot manage anymore: calming overactive children to allow concentrated learning, while risking side effects and addiction . . . Scientists are divided on what causes the syndrome of ADHD, which is why it is discussed whether ADHD is merely a fashionable disease" (Bundesdrucksache 2002: 2).[6] Twelve different advocacy groups reacted in a joint statement, trying to rebut the critical assessment, using references to the latest scientific studies and demanding to be included in future consultation and decision-making processes. The Bundsministerium für Gesundheit reacted by calling a consensus conference, bringing together representatives from psychiatry, psychology, politics, and lay advocacy groups.[7] The outcome was a clear message to the media to refrain from "wrong and irresponsible messages about the medical treatment of ADHD"[8] and an overall reinforcement of the voice and involvement of advocacy groups. This led to the publication of an informational booklet issued by the Bundeszentrale für gesundheitliche Aufklärung entitled "ADHS . . . was bedeutet das?" ("ADHD, What Does It Mean?"; BzGA 2004), which now advocates the biomedical model of ADHD, the possible benefits of pharmaceutical treatment, and the support of local and national self-help groups. In 2002, Barkley et al. published a consensus statement on ADHD that was co-signed by an international consortium of scientists. It was aimed at presenting an unequivocal stand on the matter of ADHD's validity and the critical public discourse surrounding the condition (Barkley et al. 2002). The consensus statement had a vital impact on the discussion in Germany. In 2005, the support group Elterninitiative zur Förderung von Kindern mit Aufmerksamkeits-Defizitsyndrom mit/ohne Hyperaktivität (AdS e.V.) published a translation of the consensus statement that was additionally signed by 107 German-speaking professionals from Germany, Austria, and Switzerland (AdS e.V. 2005). Hence, the organization of patients in self-help and advocacy groups can be understood as social dynamics of bottom-up medicalization, in which there is a shift from a medical imperialism toward a self-governed medicalization that is indicated by the expanding influence of self-help groups and well-informed patients (see Hafferty 2006).

ADHD Diagnosis: An Avenue toward Cognitive Enhancement?

The development of a more self-governed medicalization gives the impression that Fidgety Philip learned to take care of himself over the years. In a case study that was co-conducted by the author at the University of Augsburg, Germany, within a larger collaborative research program (DFG Sonderforschungsbereich 536 "Reflexive Modernisierung") (Wehling et al. 2007; Viehöver et al. 2009; Karsch 2011a, 2011c; Viehöver and Wehling 2011),[9] everyday practices of adult ADHD patients were examined. We conducted several focus groups with a sample of adult patients—some of whom self-identified as having ADHD while most cases had been officially diagnosed with ADHD—although the specifics of the diagnosis (e.g., type of ADHD, diagnostic criteria used) were often not known. Those patients who were active in self-help groups, on the one hand, could be virtually described as lay experts with a profound knowledge of their condition. Group discussions revealed that adult patients can perceive a diagnosis of ADHD as an opportunity since it provides legitimate access to pharmaceuticals with the possibility of optimizing their cognitive performance.

If the patients were not diagnosed as children or adolescents, the diagnostic trajectory was often initiated by a diagnosis of their own children or the perusal of self-help literature or information on the Internet, followed by a consultation with a medical professional. Consequently, the process of obtaining a precise patient history was often reported as self-directed. Participants described how being confronted with a medical diagnosis can lead to a new perception of personality traits that are then understood anew as a deficit or a disorder. The intense self-inquiry may initiate a reinterpretation of one's personal history. The following comment from a female participant in one of the focus groups illustrates this context:

> A kindergarten teacher advised me that I should read a book about ADD. And then I could totally see [my child] in it, but was afraid that I just wanted to have a diagnosis for my child, wanted it to finally get a name. I then gave the book to my husband, and he also recognized himself in it . . . Yes, I then started to dive deep into the topic of ADD, read a lot . . . and I then also started to listen to myself and think about myself and I realized more and more that I am also a typical ADD person. (Karsch 2011c: 280)[10]

This process of the "contextualization of the self" (Karsch 2011c: 283) is followed by an official medical diagnosis in most cases, but the group discussions indicated that the diagnosis is handled very differently and individually among the patients.

One patient may be convinced that she has a biological disadvantage and accept taking medication largely as a treatment for a morbid deficit. From this perspective, pharmaceutical treatment seems mandatory to leading a "normal," independent life. Since the professional medical definition is in this case a central element in the appropriation process of the label "ADHD," the compliance with the physician's advice seems distinctive, making this type of patient most closely match the concept of the classic sick role, as described by Parsons (1951). The following statement from a male focus group participant helps to illustrate that patient type:

> When I got the diagnosis, the [doctor] said to me very clearly, it is a deficiency of neuro-transmitters, which is not curable in the sense that one could make my brain reproduce the chemical messengers that I do not produce myself. My only chance would be to learn to live with it. For this, there are also behavioral therapies, but that would not make sense in my case as long as I am not adjusted with medication. After a long phase of experimentation with various drugs . . . I was now set to 56 milligrams of Concerta. It lasts approximately 8–9 hours and I think I owe it to the medication that I still have my job today. (Karsch 2011c: 281)[11]

Other participants correspondingly reported taking the drugs because of the performance-enhancing effects, but much more independently of the physician's recommendations. This type of consumer only sporadically takes the prescribed drugs and does so mostly in certain situations in which increased performance and attention are required. The actual clinical significance of the diagnosis hardly plays a role in the everyday handling of the condition and is merely a necessity to ensure legal access to the needed medication.

In certain cases, the described behavioral patterns even suggest explicit strategies of cognitive enhancement,[12] although taking the performance-enhancing psychotropic drugs is actually framed in the context of ADHD treatment. Patients often reported using their children's medications when they were out of their own prescription or were otherwise not able to access medication but felt the need for a more focused mind. The selective drug use in specific situations indicates a more enhancement-oriented usage that differs from common forms of treatment. It is remarkable that some participants describe a distinct enhancement effect when taking the stimulants, while others feel that by taking the medication, they are restored to a "normal" state and experience that state as "authentic" and "self-determined" and as their "real self." Others, however, characterize the effect of the medication as "unnatural"; they feel their identity

Table 5.1.   Patient Types and the Processing of ADHD Diagnosis and Treatment

	Acceptance of drug treatment	Repudiation of drug treatment
Acceptance of the diagnosis	Type 1: classical patient role; implicit neuro-enhancement	Type 3: classical patient role; critical of neuro-stimulants
Repudiation of the diagnosis	Type 2: self-directed patient; may include explicit neuro-enhancement	Type 4: medicalization critic; critical of both the medical labeling and neuro-stimulants

threatened or displaced by the ingestion of the drugs. Table 5.1 presents a classification of patient types in our study and the way in which they process ADHD
diagnosis and treatment.

Type 1: For type 1 patients, ADHD is understood as an illness-related deficit.
Drug therapy is accordingly understood as the restoration of health status. The
patients remain closest to a classical sick role. Due to the nature and goals of the
stimulant treatment and the disease-oriented frame of interpretation, the use of
drugs can be described as implicit neuro-enhancement.

Type 2: For type 2 patients, diagnosis is only relevant as an institutional gateway. Medication is more specifically used for performance enhancement. Since
the medical model is not the determining framework, but the effects and the efficiency of the used drugs are of more overall importance, the drug usage tends
toward explicit neuro-enhancement.

Type 3: For type 3 patients, it is notable that the medical interpretation of the
condition is accepted, but pharmaceutical treatment is refused. The patients remain close to a classical sick role but are critical of taking neuro-stimulants.

Type 4: Type 4 patients are mainly critics of medicalization and, despite the
acknowledgment of certain symptoms (or impairments), reject the disease-
oriented model of interpretation and any means of pharmaceutical treatment.

This typology is purely analytical in nature, while the actual empirical types
will more often be characterized by diverse shades of gray. It is the gray areas that
define living with ADHD symptoms. ADHD is a condition that points out that it
is not sufficient to understand cognitive enhancement as a practice performed by
undiagnosed individuals. Just because a certain field of social practice is successfully medicalized, cognitive enhancement does not suddenly transform into medical treatment. Medicalization dynamics are thus better understood as dynamics
that legitimize certain social practices of enhancement.

Whether it is attention-deficit, burnout, sadness, or shyness, there are quite a few conditions that are today understood as symptoms with definitional fuzziness that puts them in a gray area where an exact scientific boundary between a healthy state and a state of illness becomes increasingly unachievable (see Horwitz and Wakefield 2007; Wehling 2010; Karsch 2011a; Viehöver and Wehling 2011; Lane 2014). Yet the precise differentiation and a certain unambiguousness are often needed for institutional decision-making and cultural processes of interpretation. "ADHD" is today successfully codified and institutionalized as a disease category in Germany. Yet it is not only contested publicly but also within the groups of those affected. For them, the diagnosis might just function as a gateway toward medical enhancement of cognitive abilities. But everyday practice suggests that a clean distinction between drug therapy and enhancement does not seem productive or even possible.

Conclusion

Fukuyama (2003) once warned about the biotechnological revolution. He pointed out the variety of potentially dangerous forms of intervening in human nature—for example, by artificially prolonging the lifespan, genetic engineering, and the increased importance of the neuro-sciences and new forms of neuro-pharmacology—which would allow manipulation of emotion and behavior (Fukuyama 2003). More than a decade later, it can be argued that we did not enter the "Posthuman" era and that the "Consequences of the Biotechnological Revolution" haven't been as radical as predicted.

Nevertheless, there seems to be an overall increase of "sociomedical disorders" (Dumit 2000) that are characterized by "soft" criteria of diagnosis and by treatments that focus on the improvement of emotional states, cognitive efficiency, or (deviant) social behavior. It is to Fukuyama's credit that he realized the substantial and lasting importance of the subject. The possible consequences of biotechnology and the expansion of the medical realm are still widely discussed, not only in the social science and bioethics fields, but increasingly in the public sphere. The usage of psychopharmeceuticals beyond therapeutic means, often labeled "brain-doping," has become a permanent issue in the German mass media and is often linked to methylphenidate use and ADHD. "The greatest increase in drug use" as the sociologist Irving Zola noted back in the 1970s, "has not been in the realm of treating any organic disease but in treating a large number of psycho-social states. Thus we have drugs for every mood" (Zola 1972: 495). Various types of antidepressants or stimulants such as methylphenidate or modafinil are known as potential neuro-enhancing drugs. But these drugs are commonly used for the treatment of specific diseases. In other words, the usage is medically indicated most of the time—even though the indication itself might be contested. Critics often complain about the seemingly ever-rising number of ADHD cases. However, epidemiological studies on ADHD (or hyperkinetic disorder) in Germany come to conclusions similar to those of most international studies, showing an average prevalence of approximately 5%, with boys being diagnosed around three times more often than girls. With a strict application of the more stringent *ICD-10* criteria, the prevalence would probably drop significantly, but although physicians are obliged to encode their diagnosis via the *ICD* system, they may also encode *DSM* diagnoses, which seems to occur frequently. Unfortunately, there is still a lack of good data regarding actual diagnostic practice in Germany, the use and choice of diagnostic criteria, and the application of guidelines. Furthermore, it remains unclear whether the more or less constant diagnostic rates and the by now apparently stagnating trend of methylphenidate prescriptions actually point toward a finalized backlog. They could also have stagnated at high levels for other reasons, such as a cultural or political climate that is resistant or even counterproductive to further medicalization.

Besides the critical public view of medicalization dynamics and the critical mass media coverage, powers of bottom-up medicalization are growing in strength and are a significant social process within the realm of ADHD. Current discourses on ADHD in Germany show that patients are craving for their condition to be accepted and are struggling for better access to medication. Although the biomedical interpretation of ADHD still appears ambiguous and contested, the usage of medications (mostly methylphenidate) is deemed to be an integral part of coping with ADHD symptoms. It is in this regard that physicians seem to be reduced to the role of gatekeepers (e.g., to legally establish access to diagnosis and medication). Biosocial communities, on the other hand, are becoming the main engines and sites of self-medicalization practices.[13] In Germany, the definition of ADHD as a disease category remains an important factor, especially when it comes to institutional decision-making or to legitimizing certain forms of action, while in everyday practice, the usage of methylphenidate can often be interpreted as a certain means of explicit or implicit neuro-enhancement. Accordingly, in the realm of ADHD, boundaries between health and illness as well as treatment and enhancement seem to blur more and more.

Dominated by critical views for a long time, the discourse on neuro-enhancement recently became more and more liberal in Germany and has thus shifted toward a greater variety of assessments, with some even decidedly advocating for the usage of medical-enhancement methods. In 2008, a statement by a group of distinguished authors and scientists in the journal *Nature* (Greely et al. 2008) endorsed the idea that mature and responsible consumers should be able to acquire certain neuro-enhancing drugs to benefit from their effects. In Germany in 2009, a group of ethicists and scientists took a similar approach and published a consensus statement to open the discussion on a liberal approach toward medical enhancement (Galert et al. 2009). This shift in discourse may be a result of the highly restricted availability of neuro-enhancement opportunities (Karsch 2011a). The debate on ADHD shows that, for the most part, the practice of neuroenhancement takes place within the medical realm. It is still the medical profession that has the strongest impact in defining physiological states, and it is physicians who act solely as gatekeepers to provide access to diagnoses and treatments, including drugs. Thus, legitimized forms of cognitive enhancement take place in a completely medicalized field of action.

NOTES

1. The concept of the sick role was introduced by Talcott Parsons (1951, 1975). Parsons stated that sickness is not merely a physical condition but also a social role surrounded by a certain set of norms. These not only include responsibilities but also exemptions from social responsibilities and expectations.

2. The German modification (*ICD-10* GM) has been adapted to the requirements of the German health care system. https://www.dimdi.de/dynamic/de/klassi/downloadcenter /icd-10-gm/.

3. The *DSM* has been translated and published in German (APA 2015).

4. Translation by the author.

5. One of the earlier examples can be found in the archives of a large German regional daily in 1988, featuring the headline: "Der chemische Krieg gegen die Kinder" ("Chemical Warfare against Our Children"). http://www.abendblatt.de/archiv/1988/article 203742105/Der-chemische-Krieg-gegen-die-Kinder.html.

6. Translation by the author.

7. Key points are accessible at http://www.zentrales-adhs-netz.de/fileadmin/ADHS /Aktuelles/Eckpunktepapier.pdf.

8. As stated by former state secretary to the federal minister for health Marion Caspers-Merk. Translated by the author (see Drüe 2007: 187).

9. The research group was led by Peter Wehling and Willy Viehöver, University of Augsburg.

10. Translation by the author.

11. Translation by the author.

12. Cognitive enhancement may be defined as a medical intervention the goal of which is not therapeutic but aims at optimizing cognitive abilities, performance, or efficiency. For a broader discussion, see Parens (2000).

13. The idea of biosocial communities is drawing on Paul Rabinow's concept of "biosociality," which describes the emergence of new forms of identity and sociality on the basis of biological, technoscientific knowledge (see Rabinow 1996; Lemke 2015).

REFERENCES

American Psychiatric Association (APA). 1980. *Diagnostic and Statistical Manual of Mental Disorders (DSM-III)*. 3rd ed. Washington, DC: American Psychiatric Association.
———. 2000. *Diagnostic and Statistical Manual of Mental Disorders (DSM-IV)*. 4th ed. Washington, DC: American Psychiatric Association.
———. 2013. *Diagnostic and Statistical Manual of Mental Disorders (DSM-5)*. 5th ed. Washington, DC: American Psychiatric Association.
———. 2015. *Diagnostisches und statistisches Manual psychischer Störungen (DSM-5)*. Göttingen: Hogrefe.
Barkley, Russell A., et al. 2002. "International Consensus Statement on ADHD." *Clinical Child and Family Psychology Review* 5 (2): 89–111.
Bartholomäus, Ulrike. 2002. "Koks für Kinder." *FOCUS Magazin* 11.
Bundesdrucksache. 2002. "Methylphenidat bei ADHS verantwortungsbewußt einsetzen." Deutscher Bundestag. 14/8912. Wahlperiode: 24.04.2002. http://dip21.bundestag.de/dip21/btd/14/089/1408912.pdf.
Bundesinstitut für Arzneimittel und Medizinprodukte (BfArM). 2011. "Methylphenidat auch für Erwachsene: BfArM erweitert Zulassung." http://www.bfarm.de/DE/BfArM/Presse/mitteil2011/pm02-2011.html.
———. 2014. "Erstmals seit 20 Jahren kein Anstieg beim Methylphenidat-Verbrauch." http://www.bfarm.de/SharedDocs/Pressemitteilungen/DE/mitteil2014/pm05-2014.html.
Bundeszentrale für gesundheitliche Aufklärung (BZgA). 2004. *ADHS. Aufmerksamkeitsdefizit/hyperaktivitätsstörung . . . was bedeutet das?* Selbstverlag Bachem: Köln. http://www.bzga.de/botmed_11090100.html.
Clements, Sam D. 1966. *Minimal Brain Dysfunction in Children: Terminology and Identification*. Washington, DC: US Department of Health, Education, and Welfare.
Conrad, Peter. 1983. "Die Entdeckung der Hyperkinese: Anmerkungen zur Medizinierung abweichenden Verhaltens." In *Pillen für den Störenfried? Absage an eine medikamentöse Behandlung abweichender Verhaltensweisen bei Kindern und Jugendlichen*, edited by Reinhard Voss, 93–106. Hamm: Hoheneck.
Corboz, Robert. 1977. "Psychiatrische Aspekte des Streß beim Kind und beim Jugendlichen." *Schweizer Archiv für Neurologie, Neurochirurgie und Psychiatrie* 121: 81–89.
Deutsche Gesellschaft für Kinder- und Jugendpsychiatrie (DGKJP). 2007. *Leitlinien zur Diagnostik und Therapie von psychischen Störungen im Säuglings-, Kindes- und Jugendalter*. Köln: Deutscher Ärzte Verlag.
Doyle, Robert. 2004. "The History of Adult Attention-Deficit/Hyperactivity Disorder." *Psychiatric Clinics of North America* 27 (2): 203–14.

Drüe, Gerhild. 2007. *ADHS kontrovers: betroffene Familien im Blickfeld von Fachwelt und Öffentlichkeit.* Stuttgart: W. Kohlhammer Verlag.

Dumit, Joseph. 2000. "When Explanations Rest: 'Good-Enough' Brain Science and the New Sociomedical Disorders." In *Living and Working with the New Medical Technologies: Intersections of Inquiry,* edited by Margaret Lock, Allan Young, and Alberto Cambrioso, 209–32. Cambridge: Cambridge University Press.

Elterninitiative zur Förderung von Kindern mit Aufmerksamkeits-Defizitsyndrom mit/ohne Hyperaktivität (AdS e.V.). 2005. "Zur Medienberichterstattung über ADHS. Gemeinsame Erklärung internationaler Wissenschaftler (Übersetzung aus dem Englischen)." http://www.adhs-deutschland.de/ResourceImage.aspx?rid=328.

Enseroth, Timo. 2011. *Konstruktion und Validierung der MCD-Skala zur Erfassung unterschwelliger organischer Psychosyndrome (Minimale Cerebrale Dysfunktion, MCD) im Erwachsenenalter.* PhD diss., Medizinische Fakultät Charité—Universitätsmedizin Berlin.

Fangerau, Heiner. 2006. "Psychische Erkrankungen und geistige Behinderung." In *Geschichte, Theorie und Ethik der Medizin,* edited by Heiner Fangerau, Norbert Paul, Stefan Schulz, and Klaus Steigleder, 368–99. Frankfurt am Main: Suhrkamp.

Fayyad, John, R. De Graaf, R. Kessler, J. Alonso, M. Angermeyer, K. Demyttenaere, G. De Girolamo, J. M. Haro, E. G. Karam, C. Lara, J.-P. Lépine, J. Ormel, J. Posada-Villa, A. M. Zaslavsky, and R. Jin. 2007. "Cross-National Prevalence and Correlates of Adult Attention–Deficit Hyperactivity Disorder." *British Journal of Psychiatry* 190 (5): 402–9.

Fukuyama, Francis. 2003. *Our Posthuman Future: Consequences of the Biotechnology Revolution.* New York: Macmillan.

Galert, Thorsten, Christoph Bublitz, Isabella Heuser, Reinhard Merkel, Dimitris Repantis, Bettina Schöne-Seifert, and Davinia Talbot. 2009. "Das optimierte Gehirn. Ein Memorandum zu Chancen und Risiken des Neuroenhancements." *Gehirn und Geist* 11: 40–48.

Gemeinsamer Bundesausschuss (G-BA). 2010. "Zum Schutz von Kindern und Jugendlichen—Verordnung von Stimulantien nur in bestimmten Ausnahmefällen." https://www.g-ba.de/downloads/34-215-351/27-2010-09-16-Stimulantien-AMR.pdf.

Göllnitz, Gerhard. 1954. *Die Bedeutung der frühkindlichen Hirnschädigung für die Kinderpsychiatrie.* Leipzig: Thieme.

———. 1970. *Neuropsychiatrie des Kindes- und Jugendalters.* Jena: Gustav Fischer Verlag.

Greely, Henry, Barbara Sahakian, John Harris, Ronald C. Kessler, Michael Gazzaniga, Philip Campbell, and Martha J. Farah. 2008. "Towards Responsible Use of Cognitive-Enhancing Drugs by the Healthy." *Nature* 456: 702–5.

Grobe, Thomas, Eva Bitzer, and Friedrich Schwartz. 2013. *BARMER GEK Arztreport 2013.* Siegburg: Asgard.

Hafferty, Frederic W. 2006. "Medicalization Reconsidered." *Society* 43 (6): 41–46.

Horwitz, Allan V., and Jerome C. Wakefield. 2007. *The Loss of Sadness.* Oxford: Oxford University Press.

Karsch, Fabian. 2011a. "Enhancement als Problem der soziologischen Medikalisierungsforschung." In *Herausforderung Biomedizin—Gesellschaftliche Deutung und soziale Praxis,* edited by Sascha Dickel, Martina Franzen, and Christoph Kehl. Bielefeld: transcript.

———. 2011b. "Neuro-Enhancement oder Krankheitsbehandlung? Zur Problematik der Entgrenzung von Krankheit und Gesundheit am Beispiel ADHS." In *Entgrenzung* der Medizin: Von der Heilkunst zur Verbesserung des Menschen? edited by Willy Viehöver and Peter Wehling. Bielefeld: transcript.

———. 2011c. "Die Prozessierung biomedizinischen Körperwissens am Beispiel der ADHS." In Körperwissen, edited by Reiner Keller and Michael Meuser. Wiesbaden: VS Verlag.

Kramer, Franz, and Hans Pollnow. 1932. "Über eine hyperkinetische Erkrankung im Kindesalter." European Neurology 82 (1–2): 1–20.

Krause, Johanna, and Klaus-Henning Krause. 2014. ADHS im Erwachsenenalter: Symptome-Differenzialdiagnose-Therapie. Stuttgart: Schattauer Verlag.

Lane, Christopher. 2014. "Social Anxiety Disorder and Shyness." In The Wiley Blackwell Encyclopedia of Health, Illness, Behavior, and Society, edited by William Cockerham, Robert Dingwall, and Stella R. Quah, 2133–36. Oxford: Wiley.

Lange, Michael, H. G. Butschalowsky, F. Jentsch, R. Kuhnert, A. Schaffrath Rosario, M. Schlaud, and P. Kamtsiuris. 2014. "Die erste KiGGs-Folgebefragung (KiGGs Welle 1)." Bundesgesundheitsblatt-Gesundheitsforschung-Gesundheitsschutz 57 (7): 747–61.

Lehmkuhl, Gerd, and Ingrid Schubert. 2013. "Versorgung bei ADHS im Übergang zum Erwachsenenalter aus Sicht der Betroffenen." Barmer GEK, Bertelsmann Stiftung. http://www.bertelsmann-stiftung.de/cps/rde/xbcr/SID-BDC29145-FC1407F7/bst/2013.pdf.

Lemke, Thomas. 2015. "Patient Organizations as Biosocial Communities? Conceptual Clarifications and Critical Remarks." In The Public Shaping of Medical Research: Patient Associations, Health Movements and Biomedicine, edited by Peter Wehling, Willy Viehöver, and Sophia Koenen, 191–97. London: Routledge.

Lempp, Reinhart. 1973. "Das hirnorganische Psychosyndrom im Kindesalter." Deutsche Medizinische Wochenschrift 98 (39): 1817–21.

Neumärker, Klaus-Jürgen. 2005. "The Kramer-Pollnow Syndrome: A Contribution on the Life and Work of Franz Kramer and Hans Pollnow." History of Psychiatry 16 (4): 435–51.

Parens, Eric, ed. 2000. Enhancing Human Traits: Ethical and Social Implications. Washington, DC: Georgetown University Press.

Parsons, Talcott. 1975. "The Sick Role and the Role of the Physician Reconsidered." Health and Society 53 (3): 257–78.

———. 1951. The Social System. London: Routledge.

Porter, Michael E., and Clemens Guth. 2012. Redefining German Health Care: Moving to a Value-Based System. Berlin: Springer.

Rabinow, Paul. 1996. Essays on the Anthropology of Reason. Princeton, NJ: Princeton University Press.

Rothenberger, Aribert, and Klaus-Jürgen Neumärker. 2005a. "ADHS—Allgemeine geschichtliche Entwicklung eines wissenschaftlichen Konzepts." In Wissenschaftsgeschichte der ADHS. Kramer-Pollnow im Spiegel der Zeit, edited by Aribert Rothenberger and Klaus-Jürgen Neumärker. Darmstadt: Steinkopff.

———. 2005b. Wissenschaftsgeschichte der ADHS. Kramer-Pollnow im Spiegel der Zeit. Darmstadt: Steinkopff.

Schlack, Robert, H. Hölling, B.-M. Kurth, and M. Huss. 2007. "Die Prävalenz der Aufmerksamkeitsdefizit-/Hyperaktivitätsstörung (ADHS) bei Kindern und Jugendlichen in Deutschland." *Bundesgesundheitsblatt-Gesundheitsforschung-Gesundheitsschutz* 50 (5): 827–35.

Schlander, Michael, Götz Erik Trott, and Oliver Schwarz. 2010. "Gesundheitsökonomie der Aufmerksamkeitsdefizit-/Hyperaktivitätsstörung in Deutschland." *Der Nervenarzt* 81 (3): 301–14.

Schubert, Ingrid, I. Köster, Ch. Adam, P. Ihle, L. V. Ferber, and G. Lehmkuhl. 2003. "Hyperkinetische Störung als Krankenscheindiagnose bei Kindern und Jugendlichen— eine versorgungsepidemiologische Studie auf der Basis einer Versichertenstichprobe. Abschlussbericht an das Bundesgesundheitsministerium für Gesundheit und soziale Sicherung, 2003." https://www.bundesgesundheitsministerium.de/fileadmin/redaktion /pdf_publikationen/forschungsberichte/Hyperkinetische_Storrung_als _Krankenscheindiagnose.pdf.

Seidler, Eduard. 2004. "Zappelphilipp und ADHS. Von der Unart zur Krankheit." *Deutsches Ärzteblatt* 101 (5): 239–43.

Stiehler, Miriam. 2007. *Konzentrationserziehung statt AD(H)S-Therapie: ein Modell nach Paul Moor.* Bad Heilbrunn: Julius Klinkhardt.

Viehöver, Willy, and Peter Wehling, eds. 2011. *Entgrenzung der Medizin. Von der Heilkunst zur Verbesserung des Menschen?* Bielefeld: transcript.

Viehöver, Willy, P. Wehling, F. Karsch, and S. Böschen. 2009. *Die Entgrenzung der Medizin und die Optimierung der menschlichen Natur. Biopolitische Strategien und Praktiken des Enhancements und ihre Aneignung durch die Individuen, illustriert anhand der Beispiele ADHS und Anti-Aging-Medizin.* Berlin: Büro für Technikfolgen-Abschätzung beim Deutschen Bundestag (TAB).

Voss, Reinhard, ed. 1983. *Pillen für den Störenfried? Absage an eine medikamentöse Behandlung abweichender Verhaltensweisen bei Kindern und Jugendlichen.* Hamm: Hoheneck.

Watters, Ethan. 2010. *Crazy Like Us: The Globalization of the American Psyche.* New York: Free Press.

Wehling, Peter. 2010. "Schüchternheit—nur ein lästiges Hindernis auf dem Weg zu emotionaler Expressivität?" In *Unsichere Zeiten. Verhandlungen des 35. Kongresses der Deutschen Gesellschaft für Soziologie in Jena,* edited by Hans-Georg Soeffner. Wiesbaden: VS Verlag.

Wehling, Peter, W. Viehöver, R. Keller, and Ch. Lau. 2007. "Zwischen Biologisierung des Sozialen und neuer Biosozialität: Dynamiken der biopolitischen Grenzüberschreitung." *Berliner Journal für Soziologie* 17 (4): 547–67.

World Health Organization (WHO). 1992. *The ICD-10 Classification of Mental and Behavioural Disorders: Clinical Descriptions and Diagnostic Guidelines.* Geneva: World Health Organization.

Zola, Irving. 1972. "Medicine as an Institution of Social Control." *Sociological Review* 20: 487–504.

Zwaan, Martina de, B. Gruss, A. Müller, H. Graap, A. Martin, H. Glaesmer, A. Hilbert, and A. Philipsen. 2012. "The Estimated Prevalence and Correlates of Adult ADHD in a German Community Sample." *European Archives of Psychiatry and Clinical Neuroscience* 262 (1): 79–86.

6

ADHD in the United Kingdom

Conduct, Class, and Stigma

Ilina Singh

If attention deficit–hyperactivity disorder (ADHD) in the United Kingdom were a word cloud that attempted to capture its status as a social object, it would be characterized most prominently by a bold assemblage of biological and developmental research and researchers, intertwined with national guidelines and epidemiological reports. The pharmaceutical industry, health economics–related terms, and media reports would appear in smaller, lesser font caught up within this bold assemblage in a minor way. Smallest of all, elements related to ADHD as a lived experience would be (if we imagine this to be a three-dimensional word cloud) sucked into the vortex of the assemblage, a tiny object in the depths of a black hole. These elements and this configuration make up ADHD in the United Kingdom in the early twenty-first century.

I start with this attempt at a three-dimensional image because the content of this chapter is unsatisfyingly two-dimensional: it provides statistics on the prevalence of ADHD in the United Kingdom and stimulant drug use, it suggests some reasons why those statistics have stayed relatively low in comparison to those in other countries, and it offers some scenes of what ADHD looks like "on the ground." The three-dimensional image should serve as a reminder that the primary power and authority in UK ADHD resides within the bold assemblage, which produces and presents ADHD primarily in the form of genetic and brain biomarkers, complex cognitive endophenotypes, and lots of numbers. What is most interesting, perhaps, is that the authority of ADHD in this empiricist form has not translated into widespread, positive public uptake of the diagnosis or its treatments in the United Kingdom. This is not good news for families and children struggling with access to ADHD evaluations and support, ADHD stigma, and ADHD identity concerns. On the other hand, it does mean that diagnosis of ADHD and use of stimulant drug treatment are not (despite occasional media hype) at "epidemic" proportions in the United Kingdom. In fact, ADHD in the United Kingdom presents an object lesson in how powerfully national values can operate both at the level of public engagement with ADHD diagnosis and treatment and, less transparently, in the production of national guidelines and in the management of children in schools, families, and clinics.

This chapter also includes some personal observations and experiences. I have spent the past decade working on ADHD in and around scientists, clinicians, patients, and parents in the United Kingdom, and my research has, in both explicit and implicit ways, become part of the national discourse on ADHD. I do not develop a sustained critical analysis of my role or engagements; instead, I use my experiences to illuminate dynamics and actors that have informed the development of ADHD in the United Kingdom outside the formal processes of the National Health Service (NHS), the evidence base, and public groups and discussions.

ADHD Prevalence in the United Kingdom

Prevalence estimates for ADHD in any country are difficult to interpret because the methods for obtaining them vary across studies. In the case of ADHD estimates, data can be derived from parent reports, physician databases, population studies, and so forth. The data frequently do not differentiate among types of ADHD diagnosis (mild, moderate, severe; inattentive, hyperactive, or combined type); diagnostic criteria used by the clinician (different versions of the American *Diagnostic and Statistical Manual of Mental Disorder* [*DSM*] or the *International Classification of Diseases* [*ICD*]); or diagnostic methods used in the clinical evaluation process (parent report, teacher and parent report, child interview, developmental history interview, etc.). Even when the same diagnostic methods are used, those methods can be applied differently. On the ground, approaches to ADHD diagnosis frequently vary (to a greater or lesser degree) according to clinician, service, location, and the type of health service coverage

(NHS or private). These complexities are why prevalence estimates often include wide statistical ranges. These caveats invite a critical reading of ADHD diagnosis and stimulant drug treatment reports in any country, but this orientation should not necessarily discount epidemiological estimates.

In the United Kingdom, a recent systematic analysis provides an estimate of 1.9% to 5% of UK children who meet criteria for an ADHD diagnosis—interestingly, this most recent analysis was performed by a group of US researchers (Murphy et al. 2014). A footnote on the sources used for this analysis notes that "UK clinicians and researchers commonly use hyperkinetic disorder instead of ADHD" (Murphy et al. 2014: 189). Hyperkinetic disorder is the international kin of ADHD, described in the tenth revision of the *ICD* (http://www.wolfbane.com /icd/) as a more severe form of ADHD, characterized by significant psychosocial impairments. The *ICD* is a World Health Organization (WHO) compilation used to classify and manage psychiatric disorders around the world, except in the United States, which uses the *DSM*. In the United Kingdom, clinical practice is governed by the National Institute for Clinical and Care Excellence (NICE). NICE performs systematic reviews of the evidence for diagnostic and treatment practices and issues guidelines for best practice. It also performs technology assessments and cost-benefit analyses for treatments. On the basis of a balance of costs, benefits, and evidence, NICE directs which treatments should be covered under the NHS. Licensed drug treatments for ADHD on the NHS are short- and long-acting forms of methylphenidate (Concerta, Equasym, Medikinet, Ritalin, or generic), dexamfetamine (generic), or lisdexamfetamine (Elvanse in the United Kingdom; Vyvanse in the United States) and atomoxetine, marketed as Strattera.

Non-UK researchers might have the impression that UK researchers use the term "hyperkinetic disorder" instead of "ADHD"; in practice, however, it is not clear that the use of "hyperkinetic disorder" instead of "ADHD" is so "common." *ICD* criteria represent an international consensus in relation to ADHD. In the United Kingdom, NICE describes the use of both systems of classification of ADHD, and characterizes ADHD along "mild," "moderate," and "severe" dimensions. In generating guidelines for UK practitioners on ADHD diagnosis and treatment, NICE specifies that it uses *DSM* criteria, not *ICD* criteria (https:// www.nice.org.uk/guidance/cg72). The *ICD* and the *DSM* are, respectively, associated with lower and higher estimates of ADHD in the population. In 2013, NICE estimated that, based on the narrower criteria of *ICD-10*, hyperkinetic disorder occurred in about 1% to 2% of children in the United Kingdom (Green et al. 2004). Using the broader criteria of *DSM-IV*, NICE estimated that about 3% to 9% of school-age children met criteria for ADHD (https://www.nice.org.uk/guidance/qs39).

In my observation of clinic interactions and participation in national conference presentations, clinicians and clinician-researchers are more likely to refer to *DSM* criteria for ADHD than to *ICD* criteria. The new emphasis on psychiatric biomarker discovery initiated by the US National Institutes of Mental Health (called Research Domain Criteria, or RDoC) is also starting to affect how researcher-clinicians conceptualize ADHD (http://www.nimh.nih.gov/about /director/2012/research-domain-criteria-rdoc.shtml). ADHD comorbidities and theories of common biological risk factors in neurodevelopmental pathways are increasingly emphasized in research designs and in discussion of therapeutics. In summary, it would appear that NICE UK ADHD is influenced in explicit ways more by shifts in American research orientation, funding, and theories than by international classification or trends.

ADHD Treatment in the United Kingdom

It is possible that the historic use of the term "hyperkinetic disorder" in the United Kingdom lingers at an unconscious level among clinicians trained there. This history, combined with emphasis in the NICE guidelines on severity and impairment in ADHD diagnosis, might shift the normal distribution of ADHD diagnosis in the United Kingdom toward the more severe end. However, the data on the use of stimulant drugs in the United Kingdom undermine this inference, as one might assume that if a more severe form of ADHD is being diagnosed in the United Kingdom, then there would be proportionately high use of stimulant drug treatments (which would follow NICE guidelines). NICE specifies that stimulant drugs should only be used as a first-line treatment for severe ADHD. Available data on use of ADHD medications indicate that use in the United Kingdom, ranging from 0.02% to 1.3% among 3- to 18-year-olds, is consistently estimated to be among the lowest in the world, and is low relative to overall UK ADHD prevalence estimates (INCB 2012; Murphy et al. 2014; Beau-Ledjstrom et al. 2016). However, this range does fit well with the NICE estimate of severe ADHD prevalence in the United Kingdom (1% to 2% of the child population), so it may be that the proportion of diagnosed children who have severe ADHD, or hyperkinetic disorder, in the United Kingdom are being treated appropriately with stimulant medication according to NICE guidelines. But this is conjecture: there are no data available that match ADHD medication prescription to the type of ADHD diagnosis recorded for a child.

The relatively low estimates of ADHD drug treatment also signal general concerns on the part of doctors about treating children with stimulant drugs. These concerns can be mapped in part to the influence that NICE has had in shaping UK clinical practice and in publicizing views on ADHD diagnosis and stimulant drug treatments. In the 2008 ADHD Guidelines, NICE emphasized that the first line of treatment for mild to moderate ADHD should be parent training, and that drug treatment should be used only in severe cases (https://www.nice .org.uk/guidance/cg72). In 2013, NICE published a Quality Standard on ADHD (https://www.nice.org.uk/guidance/qs39/chapter/Introduction). A Quality Standard can be interpreted as a response to a perceived lack of good practice in national clinic settings, or, more generally, concerns about rising rates of diagnosis and drug treatments. The ADHD Quality Standard outlined seven criteria for quality diagnosis and assessments; these criteria again underscored the use of parent training as the first-line treatment for ADHD and introduced psychological treatments for children into the ADHD treatment package.

Soon after the Quality Standard was published, the Care Quality Commission (CQC) published an annual report on the management of controlled drugs in England (http://www.cqc.org.uk/content/annual-report-201314). The report found that prescription of methylphenidate in NHS primary care had increased by 56% in the past six years (http://www.cqc.org.uk/content/report-warns-need -continued-vigilance-and-monitoring-controlled-drugs). NICE responded with a brief story on its website entitled "Avoid Drug Treatment for Children and Young People with Moderate ADHD" (https://www.nice.org.uk/news/article/avoid -drug-treatment-for-children-and-young-people-with-moderate-adhd). The story goes on to suggest that the level of prescribing indicated that ADHD drugs were being "abused." Tim Kendall, director of the National Collaborating Centre for Mental Health (the group that leads the development of NICE Clinical Guidelines), was quoted by the British Broadcasting Service (BBC): "I think there's also increasing evidence that [use of ADHD drugs] precipitates self-harming behavior in children, and in the long-term we have absolutely no evidence that the use of Ritalin reduces the long-term problems associated with ADHD." When asked whether there were any long-term risks among people who take methylphenidate drugs, Kendall said: "In children, without doubt. If you take Ritalin for a year, it's likely to reduce your growth by about three-quarters of an inch"

(https://www.nice.org.uk/news/article/avoid-drug-treatment-for-children-and
-young-people-with-moderate-adhd).

As a director of NICE and as lead for the ADHD Clinical Guideline Group in
2008, Kendall's voice carries significant medical and even political authority.
One might argue that on a public website accessed by families looking for support and information, this voice should provide a more balanced account of the
evidence on risks and benefits of ADHD drug treatments (see Poulton 2005;
Vitiello 2008; Bushe and Savill 2013). On the other hand, it may be that firm application of the precautionary principle has helped to keep use of ADHD drugs in
the United Kingdom from escalating to levels seen in other countries.

A concrete way in which NICE may help to keep control over rates of ADHD
drug prescribing is by limiting the number of NHS-approved ADHD medications. This creates an interesting situation in which families who want drugs
that are not available on the NHS must obtain them from elsewhere. For example, Adderall is widely used in the United States but it is not licensed for treatment of ADHD in the United Kingdom. A little noted detail in the CQC report is
that the second most commonly prescribed drug in the UK private care system
(non-NHS) was dexamfetamine. Dexamfetamine is a central nervous stimulant
and a main ingredient in Adderall. Dexamfetamine did not appear at all on the
list of commonly prescribed schedule II drugs in the NHS. The report did not
make the association between prescription of dexamfetamine and ADHD diagnosis, and the drug is prescribed for conditions other than ADHD. However,
the difference between rates of NHS and private prescribing of dexamfetamine
could mean that families with the resources are turning to the private care system for ADHD prescriptions, where they are also able to access a wider range of
drug treatments for ADHD.

The 2013 Quality Standard on ADHD also included emphasis on the best
practice pathway to ADHD diagnosis and treatment, and urged adherence to
the recommended guidelines for follow-up of children treated with stimulant
drugs. In the NHS, initial diagnosis of ADHD must be performed by an
"ADHD specialist," defined as a "psychiatrist, pediatrician or mental health
specialist with training and expertise in the diagnosis and treatment of ADHD.
For the assessment and diagnosis of ADHD in children and young people this
will be a child psychiatrist, pediatrician or specialist ADHD nurse" (https://www
.nice.org.uk/guidance/qs39/chapter/Quality-statement-1-Confirmation-of
-diagnosis). In practice, most children are referred to a specialist ADHD service.
The service is headed by a child psychiatrist and supported by a multimodal team

composed variously of pediatricians, psychologists, social workers, and mental health nurses. Online support group chatter suggests that there is significant variation (between 12 weeks and 2 years) in waiting times across the NHS for children and adult assessments (http://www.leicspart.nhs.uk/Library/Library FOI1213376.pdf; https://www.reddit.com/r/ADHD/comments/1chqpt/anybody _have_any_experience_of_a_recent_adult_add/). Depending on the service, a child presenting for an ADHD assessment may be evaluated in two visits (the first to take a developmental history from parents, and the second to evaluate the child in the context of family and environment) or in one visit. The Quality Standard also emphasized taking a period of time to properly titrate the dose of ADHD medication, if a child was prescribed it, and the importance of an annual follow-up of children taking medication for ADHD. It is too soon to know whether these recommendations are making a difference in the quality of care received by children and families who are in the system for diagnosis and treatment of ADHD.

Social Factors Associated with ADHD in the United Kingdom
Social Class

A valuable report investigating the demographic features associated with mental disorders in children in the United Kingdom, including "hyperactivity," was published by Meltzer and colleagues in 2000. The report found that social class was associated with significant differences in the rates of diagnosed mental disorder in children, with those in social class V (unskilled occupations) about three times more likely to have a mental disorder than those in social class I (professionals)—14% compared to 5%, and about twice as likely as those in social class II (managerial and technical workers). Both conduct disorders and hyperactivity showed significant class trends in diagnosis, and were also significantly comorbid. Conduct disorder was then, and is now, the most prevalent child psychiatric diagnosis in the United Kingdom (https://www.nice.org.uk /guidance/cg158/evidence/cg158-conduct-disorders-in-children-and-young -people-full-guideline3). High comorbidity between conduct disorder and ADHD was confirmed in both the 2008 ADHD NICE Guideline and the 2013 Conduct Disorder NICE Guideline. In Meltzer and colleagues' survey, 10% of children 5 to 15 years of age in social class V families had been diagnosed with conduct disorder as compared to 2% of the same age children in social class I. Elspeth Webb has argued on the basis of this data that "if all child populations in the United Kingdom had the same prevalence of ADHD as seen in the wealthiest quintile, we would have a 54% decrease in ADHD prevalence overall" (http://www.med scape.com/viewarticle/804142_3).

The association between ADHD and poverty has recently been confirmed in a number of studies available in the United Kingdom. In 2014, Russell et al. reported findings based on the Millennium Cohort Study that ADHD diagnosis in the United Kingdom was associated with a range of indicators of social and economic disadvantage, including poverty, low levels of maternal education, low income, single parenthood, and younger motherhood. A local authority study confirms what is found in the national cohort study: based on data from Liverpool, a major urban center in northwest England, authors found significant associations between the degree of deprivation in residential areas and ADHD diagnosis rates, concluding that "an improved socio-economic environment may significantly improve the overall outcome of childhood ADHD" (Ogundele and De Doysa 2011: A25).

Schooling

The average British child attends mandatory schooling until age 16. In the United Kingdom, a good deal of a child's life is spent in school, and school is where behaviors associated with ADHD are often first identified as problematic. Therefore, schooling and children's experiences in a particular school within a particular community make up an important proximate factor in a child's development (Singh 2006). Approximately 93% of UK children attend state-funded schools or academy (public-private partnerships) or religious schools. The remaining small minority of children attend fee-paying "public" schools. School quality is a much-debated subject in the United Kingdom (see, e.g., http://www .lrb.co.uk/v37/n09/dawn-foster/free-schools). A recent report on school performance standards revealed that 30% of state schools in the United Kingdom are judged not to deliver a quality education (https://www.gov.uk/government/news /ofsted-annual-report-201314-published). School quality also varies widely according to geographic region, with children in some areas having a less than 50% chance of getting a good education and children in other areas having a greater than 90% chance of a good education in the state system (http://www.lrb.co.uk /v37/n09/dawn-foster/free-schools).

A UK child's opportunities beyond the period of mandatory schooling are contingent on social class: social and geographic mobility in the United Kingdom are still low (http://www.swslim.org.uk/downloads/sl2003.pdf), and there are wide achievement gaps between advantaged and disadvantaged children. At least one study has shown, however, that bad schools are not entirely to blame for the relatively poor performance of disadvantaged children (http://theconver sation.com/even-at-best-schools-kids-on-free-school-meals-are-performing-worse -than-their-peers-32006). Disadvantaged children who attend outstanding schools also achieve poorly, relative to their peers. Therefore, additional social factors such as the stress of low-resource environments and peer and community influ-ences must be taken into account when understanding achievement differences among children.

Children diagnosed with ADHD in the United Kingdom are not recognized as having a disability, and they are not automatically eligible for special education services. Parents can apply for children diagnosed with ADHD to be recognized as having special educational needs, either through the school special education services or through a national legal mechanism called an "education, health and care plan." The former route provides support services from a trained provider in the school setting; the latter route—often referred to as "a statement"—is for children with more complex needs. A statement sets out legally mandated provi-sions for a child's education that map onto the child's development in the school setting (https://www.gov.uk/children-with-special-educational-needs/overview). For parents, both these routes are fraught with upset, difficulty, and disappoint-ment. Under the first route, many schools do not have sufficient resources to provide adequate or sufficient special educational services for all the children who need them. The second route is a legal mandate; however, in practice it is difficult to obtain a statement for a child with ADHD (see, e.g., the discussion at http://www.mumsnet.com/Talk/special_needs/1128156-ADHD-does-not-qualift -for-a-Statement).

Poverty and school resources are linked problems in the United Kingdom, with children in poor neighborhoods more likely to attend schools with lower-quality teaching, lower educational standards, and fewer resources for special educational needs. Schools with a high proportion of poor children also tend to have higher levels of students with emotional and behavioral problems. One indicator of a child's achievement in school is parental interaction with the school (http://www.cls.ioe.ac.uk/library-media/documents/Primary%20and%20 secondary%20education%20and%20poverty%20review%20August%202014 .pdf). Poor children's parents are less likely to interact with school because of a combination of factors, including lack of confidence and time. Given the diffi-culties involved in getting special educational services for children with ADHD in the United Kingdom and the expectation of parent (often maternal) advocacy on behalf of children (Blum 2014), children benefit from parents who establish and maintain good connections to teachers and schools. Parental communication and involvement increase the chances that children's behaviors will be understood and managed appropriately at home and at school. This is particularly true for children with behavioral difficulties, who are heavily stigmatized in the United Kingdom as "naughty" or "bad" children (see "Conduct" below). For all these reasons, children diagnosed with ADHD living in poor neighborhoods in the United Kingdom are likely to be worse off in educational terms than children diagnosed with ADHD living in wealthier neighborhoods.

CONDUCT

Conduct is a live issue in UK schools and in UK politics. In national reports and in interviews with children, two features of UK schools frequently stand out: widespread evidence of poorly run classrooms, in which teachers are unable to control children's behavior, and a culture of verbal and physical bullying among peers. The problem of classroom behavior management was documented in 2009, in the Good Childhood Report (Children's Society 2009). In a survey of children 11 to 14 years of age, 29% said that other children tried to disrupt lessons on a daily basis and 43% said other children were "always" or "often" so noisy that they found it difficult to work. A 2008 survey of teachers found that 43% experienced disruption in their lessons on a daily basis and 12% found themselves pushing/touching students on a weekly basis (http://www.publications .parliament.uk/pa/cm201011/cmselect/cmeduc/writev/behaviour/we39.htm). In 2015, UK Prime Minister David Cameron found the issue sufficiently urgent to appoint a "school behavior management tsar" to tackle the crisis on a national level (www.ofsted.gov.uk/resources/140157; http://www.theguardian.com/edu cation/2015/jun/16/school-behaviour-tsar-classroom-disruption).

Data on bullying behavior are difficult to come by in the United Kingdom because of a lack of good systematic data, poor methodology (including varying definitions of bullying), and accusations of biased reporting by all involved. Outside official reports, one indication of the importance of the topic on a national level is the level of attention it has received from prominent individuals. In 2015, the Duke and Duchess of Cambridge, arguably the two most prominent and popular national figures in the United Kingdom, declared bullying to be a royal priority over the next few years, particularly in the context of the development of mental illness in young people (http://www.thetimes.co.uk/tto/news/uk/royal family/article4522183.ece).

Of the official reports available, it appears that bullying is more prevalent in primary school as compared with secondary school, but that in secondary school cases of bullying accompanied by physical aggression are more frequent. The 2003 Tackling Bullying survey reported that, in year 5 (when most children are 9 to 10 years old), 44% of students said they had been pushed by another child, 37% said they had been hit on purpose, and 35% said they had been kicked (http://www.antibullying.net/documents/Childline%20DP%20Bullying.pdf). A new and fast-rising anti-bullying charity called Ditch the Label provides data that give some insight into the experience of bullying in the United Kingdom (http://www.ditchthelabel.org). The charity surveyed young people at a limited sample of schools over a three-year period, using transparent and fairly rigorous methods. In 2014, they surveyed 3,600 students, finding that 45% of young people 13 to 18 years of age surveyed had experienced bullying before the age of 18. Of those who reported having been bullied, 61% said they had been physically attacked and 55% reported having been cyberbullied. Twenty-six percent of bullied students said that bullying occurred on a daily basis. Thirty-four percent reported that bullying occurred because of discrimination or prejudice, including disability, and 51% were dissatisfied with how teachers handled reports of bullying (http://www.ditchthelable.org).

Children's Experiences of ADHD

Urie Bronfenbrenner's ecological model of child development argues that macro-level features of social class, schooling, and bullying interact with micro-level, or "proximate," features of children's daily lives, such as family and community life and friendships (Bronfenbrenner 1979). A child's development must be seen as a process of adjustment and adaptation to her "ecological niche." On the basis of the Bronfenbrenner model, one would expect to hear experiences from children with conditions such as conduct disorder and ADHD that map the broader ecological dynamics surrounding and informing children's behavioral norms and expectations.

In the VOICES (Voices on Identity Childhood, Ethics and Stimulants: Children Join the Debate) study, a major study of children's experiences of ADHD diagnosis and treatment in the United Kingdom, we discovered that there were distinctive ways in which the ecological dynamics described above informed perceptions and experiences of ADHD diagnosis (see www.adhdvoices.com).[1] We found that ADHD was widely viewed as a "disorder of anger and aggression" (Singh 2011). Children diagnosed with ADHD, as well as their peers, teachers, and family members, consistently described ADHD symptoms—particularly the difficulty with self-control—as "an exploding volcano," "hot," and "boiling." Peers referred to children diagnosed with ADHD as having "an anger problem." Children diagnosed with ADHD were subjected to stigmatizing assumptions and activities, primarily in the school context. On the playground, they were frequently drawn into bullying encounters in schools, both as victims of bullying and as victimizers of other children. These experiences tended to be more aggressive, to be more sustained, and to have more negative consequences (such as school expulsion) for students from lower social class categories. In the VOICES study sample of 82 UK children, we found that the focus on ADHD as a problem of poorly controlled anger meant that behavior, rather than academic performance, was the primary target of concern among adults and children and of treatment following diagnosis. In this way, both the embodied and the performative dimensions of ADHD mapped the broader ecological preoccupation with children's conduct and behavior.

PARENTAL ATTITUDES AND ADHD

In the United Kingdom, good behavior in children, and its opposite "naughtiness," are major preoccupations in parenting discourse; naughtiness in a child is seen to be a key responsibility of parents and a target of intervention. As we have seen, good behavior is also foregrounded as a key developmental value in social policies. "Naughtiness," whether as part of a diagnosis or not, is a label that confers stigma and signals that a child is unlikely to have good outcomes. However, in the context of ADHD, attitudes on parental responsibility for good behavior in children integrate some other more general social values, which are elaborated frequently in discussions with parents. These values hold that one should "sort things out" on one's own and "not make a fuss." Parents used such language to explain a lack of interaction with the school over a child's difficulties (parents would attend school meetings when a child got into trouble, but not to discuss general difficulties) and to explain their reluctance to seek expert advice and treatments for a child. Such attitudes may be pervasive across social class categories, but they may have more negative consequences for children in lower social classes because they further inhibit parental interactions with teachers and schools.

In our research on ADHD in the United Kingdom, a subset of children in the study had what was called "teacher-identified ADHD." In schools, this group was managed primarily by the learning disabilities staff. Staff tended to frame these children as having symptoms of ADHD with associated learning difficulties. Parents reported that they were grateful for school support and for what they considered to be a safe place for their children to go when they were "stressed." In many cases we encountered, ADHD was not discussed explicitly with parents whose children were being managed in these ways. Thus, the value of good behavior in children was effectively enacted through alternative means to ADHD diagnosis, allowing parents to avoid "a fuss" and school personnel to "sort things out" without medical intervention. While this approach may be preferable to diagnosis and medication to some observers, parents, children, and school staff reported that these school-based interventions were not wholly effective in preventing escalation of social and academic impairments and more severe behaviors.

The values of independence ("I'll sort it out") and emotional reticence ("don't make a fuss") uncovered in the VOICES research may track more generally across the United Kingdom to help explain consistently lower rates of ADHD diagnosis and use of drug treatments in the United Kingdom, as compared with other Western countries. But it is important to avoid simplistic deployment of national clichés in the attempt to explain ADHD diagnosis rates and treatment uptake. The role of national attitudes and values in ADHD should be investigated using conceptual and methodological tools that enable refinement of hypotheses and more in-depth understanding. Only then can claims about the importance of one factor or another in ADHD diagnosis and treatment be taken seriously.

ADHD Advocacy

Perhaps due in part to the values of independence and emotional reticence, ADHD advocacy in the United Kingdom is a relatively quiet space.[2] The most prominent and probably the oldest national advocacy organization is ADDISS (Attention Deficit Disorder Information and Support Service, http://www.addiss .co.uk). Its director has close relationships with some key ADHD researchers in the United Kingdom, but the primary role of ADDISS is to function as an information distribution center. More recently, ADDISS has started offering training for practitioners and educators in ADHD diagnosis and management. ADDISS is a registered charity, but there is no information available on its website about its sources of income or annual budget. It raises money through fundraisers, sales at its bookstore, and training sessions. Its website suggests a low-budget enterprise with limited resources for upkeep. ADDISS representatives frequently participate in UK ADHD scientific meetings, and the organization is known and appreciated by UK researchers and parents alike. Publicly, ADDISS has carved out a successful, neutral stance on most controversies in ADHD, maintaining its profile as a supportive resource for those grappling with ADHD from any perspective.

In 2009, a group of prominent mental health professionals created UKAAN (UK Adult ADHD Network). The UKAAN website states that the network was a specific response to the NICE 2008 ADHD Guidelines and further guidelines established by the British Association for Psychopharmacology (http://www .ukaan.org/what-is-ukaan.htm), which found there to be a lack of resources for adult ADHD in the United Kingdom. UKAAN holds a well-attended international conference each year and sees education of clinical professionals as its central remit. It is funded largely and transparently by the pharmaceutical industry and, as a consequence (which is not at all unusual in UK medicine), UKAAN conferences have an active pharmaceutical industry presence.

In the past two years, another advocacy organization has entered the frame: the ADHD Foundation (http://www.adhdfoundation.org.uk). Its remit is to promote "inclusion in mental health, education and employment." The ADHD Foundation is a multipartner public-private organization that lists the NHS as a partner. As of 2017, the Foundation's corporate sponsors included two pharmaceutical companies (Shire and Flynn Pharma Ltd), as well as universities and third-sector organizations. A main objective of the organization is to deliver training to educators and employers, as the tagline suggests. In contrast to ADDISS, the Foundation's website is sleek, user-friendly, and confident, suggesting more resource inputs and a clearer strategy for advocacy.

Pharmaceutical companies have played an active role in ADHD education and training over the past decade. The industry players have shifted over the years, from the turn of the century, when Janssen was marketing Concerta; to 2005–7, when Eli Lilly was marketing Strattera; to the present day, when Shire put through a big push for Elvanse (Vyvanse), approved in the United Kingdom in 2014. Throughout this time, clinicians' offices have been peppered with information leaflets from the industry about ADHD diagnosis and management. These leaflets are generally beautifully made, highly attractive, and informative, and they offer families a wealth of advice beyond the treatment offered by the drug company; examples include child behavior management techniques, ways to deal with parental stress, school and teacher discussions, homework routines, and organizational management of child and family.

UK rules on industry promotional activities in the context of prescription medicines are fairly strict: no marketing of a drug is allowed prior to the license being approved; no direct-to-consumer (DTC) advertising is allowed at any time; and promotional activities, for example, to health care professionals following drug licensing, are subject to governance and audit (PMCPA 2015). One might argue, of course, that in the Internet age, restrictions on industry marketing activities are relatively meaningless, from the consumer's point of view, unless they are globally enforced. At the moment, consumers looking for information about a drug like Adderall, which is not licensed in the United Kingdom, can just go to the Shire website. On the other hand, in my experience, PMCPA restrictions have had positive effects on decreasing the number and type of pharmaceutical industry products found in clinical settings.

The restriction on pre-licensing activities in the United Kingdom has led to some creative ways of providing information on a new drug. For example, in the years preceding the approval of Elvanse in the United Kingdom, Shire Pharmaceuticals was active in ADHD education for teachers and medical professionals, sponsoring a variety of educational and informational forums for educators and clinicians. In meetings in which I participated, the program advocated a multimodal approach to ADHD; there was no explicit recommendation for psychotropic treatments over other treatments, nor was there specific mention of Shire-owned drug treatments for ADHD.[3] Substantive, well-resourced pharma-booklets on a range of non-drug-related topics, from coping in school to parenting strategies, are ubiquitous at ADHD educational and scientific meetings, and in clinical settings in the United Kingdom. It is easy, even for a skeptic, to understand why educators and health care professionals would hand over these beautifully produced, child-friendly materials when families ask for more information. The NHS does not provide comparably attractive and user-friendly resources.

Post-licensing, the dissemination of pamphlets and other materials across a range of institutional contexts continues to have normalizing effects. A case from the VOICES study illustrates the point. During an interview, a father reported having gone to the local library to look for more information about ADHD. The family was working class and had few professional or peer resources to draw on for information; they had found the information they received from the NHS to be lacking in substance and details, particularly in the context of treatment options. In the library, the father found a pamphlet on ADHD stuck between some medical books, and he asked to take it home. He found the information useful and dialed the information number on the pamphlet. A "really helpful lady" answered his questions patiently for about 20 minutes; he was impressed with the service. The father could not recall where the pamphlet was from, but he was sure it was an ADHD support service of some sort. He eventually found the pamphlet and showed it to the researcher. The father had been speaking to an Eli Lilly representative, who was, in fact, in violation of the UK PMCPA, which states that "requests from individual members of the public for advice on personal medical matters must be refused [by drug maker representatives] and the enquirer recommended to consult his or her own doctor or other prescriber or other health professional" (PMCPA 2015). The reality needs to be conceded: in conditions of relatively scarce resources—such as NHS child mental health services—parents, researchers, educators, and clinicians find financial and emotional support in industry partners. The problematics of these engagements have been extensively documented (see Angell 2005), and the PMCPA cannot keep all of these at bay, particularly since UK drug research depends on big pharma's continued financial input. Instead of once again critiquing the role of industry in ADHD, it may be more useful to indicate where that role does the most potential harm and to consider how that harm might be minimized.

Many actors are brought together in the long game played by industry in the pre-licensing period: scientists, clinicians, parents, children, and teachers. In the United Kingdom, this game is known to researchers and clinicians, and their participation is informed by an awareness of where they fit in this work, along with its risks and benefits. However, this sort of informed analysis is less likely to characterize the involvement of educators in pharmaceutical company activities, and many parents who find themselves involved in a pharma-supported information network are almost certainly unaware of the background to the network. Parents are sometimes desperate for information, and because of the stigma surrounding ADHD, the lack of NHS resources, and the lack of awareness of pharmaceutical industry activities, they are less likely to take a critical view of what is on offer. Parents who experience the challenges of low-resource settings are particularly vulnerable to parental stigma (bad children are thought to be caused by bad parents, especially bad mothers) and this combination of factors may mean that they are more susceptible to misunderstanding pharmaceutical marketing techniques as bona fide efforts to promote good child outcomes. Therefore, parents and educators in low-resource settings are likely to be most vulnerable to pernicious pharmaceutical industry activity but, paradoxically, also most likely to benefit from constructive industry activities.

ADHD Contestation

It may be a peculiarly British phenomenon that the interactions between the critics of ADHD and researchers in biological psychiatry who uphold the diagnosis are generally courteous. It is also notable that there is only one major public critic of ADHD. Sami Timimi, a psychiatrist, has written several widely read books that include criticisms of ADHD diagnosis and stimulant drug treatments (Timimi 2005, 2007). Timimi has also initiated an international group called CAPSID (Campaign to Abolish Psychiatric Diagnostic Systems such as ICD and DSM). The group's claims are as follows (http://www.criticalpsychiatry.net/wp -content/uploads/2011/05/CAPSID12.pdf):

1. Psychiatric diagnoses are not valid.
2. Use of psychiatric diagnosis increases stigma.
3. Use of psychiatric diagnosis does not aid treatment decisions.
4. Long-term prognosis for mental health problems has gotten worse.
5. It imposes Western beliefs about mental distress on other cultures.
6. Alternative evidence-based models for organizing effective mental health care are available.

The group argues that the scientific paradigm that looks to the causes and solutions to mental distress in underlying biology is ineffective. Nonmedical paradigms that take account of contextual factors and degrees of impairment, without trying to link these to stigmatizing psychiatric categories, are likely to be more useful in generating knowledge about the causes of mental distress and better at specifying effective treatments. On the website, UK membership of CAPSID stands at six people, including Timimi. This is not indicative of the number of mental health practitioners who might agree, in some part, with some of these claims. The problems of validity in psychiatric diagnosis and stigma associated with mental illness diagnoses are consistently raised in meetings organized by the Royal College of Psychiatrists (RCP), whose members are a representative field of UK psychiatry. And although support for CAPSID is not overtly strong, some of its messages are echoed in a number of other communities in the United Kingdom, notably in the recovery movement, the neurodiversity movement, and psychiatric user communities.

It is also important to distinguish between CAPSID and Scientology-related anti-ADHD advocacy. Scientology in the United Kingdom is more anti-psychiatry than critical-psychiatry, and the arguments advanced in support of this position are significantly less sophisticated and informed than those of critical-psychiatry movement supporters. Scientology remains primarily in the background in the context of UK psychiatry; there are no prominent celebrities or national campaigns. However, the group does make its presence known to prominent psychiatrists in the Twittersphere and helps to organize protests online and in-person ahead of high-level conferences.

As noted at the beginning of this chapter, the collective impact of movements and groups critical of psychiatry in general, and of ADHD in particular, is marginal when viewed against the authority of the biomedical model of ADHD. Nevertheless, perhaps in part because many members of the critical-psychiatry movement are psychiatrists and psychiatric service users, the voices of this group are not ignored in the United Kingdom (although it is going too far to say that they are fully welcomed in biomedical psychiatry). For example, Timimi was invited as an expert advisor on the NICE ADHD Guideline, and his points about the lack of evidence for diagnosis and treatment were included, although not without challenge by biologically oriented researchers.[4] A widely read dialogue in the *British Medical Journal* between Timimi and a prominent ADHD researcher, Eric Taylor, also helped to clarify areas of disagreement as well as overlapping concerns (Timimi and Taylor 2004).

In some countries, print media and individual journalists are playing a key role in raising concerns about rates of ADHD diagnosis and use of stimulant drug treatments (see, e.g., a series of articles in *The New York Times* by the journalist Alan Schwarz: http://topics.nytimes.com/top/reference/timestopics/people/s/alan_schwarz/index.html). In the United States, these stories are frequently framed as investigative human-interest stories, in which a central character (often a child or a doctor) performs illegal or immoral acts or is the victim of such acts. Against the backdrop of escalating rates of ADHD diagnosis and stimulant drug use in the United States, these stories have had an impact: prominent American ADHD researchers have publicly admitted regret over a potential role in encouraging careless diagnosis and use of ADHD drugs (http://www.nytimes.com/2013/04/01/health/more-diagnoses-of-hyperactivity-causing-concern.html).

In contrast, the UK print media has not taken on a consistent ADHD or stimulant drug agenda. Newspapers are fairly predictable in the degree of negative bias shown in articles about ADHD diagnosis and drug treatments. The papers associated with a more liberal readership tend to have more balanced reports, while newspapers with a more conservative readership tend toward more hype and scaremongering (https://researchtheheadlines.org/2015/12/01/stimulant-medi cation-for-children-with-attention-deficit-hyperactivity-disorder-adhd/). Articles will occasionally make frightening claims about new epidemiological statistics on ADHD diagnosis and drug treatment, with headlines about "drugging children" (http://www.dailymail.co.uk/health/article-443431/The-children-drugged -naughty.html). Such articles have not been widely influential in an observable way, but in open comments associated with some of these articles online, it is clear that there is substantial public skepticism about the role of psychiatry in the management of child behavior and about the validity of psychiatric diagnosis. Social stigma related to mental health constitutes a major barrier to service access (Clement et al. 2014). This may be one reason why some clinicians and researchers believe that the benefits of partnering with pharmaceutical companies in some educational activities outweigh the risks.

Conclusion

In the United Kingdom, ADHD is a complex assemblage that has strong biomedical investment, alongside substantial, but subtle public skepticism in relation to mental disorders and treatments in general. Using an ecological model, this chapter has highlighted social dynamics and factors that influence child development at proximate and distal levels, in order to illustrate key sociological and experiential features of ADHD in the United Kingdom. Inadequacies in schooling and in mental health services mean that children and parents are particularly vulnerable to stigma and, indirectly, to the influence of pharmaceutical company marketing activities. The experiences of children diagnosed with ADHD suggest that perceptions of the disorder are entangled with a national preoccupation with the conduct of young people. Consequently, ADHD is viewed as an "anger problem" more than as a problem of academic performance. National statistics on the relationship between ADHD diagnosis and social class suggest that this social model of ADHD may instantiate and have more harmful consequences for children in low-resource settings.

Public and policy skepticism over child psychiatric diagnosis and treatments and cross-party political emphasis on managing child conduct as a social rather than a medical issue suggest that rates of ADHD diagnosis and stimulant drug use are likely to stay relatively low over the next 5 to 10 years. In the biopsychiatric research realm, a change of emphasis from managing and treating disorders to early identification and prevention of disorders is likely to interact positively with public skepticism and with policy interests in managing child conduct as a social issue. Prominent teams of researchers in the United Kingdom are developing studies to investigate prodromal ADHD and related disorders, such as autism, in high-risk baby and toddler groups (Geddes 2015). High-level research into the developmental mechanisms and pathways of ADHD, and preventive psychosocial interventions at the prodromal or preclinical stage, may well characterize the landscape of UK ADHD research and treatment in the near future.

NOTES

1. I was the principal investigator in the VOICES study, conducted between 2008 and 2012 and funded by the Wellcome Trust. Numerous outputs, including a report, videos, and publications are available on the VOICES website: www.adhdvoices.com.

2. This section is informed in part by my own participation in some of the groups mentioned below. I have participated as a speaker in conferences organized by ADDISS and UKAAN, and I have been contacted to be a speaker at an ADHD Foundation conference. I have interacted professionally and in research with many of the clinicians and researchers involved in these organizations.

3. I participated in two Shire-sponsored continuing medical education conferences as a speaker. I accepted no speaking fees or other honoraria. I was reimbursed for travel expenses.

4. I was a special advisor to the 2008 NICE ADHD Guideline, and I was present at a meeting in which Timimi presented his views to the Guideline Group, special advisors, and other observers.

REFERENCES

Angell, Marcia. 2005. *The Truth about the Drug Companies and How They Deceive Us.* New York: Penguin.

Beau-Ledjstrom, Raphaelle, Ian Douglas, Stephen J. W. Evans, and L. Smeeth. 2016. "Latest Trends in ADHD Drug Prescribing Patterns in Children in the UK: Prevalence, Incidence and Persistence." *British Medical Journal Open* 6: e010508. doi:10.1136/bmjopen-2015-010508.

Blum, Linda. 2014. *Raising Generation Rx: Mothering Children with Invisible Disabilities.* New York: New York University Press.

Bronfenbrenner, Urie. 1979. *The Ecology of Human Development.* Cambridge, MA: Harvard University Press.

Bushe, Chris J., and Nicola C. Savill. 2013. "Suicide-Related Events and Attention Deficit Hyperactivity Disorder Treatments in Children and Adolescents: A Meta-analysis of Atomoxetine and Methylphenidate Comparator Clinical Trials." *Child and Adolescent Psychiatry and Mental Health* 7: 19.

Children's Society. 2009. http://www.childrenssociety.org.uk/sites/default/files/publications/the_good_childhood_report_2014_-_final.pdf.

Clement, Sarah, O. Schauman, T. Graham, F. Maggioni, S. Evans-Lacko, N. Bezborodovs, C. Morgan, N. Rüsch, J. S. Brown, and G. Thornicroft. 2015. "What Is the Impact of Mental Health-Related Stigma on Help-Seeking? A Systematic Review of Quantitative and Qualitative Studies." *Psychological Medicine* 45: 11–27.

Geddes, Linda. 2015. "The Big Baby Experiment." *Nature* 527: 22–25. http://www.nature.com/news/the-big-baby-experiment-1.18701.

Green, Hazel, Áine McGinnity, Howard Meltzer, Tamsin Ford, and Robert Goodman. 2000. *The Mental Health of Children and Adolescents in Great Britain.* London: The Stationery Office. http://www.dawba.com/abstracts/B-CAMHS99_original_survey_report.pdf.

International Narcotics Control Board (INCB). 2012. "Psychotropic Substances: Statistics for 2011." International Narcotics Control Board Report. http://www.incb.org/documents/Psychotropics/technical-publications/2012/en/Eng_2012_PUBlication.pdf.

Murphy, J. Michael, Alyssa E. McCarthy, Lee Baer, Bonnie T. Zima, and Michael S. Jellinek. 2014. "Alternative National Guidelines for Treating Attention and Depression Problems in Children: Comparison of Treatment Approaches and Prescribing Rates in the United Kingdom and United States." *Harvard Review of Psychiatry* 22: 179–92.

Ogundele, Michael O., and R. De Doysa. 2011. "Is ADHD a Disease of Affluence? A Local Authority Experience in North-West of England." *Archives of Disease in Childhood* 96: A25–A26.

Poulton, Alison. 2005. "Growth on Stimulant Medication: Clarifying the Confusion; A Review." *Archives of Disease in Childhood* 90: 801–6.

Prescription Medicines Code of Practise Authority (PMCPA). 2015. http://www.pmcpa.org.uk/thecode/interactivecode2015/Pages/default.aspx.

Russell, Ginny, Tamsin Ford, Rachel Rosenberg, and Susan Kelly. 2014. "The Association of Attention Deficit Hyperactivity Disorder with Socioeconomic Disadvantage: Alternative Explanations and Evidence." *Journal of Child Psychology and Psychiatry* 55: 436–45.

Singh, Ilina. 2006. "A Framework for Understanding Trends in ADHD Diagnoses and Stimulant Drug Treatment: Schools and Schooling as a Case Study." *BioSocieties* 1: 439–52.

———. 2011. "A Disorder of Anger and Aggression: Children's Perspectives on Attention-Deficit/Hyperactivity Disorder in the United Kingdom." *Social Science Medicine* 73: 889–96.

Timimi, Sami. 2005. *Naughty Boys: Anti-Social Behaviour, ADHD and the Role of Culture.* Basingstoke: Palgrave Macmillan.

———. 2007. *Mis-understanding ADHD: The Complete Guide for Parents to Alternatives to Drugs.* Bloomington: AuthorHouse.

Timimi, Sami, and Eric Taylor. 2004. "ADHD Is Best Understood as a Cultural Construct." *British Journal of Psychiatry* 184: 8–9.

Vitiello, Bernardo. 2008. "Understanding the Risk of Using Medications for Attention Deficit Hyperactivity Disorder with Respect to Physical Growth and Cardiovascular Function." *Child and Adolescent Psychiatric Clinics of North America* 17 (2): 459–74.

7

The Emergence and Shaping of ADHD in Portugal

Ambiguities of a Diagnosis "in the Making"

Angela M. Filipe

In 2010, under the headline "Hiperatividade é a Perturbação Mais Diagnosticada" ("Hyperactivity is the Most Diagnosed Disorder"), the president of the Portuguese association of child psychiatry said in an interview that attention deficit–hyperactivity disorder (ADHD) is, in his experience, the most common diagnosis made in school-age children and adolescents (Carreira 2010). However, he also noted that there are no exact or reliable prevalence data on this complex, variable diagnosis in Portugal; this caveat has been underlined by other clinicians as well (e.g., Rodrigues and Nuno Antunes 2014; for a debate, see Filipe 2015). This discrepancy is but one visible aspect of the shaping of this diagnosis in Portugal, where it is undergoing an ambiguous process of definition and validation in which ADHD is recognized as a prevalent yet uncharted diagnosis. In this chapter, I examine how ADHD emerged and is currently being defined in this country, and I highlight some of the challenges that those dealing with this diagnosis will face in the near future, including soaring levels of psychostimulant drug prescription and consumption. In so doing, I throw fresh light on the dynamics, contingencies, and ambiguities that characterize the case of ADHD in the Portuguese context seen as both a relevant case study, on its own terms, and a case in point for a shifting configuration of the diagnosis in the European and global contexts.

Inspired by the social studies of diagnosis and medicine (Blaxter 1978; Mol 2002; Rosenberg 2006; for a recent overview, see Jutel and Nettleton 2011), I look at the diagnosis of ADHD not as a static medical category but as a dynamic and socially situated process that varies in time and across contexts (Filipe 2016) and whose contours are, in the case of Portugal, distinctively intermediate. The term "intermediate" can be applied here to emphasize the ongoing configuration of diagnosis (i.e., a process "in the making") and the particular economic and political position that this country has historically occupied in Europe and in the global system, as proposed by the Portuguese sociologist Boaventura de Sousa Santos (1985). From this perspective, I draw attention to the ways in which the diagnosis of ADHD in Portugal intersects and is shaped by global data and diagnostic standards, local practices and contingencies, public debates and available models of care, and a unique social and political history. Empirically, I draw on a mix of documentary analysis of the medical literature and public statements on ADHD in Portugal, archival research on the history of child mental health (see Filipe 2014), and an ethnographic case study of a developmental clinic specializing in this diagnosis that I conducted as part of my doctoral research. This study included observing medical consultations and interviewing the developmental clinicians who were involved in the assessment and treatment of ADHD. In order to update this study, which involved fieldwork mainly between 2011 and 2013, I have included documentary analysis of more recent publications on ADHD (2013–16) and personal communication with the founder of the main ADHD advocacy group in the country.[1]

First, I look briefly at the history of child mental health and the emergence of the ADHD diagnosis in the 1970s and 1980s expert literature, and at the translation and popularization of the term *hiperactividade* (hyperactivity) in the Portuguese context. Second, I draw attention to the establishment of ADHD as a clinically relevant and treatable condition in the late 1990s, which was accompanied by some contention and the creation of an advocacy group. Third, I look at what I term here the two main models of care in the case of ADHD—the "medical-pharmacological" and the "psychopedagogic" models—which may provide complementary responses to the diagnosis, even though they are faced with institutional constraints as well as ethical and social challenges. These challenges include, but are not limited to, the overdiagnosis of ADHD and the overprescription of psychostimulants. Fourth, I show how the diagnosis of ADHD has been managed and framed in the past decade, despite the lack of epidemiological data and clinical guidelines. I explore how the diagnosis brought together various forms of assessment protocols, medical expertise, and emerging approaches and interventions that seem to widen its meaning and scope in important ways. Finally, I conclude the chapter by discussing the contemporary issues relating to ADHD in Portugal as well as the challenges that complex behavioral diagnoses and mental health care will face in the near future, in an age of economic austerity and social inequality.

The Emergence and Ambiguity of *Hiperactividade*

The Portuguese history of child mental health and, more generally, of medical intervention for problematic child behavior can be traced back to a complex institutional background underpinned by various medical and therapeutic approaches (including medical-pedagogy, child neuropsychiatry, psychoanalysis, and neuropediatrics) and a unique sociopolitical configuration (Filipe 2014). In this respect, the country's twentieth century and medical landscape were marked by more than four decades of dictatorship (for a historical review in English, see Sardica 2008) and by the establishment of the Portuguese national health service in the late 1970s; doctors played an active social and political role in this process (Pinto Costa 2009). This institutional landscape, alongside the belated implementation of some health policies and regulation of medical practices, is particularly notorious in the field of mental health (Hespanha 2010) and child mental health (Marques et al. 2006). Moreover, some medical reports indicate that Portuguese psychiatrists were resistant to some forms of diagnostic categorization until at least the 1980s, when the ninth edition of the *International Classification of Diseases* (ICD) was implemented in the country (Barahona Fernandes, Polónio, and Seabra-Dinis 1970; Barahona Fernandes 1982).

Given these historical circumstances, it is perhaps surprising to find that child neuropsychiatry was officially recognized in Portugal in 1959, as early as in the United States and at the height of Salazar's regime (Filipe 2014), and that some of the earliest references to behavioral criteria resembling the diagnosis ADHD in the Portuguese clinical literature date back to the late 1970s and 1980s.

In a compendium published by the then Centro de Saúde Mental Infantil de Lisboa and the Instituto de Assistência Psiquiátrica, a condition called *disfunção cerebral mínima*—minimal brain dysfunction (MBD) in English—was described as a "symptomatic cluster" (Ataíde 1977: 264) that includes impulsivity, hyperkinesis, affective liability, difficulty in maintaining concentration, behavioral immaturity, a tendency to daydream, and low tolerance for frustration. Internationally, the following decade saw the publication and revision of the third edition of the *Diagnostic and Statistical Manual of Mental Disorders* (*DSM*), which specified the symptomatic triad of inattention, impulsivity, and hyperactivity in ADHD and reshaped the global landscape of psychiatric diagnosis (Lakoff 2000). This is when the notion of *hiperactividade* (hyperactivity) gained salience in the Portuguese clinical and psychological literature. According to Rebelo (1986), hyperactive children could be described as those who have, among other characteristics, indiscriminate and impulsive reactions to different stimuli; who are restless and unable to complete tasks; and who persistently exhibit these behaviors in more than one social context (e.g., school and home) such that these behaviors have a tangible negative impact on their functioning.

What is striking in this description is that it also renders visible the weight of the term *hiperactividade* in Portugal, where it has become a functional synonym for ADHD and where several medical services and consultations specializing in ADHD are designated *consultas de hiperactividade* (for details, see Neto 2014). The fact that hyperactivity gained wider currency in this context is linked not only to the history of the diagnosis in Portugal but is also related to the translation of the category and criteria of the *DSM,* which is published by the American Psychiatric Association (APA) (for the latest edition, see APA 2013). Indeed, the adaptation and translation of the diagnostic category has implied some variations in terms of meaning, even within the same language. As discussed elsewhere (Filipe 2016), the Brazilian category for ADHD is called *transtorno do déficit de atenção com hiperatividade*, or TDAH, whereas in Portugal it is called *perturbação de hiperactividade e défice de atenção*, or PHDA. As the wording changed with the translation of the diagnostic category from English, its criteria and components were also altered, as argued by one of the clinicians that I interviewed: "I think there is still a bit of confusion about the explanation of the issue of hyperactivity. When we say this is a disorder of hyperactivity and deficit of attention PHDA, even though the name is like this, the English version was the correct one—ADHD—because the attention-deficit is the one at its core" (Interview C, pediatrician).

As this pediatrician notes, there is considerable ambiguity in the definition of ADHD because the translation of the diagnosis into Portuguese changed the category and, quite fundamentally, reversed the order of its criteria. As she suggests, because hyperactive behaviors are prioritized over inattention, this core clinical problem may eventually be overlooked. Furthermore, hyperactivity is frequently a gendered notion that is more often associated with externalizing impulsive and restless behaviors and is incarnated in the figure of the naughty boy, as documented in the social science literature (Singh 2002). Thus, in many of the consultations that I observed in my fieldwork, clinicians sought to "state the fact of ADHD" (Edwards et al. 2014: 154) and to disambiguate its meaning as a disorder of attention (Filipe 2016). These variations in the meaning and translation of ADHD do not just reveal some specious technicalities of medical taxonomy, but rather signal the ambiguities of a category that has undergone a relatively recent process of adaptation in and translation into the Portuguese context, where what is at stake is making ADHD evident (Filipe 2016). Yet, the popular notion of *hiperactividade* also confers on it a moral dimension that becomes particularly salient when the diagnosis is linked to the controversies around psychostimulant medication.

The Establishment of the ADHD Diagnosis and Its Treatment: Advocacy and Contestation

After the emergence and popularization of the notion of hyperactivity in the 1980s in Portugal, the next few decades saw the popularization of this concept and the prescription of psychostimulant treatment based on methylphenidate to children diagnosed with ADHD. This happened during the late 1990s and early 2000s and corresponded with the establishment of ADHD as a clinically relevant and treatable condition and the emergence of medical and parent advocacy. This shift was marked by the 1996 symposium on pediatric neurology (Ferreira 2014) and the 1998 special issue of the journal *Psychologica* that was dedicated to hyperactivity and attention problems (see Fonseca et al. 1998), following Russell Barkley's (1997) proposition that a unifying theory of ADHD should be constructed. A few hospital pharmacies in the Portuguese health service were then able to access methylphenidate through direct hospital importation from Switzerland, and it has been reported that some families took the prescriptions to the neighboring country of Spain when these pharmacies ran out of stock (Porfírio, Boavida Fernandes, and Borges 1998).

Shortly thereafter, a renowned pediatrician wrote a commentary provocatively titled "Bichos Carpinteiros Normalizados" ("Normalized Carpenter Bees") (Mota 1999). This commentary cautioned against the perils of psychostimulant drug treatments and the normalization of problematic child behavior using a culturally relevant trope in Portuguese for agitated behavior and restless children. This reconfiguration of hyperactivity as a medical condition and, quite important, its association with psychostimulant medication brought the validity of the diagnosis to the forefront of the medical and public debates. It was precisely during this transition period of the late 1990s and early 2000s that the mother of two children diagnosed with ADHD decided to create an advocacy group called Associação Portuguesa da Criança Hiperactiva (APdCH) with the support of a local pediatrician and, among other sponsors, the pharmaceutical company Novartis (http://www.apdch.net). Such a relationship between advocacy, health care professionals, and pharmaceutical companies has been found in a number of other advocacy and patient groups in Portugal, most noticeably in the past two decades and in cases where the public provision of care and support to families is limited (Filipe et al. 2014).

According to the founder of APdCH, the association was formed to respond to the needs of parents and families with the aim of raising public awareness of ADHD in Portugal: "It was in the beginning of 2000, when the association was created, that we started talking about hyperactivity. At that time, there was a 'boom' in terms of public debate, and in the media, about this problem and the need emerged to better understand it . . . Some parents were not able to access medication or simply couldn't afford it for their children; there were teachers who mistreated these children." During this period, the ethical and social dimensions of ADHD and psychostimulant treatment concomitant with lack of public awareness and recognition of the diagnosis seem to have placed families in an ambiguous and difficult position. On the one hand, this was the time when ADHD started to be contested, as noted in the above excerpts, by members of the medical community and schoolteachers, while access to treatment and medical information was still limited. On the other hand, it was also during this period that ADHD was gradually established as a treatable condition and that advocacy around the condition emerged, including medical advocacy in support of families. It is not surprising to find, thereafter, accounts from clinicians that rebuke comments that ascribe the causes of and blame for ADHD to the child's volition or the parents' childrearing practices (for an example, see Boavida Fernandes 2006).

This tension between advocacy and contestation is linked to the ambiguity or paradoxical aspect of the diagnosis, as Rosenberg (2006) puts it, which means that it may simultaneously legitimize people and entitle them to some form of support or treatment but also stigmatize those who are affected by or associated with it (Singh 2002; Singh et al. 2013). For this reason, the establishment of the diagnosis and treatment of ADHD in Portugal since the late 1990s and early

2000s has raised numerous issues around its diagnostic validity and legitimacy as well as the accessibility and availability of different models of care.

Available Models of Care and Their Contingencies

According to the Portuguese medical literature, in relation to ADHD, pharmacological treatment and psychological and educational interventions should always, or at least ideally, be combined, including learning strategies and adaptions in the classroom (see, e.g., Lopes et al. 2007; Cordinhã and Boavida Fernandes 2008; Padilhão, Marques, and Marques 2009). In this way, ADHD is placed right in the middle of what I call ADHD's two models of care: the medical-pharmacological model and the psychopedagogic model. For example, in the clinic that I sat in on, the diagnosis of ADHD was made by a multidisciplinary team of pediatricians and psychologists who would discuss the diagnosis with clinical psychologists, child psychiatrists, and therapists. This clinical team also had a fairly collaborative relationship with schoolteachers and school or private psychologists outside the clinic. Teachers would fill in behavioral questionnaires and checklists, and clinicians would consult with the non-clinical psychologists to gather information about specific cases and the social context of children and adolescents. However, outside the remit of the clinic, ADHD is a daily issue at school in relation to which the medical and educational models necessarily overlap and, on some occasions, place children and their parents in a challenging position, as I observed in the following two consultations:

> The schoolteacher has complained about the boy's behavior and told the mother he should comply with the medical treatment. (EQ, 10-year-old boy)

> At this follow-up consultation, the psychologist finds the girl has not been taking the medication and moved to another school (the reasons are unclear). According to the mother, her new teacher refuses to give her the medication. (MB, 8-year-old girl)

These observations illustrate two authoritative and normative positions that are assumed by teachers in relation to the psychostimulant treatment of school-age children diagnosed with ADHD and, consequently, the management of medication in school settings where those children spend most of their week. While in one case the schoolteacher refuses to give the medication to a school-age girl, in the other case it was the teacher who drew attention to the fact that EQ, a 10-year-old boy, was not following the prescribed treatment. Such normative positions could be read as an illustration of the collaborative or polarized relationships between teachers and clinicians or an example of tensions that surround the ADHD diagnosis as the symbol of an increasingly medicalized education (Singh 2002; Petrina 2006). This ostensible trend in the diagnosis has been locally contested by a group of education and health care professionals in Portugal, including psychoanalysts, who wrote a manifesto advocating a non-medicalizing and non-pathologizing approach to education (http://education medicalisation.blogspot.pt). The signatories argued that a predominantly neurobiological and pharmacological approach to ADHD not only deflects attention from its educational and social underpinnings but also contributes to the undue medicalization of school-age children and the delegation of responsibility from the state to individuals and families.

Yet the scenario is similarly complex and fragmented (for a discussion on fragmentation, see Mol 2002) in relation to the numerous institutional contingencies and limitations that impinge on special education and on psychopedagogic approaches to ADHD as a whole. For example, the revision of the Ministério da Educação 's Decreto-Lei N.° 3/2008 that redefined the terms and scope of special education in Portugal recommended that a set of educational, curricular, and pedagogic adaptations should be made. Within this legal framing, often mentioned and mobilized by the clinicians I observed, children and adolescents diagnosed with ADHD and, often, other learning difficulties could be entitled to personalized pedagogic support, an adapted examination protocol, and even an individual curriculum and adapted learning content (Ministério da Educação 2008). In order to access this support, the request to access these special educational services should be made by parents and corroborated by a clinical report that testifies to a behavioral diagnosis or learning disability and should also be approved by the schoolteacher or head teacher, as the observation below indicates:

> The teacher has written a letter to the doctor mentioning the Decreto-Lei N.°
> 3/2008 and that a 12-year-old boy did not pass the tests in several subjects. The
> doctor thinks that the original report from his psychological assessment
> should have sufficed but tells the mother: "I'll write you another so that you
> get pedagogic support."

As the observation above suggests, even though the mother of a school-age boy had a report from a psychologist attesting to his multiple learning difficulties and a diagnosis of combined ADHD, an additional report from the doctor was needed. This special education framework is fraught with numerous limitations and contingent on technical reports and forms that may not always be accessible to parents, causing delays in the provision of benefits to the families, such as the subsidy toward special education school attendance (Provedor da Justiça 2008). Additionally, the special education model was built on the premise of differentiation and may fail to respond to the complexities posed by highly variable and compounded diagnoses of ADHD and associated learning difficulties, in which a combination of behavioral, educational, and psychotherapeutic interventions has been recommended. In this respect, social scientists have argued that the differentiation and medicalization of behavioral problems deemed to be ADHD tend to elide some of the failings of contemporary models of education and schooling practices (Pais, Menezes, and Nunes 2016).

In turn, the medical-pharmacological model of intervention in ADHD also faces important challenges. Methylphenidate was licensed by the Autoridade Nacional do Medicamento e Produtos de Saúde—Infarmed—and subsidized by the state in the early 2000s (Furtado 2015). Since 2013, generic formulations of Concerta have been introduced in the Portuguese market by Sandoz, Mylan, and Farmoz (http://www.infarmed.pt/genericos/genericos_II/lista_genericos.php?tabela=spr&fonte=dci&escolha_dci=TWVoaWxmZW5pZGFobw==), followed by the introduction of atomoxetine in 2014. At the time of my study, however, there were only three kinds of methylphenidate available on the Portuguese market, Rubifen, Ritalina LA, and Concerta, varying between the cheapest formulation with a short-term effect and the most expensive formulation that offers an extended release (Infarmed 2009). Yet in a country that has undergone several years of economic recession and austerity measures, families have had to bear some of the costs of a treatment, which is only partly subsidized by the state (Diário da República 2009). Not coincidentally, before the commercialization of generic methylphenidate and when Rubifen ran out of stock in 2012, the spokesperson for APdCH and a clinician reported problems regarding the access of families to treatment and their resort to the cheapest prescription possible, which might have had to do with the cost of medication and might have led to therapeutic inadequacy or inefficacy (Palha 2012).

Conversely, some clinicians have expressed their concern regarding excessive pharmacological intervention in ADHD and the structural gaps in the provision of accessible psychological therapies and of health and social care to school-age children, claiming that Portugal is one of the countries in the world where there is more medical intervention in these cases (Borges 2006). Others have warned against the perils of inappropriate medical intervention linked to the potential "misdiagnosis" of ADHD in this age group, which may be due to a pathological (as opposed to a dimensional or relational) model of the condition (Gomes Pedro 2015). Against this backdrop and counter to the aforementioned recommendations for multimodal approaches to ADHD, it seems that pharmacological treatment may have become its dominant model of care. According to the newspaper *Jornal i* (2012), data from the agency Intercontinental Marketing Services (IMS Health) suggest that the sales of methylphenidate had increased by nearly 80% between 2007 and 2011, whereas a recent study conducted by researchers at Infarmed (Furtado 2015) shows that the measured prescription of methylphenidate for school-age children and adolescents (ages 5–19) more than doubled since 2010, reaching 13.4 defined daily doses (DDD) in continental Portugal.[2] In fact, a recent report from the International Narcotics Control Board (INCB 2016) that details the world consumption of methylphenidate in 2011–13 shows Portugal in the "red zone" of 3–10 DDD, together with high-consuming and high-producing countries such as Germany and Spain.

Added together, these data suggest that Portugal rapidly became a major prescriber and consumer of this psychostimulant medication in Europe, despite its cost and relatively recent commercialization. Hence, the available responses to ADHD in Portugal, be they mainly pharmacological or be they "psychopedagogic," are contingent on and pose numerous challenges to clinical and educational practice, pharmaceutical regulation, and health and social care policy, to name a few. In turn, these challenges raise pressing questions about the framing of the diagnosis, epidemiology, and meaning of ADHD. I explore some of these issues in the following section.

(Re)Framing the Diagnosis and Meaning of ADHD

Official reports on mental health and illness in Portugal have highlighted the absence of systematic data collection and information from the field, especially in the domains of psychiatric epidemiology and child mental health (see Marques et al. 2006; Caldas de Almeida et al. 2007). The first national report on the prevalence of mental disorders in Portugal, published in 2013 and sponsored by the World Mental Health Surveys Initiative, mentions an estimated prevalence of ADHD of 0.4% and a lifetime prevalence of 1.5% in Portugal (Caldas de Almeida et al. 2013). The study encountered, nevertheless, numerous difficulties in the field and only surveyed the adult population in which the diagnosis has been less frequently made and for which the prescription of psychostimulants was autho-rized as recently as 2011 (Furtado 2015). By force of these circumstances, clinicians have relied either on localized studies or on worldwide prevalence estimates. For instance, a recent book on ADHD indicates estimated prevalence rates of 4% to 5% (Rodrigues and Nuno Antunes 2014) based on two studies conducted in the 1990s and early 2000s, whereas a second book published in the same year claims that there are 80,000 school-age children with ADHD in Portugal (Neto 2014) based on a reported estimate rate of 5% to 8%. It is difficult to assess, therefore, to what extent these numbers provide a reliable, up-to-date estimate of the prev-alence of ADHD in Portugal.

Unlike in the United Kingdom, where the National Institute for Clinical Ex-cellence (NICE 2008) issued a national guideline for the diagnosis and treatment of ADHD, there is no such cohesive guideline in Portugal. Available recommen-dations for the practice of child mental health in primary health care in Portugal (Marques and Cepeda 2009) are discretionary. These recommendations mainly provide general practitioners with a referral system for the diagnosis and treat-ment of ADHD whose prerogative has lain with the medical specialties of child psychiatry and (neuro)pediatrics in secondary care. In this seemingly loose diag-nostic framing, a significant proportion of ADHD diagnoses in school-age children in Portugal has been made by developmental clinicians outside the re-mit of specialist mental health services, similar to what has been described in the United States (Parens and Johnston 2009). A survey that covered 2008 and 2009 showed that a significant number of pediatric hospitals and developmental clinics in the national health service offered specialized consultations for the assessment and treatment of ADHD (Oliveira et al. 2012). And, in the private health care sector, several developmental clinics and units are now offering those consultations as well. For example, in the metropolitan area of Lisbon alone, there are three large developmental centers (CADin, Diferenças, and Sei), and a developmental unit in a private hospital that also specializes in ADHD (Cuf Descobertas).[3]

According to recent data on the prescription of methylphenidate in continen-tal Portugal, private clinics account for 39% of prescriptions for children and adolescents who are 5 to 19 years of age (Furtado 2015), which may indicate a growing number of specialized ADHD clinics and consultations. Some of these private practices have also taken the lead in non-pharmacological, (neuro)psycho-logical, and cognitive-behavioral interventions, however, filling in gaps left by the state services, as mentioned in the previous section. Experts in these private practices have been working, for instance, on a variety of techniques and interventions for ADHD that include neurofeedback and cognitive-behavioral therapy (Neto 2014) as well as family interventions and parental training (Rodrigues and Nuno Antunes 2014). Relevant work on parental training and early intervention has also been done outside the clinic and in relation to the wider spectrum of behavioral, cognitive, and learning difficulties, inspired by the North American training series The Incredible Years, with a specific focus on health and social inequalities (for a local example, see Santos and Gaspar 2015). Other experts have also taken the lead in efforts to increase recognition of ADHD as a lifelong condition (see Filipe 2004) and have been involved in the revisions and translation of the *Diagnostic Interview for ADHD in Adults* (Kooij and Franken 2010) into Portuguese.

The establishment of the diagnosis of ADHD in Portugal has depended, moreover, on a process of adaptation and localization of the diagnosis and its global data and standards, across clinical and research settings. Neuropsychology has played a particularly important role by working toward the validation of psychological and cognitive diagnostic instruments for the Portuguese population (see, e.g., Simões, Gonçalves, and Almeida 1999). More specifically and in the case of pediatric ADHD, this included the standardization of the Conners questionnaires (Rodrigues 2007) and the validation of other neuropsychological and cognitive tests in clinical trials (Alfaiate 2009) locally. Thus, in those clinical sites where there are significant collaborations with research, new diagnostic techniques and assessment protocols have been adapted and developed by building on that expertise. In my clinical ethnographic case study, in which the diagnosis of ADHD was made by pediatricians and psychologists, school-age children were assessed with the use of a specific assessment protocol that included the simplified *DSM* interview and the Conners checklists, as mentioned in the American Academy of Pediatrics (AAP) (AAP 2011), and the Wechsler Intelligence Scale for Children and Self-Concept Scales (for further details, see Filipe 2016).

Although some of these instruments do not specifically relate to the *DSM* criteria for the diagnosis of ADHD, they seem to provide developmental clinicians with a grasp of its associated emotional, learning, and psychological dimensions for the purpose of a differential or more granular diagnosis. This peculiarity is highlighted in the following argument made by a pediatrician at a conference: "ADHD [is not only] a triad of hyperactivity, impulsivity, attention-deficit . . . it involves other neurocognitive deficits, other psychological competences . . . [These tests] help us to understand that there is more in ADHD than what the *DSM* says." These clinic-based definitions can be found in other expert literature in which ADHD has also been described as the expression of broader neurocognitive "deficits" (Cabral 2006) and as a multifaceted problem in which relational problems (Lopes et al. 2007), low self-esteem (Maia et al. 2011), parenting stress (Pimentel et al. 2011), and emotional liability (Rodrigues and Nuno Antunes 2014) are more often present than not. In practice, the clinical meaning and scope of the diagnosis shift from the *DSM* criteria of hyperactivity, impulsivity, and inattention toward a wider, multifactorial definition of the condition that is grounded in empirical research, multidisciplinary clinical practice, and a dimensional approach to ADHD.

Discussion: Current Issues and Future Challenges of ADHD

The case study of ADHD in Portugal allows us to better understand the diagnosis as an ongoing, situated process wherein multiple medical disciplines and popular meanings, models of care and institutional frameworks, and overlapping global trends in the diagnosis and local practices play a role. Through a combination of documentary analysis and historical and ethnographic data, I have examined several of the ambiguities and complexities that characterize the case of ADHD in Portugal. Salient among these aspects were the following: first, the meaning of ADHD as a prevalent yet uncharted diagnosis; second, the meaning and framing of the diagnosis that is commonly known as *hiperactividade* vis-à-vis a disorder of attention that may signal more than what the *DSM* says; third, the establishment of the diagnosis and its treatment with psychostimulant medication that, counter to medical critique and recommendations for multimodal intervention, seems to have become the first-line therapeutic response to ADHD; and, fourth, the rapid increase in psychostimulant drug sales and prescriptions, despite the costs of this medication and its relatively recent commercialization. This ambiguous, intermediate configuration of ADHD in Portugal illustrates a process that is, by definition, in the making and entangled in seemingly universal issues of care, stigma, policy, and responsibility, albeit contingent on and situated in particular institutional and sociopolitical circumstances.

The diagnosis of ADHD has been made for several decades in Portugal by multidisciplinary clinical teams, including pediatricians, psychologists, and child psychiatrists, and has involved several other participants, such as parents, schoolteachers, and therapists, and has also been the object of controversy and debate. While it has been generally recognized that the current models of care in

ADHD are, in Portugal, hampered by numerous gaps, clinicians have specifically voiced their concerns regarding a pharmacological approach to these behavioral problems as the first line of treatment, which is part of the medical critique of overprescription in this country. Others have warned against the perils that lie in the medicalization of childhood and education, an issue that was raised in the Portuguese parliament in 2015 (Soeiro 2015). In the coming years, one of the challenges posed by the diagnosis of ADHD in Portugal will be dealing with the inherent ambiguities of a complex, multifactorial condition that, paradoxically, may have been overdiagnosed and overmedicated but that may also have gone under- or misdiagnosed (for a debate, see Singh et al. 2013). Similarly, and related to this aspect, tensions are likely to emerge in the field between those who advocate a more dimensional and relational understanding of ADHD and its associated problems and those who describe it as a brain disorder, as defined by the US National Institute of Mental Health (NIHM) (2012). The reconfiguration of the diagnosis in Portugal has also meant an increasing demand for recognition of the diagnosis of both child and adult ADHD as well as a proliferation of private clinics and new forms of intervention that require longer-term commitment and financial investment on the part of both public services and families.

It is expected that these developments will continue to raise challenges in relation to the provision of integrated care for people with ADHD and associated problems over their life course, putting at stake issues such as the accessibility and availability of alternative responses to multiple, often concurring, forms of individual, familial, and social distress. The problem is that in a scenario of economic recession and the numerous austerity measures that were imposed in Portugal, as elsewhere in Europe, service users and families have been affected by the lack of access to health services and social care associated with cuts in public spending, as suggested in a recent, independent report by Observatório Português dos Sistemas de Saúde (OPSS) (2013). In the near future, one of the key challenges posed by but not exclusive to the diagnosis of ADHD is how to respond to increasingly prevalent behavioral, learning, and mental health problems, or other forms of distress, in the face of seemingly scarce resources and widening inequalities in accessing health care. These are challenges that warrant further anthropological and sociological research in Portugal to explore the social dynamics and inequalities that shape the diagnosis and treatment of ADHD (Blum 2014), the increase of psychoactive drug prescriptions in times of economic recession (Lakoff 2004), and, more broadly, the detrimental effects of austerity measures on the health and mental health of the Portuguese (Augusto 2014; Legido-Quigley et al. 2016). I would therefore argue that the engagement of the various stakeholders in a meaningful public debate is of crucial importance in the case of ADHD, as is the inclusion of social scientists, ethicists, policymakers, teachers, young people, and families in the wider debate on health and mental health care in Portugal. For all these reasons, an empirically informed and culturally sensitive account of complex behavioral diagnoses, such as ADHD, calls for the consideration of these wider diagnostic situations (Filipe 2015) in light of their historical, socioeconomic, and political dimensions.

NOTES

1. The quotations are my translations. All personal data and sites relative to my clinical ethnography were anonymized and identifying features removed or altered to ensure the privacy of the study's direct and indirect participants. Observations of the consultations were simply noted down in writing and coded through generic descriptors and letter codes (i.e., XT, 7-year-old boy). Ethics approval was negotiated with the local clinical management team and obtained on November 4, 2011, from the London School of Economics and Political Science, where this project began.

2. The defined daily dose (DDD) is a statistical measure of drug consumption, defined by the World Health Organization. One DDD of methylphenidate equals 30 mg: http://www.whocc.no/atc_ddd_index/?code=N06BA04.

3. I am referring to the developmental centers Sei—Centro Desenvolvimento e Aprendizagem (see http://sei-online.net), CADIn—Centro de Apoio ao Desenvolvimento Infantil (see http://www.cadin.net), Diferenças—Centro de Desenvolvimento Infantil (see http://www.diferencas.net), and the developmental clinic of the private hospital Cuf Descobertas (https://www.cufdescobertas.pt).

REFERENCES

Alfaiate, Cláudia. 2009. "Impacto da Perturbação de Hiperactividade com Défice de Atenção (subtipo Combinado) no Funcionamento Neuropsicológico: Estudos de Validade com a Bateria de Avaliação Neuropsicológica de Coimbra (BANC)." Master's thesis, Universidade de Coimbra.

American Academy of Pediatrics (AAP). 2011. "ADHD: Clinical Practice Guideline for the Diagnosis, Evaluation, and Treatment of Attention-Deficit/Hyperactivity Disorder in Children and Adolescents." *Pediatrics* 128: 1007–22.

American Psychiatric Association (APA). 2013. *Diagnostic and Statistical Manual of Mental Disorders (DSM-5)*. 5th ed. Washington, DC: American Psychiatric Association.

Ataíde, José Schneeberger de. 1977. *Elementos de Psiquiatria da Criança e do Adolescente*. Lisbon: Instituto de Assistência Psiquiátrica e Centro de Saúde Mental Infantil de Lisboa.

Augusto, Gonçalo. 2014. "Mental Health in Portugal in Times of Austerity." *The Lancet Psychiatry* 1: 109–10.

Barahona Fernandes, Henrique. 1982. "Classificações Internacionais e Diagnóstico individual estruturado e personalizado. A propósito de um caso de 'fronteira.'" *O Médico* 1591: 857–75.

Barahona Fernandes, Henrique, Pedro Polónio, and Joaquim Seabra-Dinis. 1970. "Classificação Internacional das Doenças Mentais. Proposta de Adaptação Portuguesa." *Jornal do Médico* 1428: 300–308.

Barkley, Russell. 1997. "Behavioral Inhibition, Sustained Attention, and Executive Functions: Constructing a Unifying Theory of ADHD." *Psychological Bulletin* 121: 65–94.

Blaxter, Mildred. 1978. "Diagnosis as Category and Process: The Case of Alcoholism." *Social Science & Medicine* 12: 9–17.

Blum, Linda. 2014. *Raising Generation Rx: Mothering Children with Invisible Disabilities.* New York: New York University Press.

Boavida Fernandes, José. 2006. "Editorial: Hiperactividade Ou Má 'educação'?" *Saúde Infantil* 28: 3–5.

Borges, Luís. 2006. "Faltam Estruturas para Tratar Hiperactividade e Défice de Atenção em Portugal." *Notícias da Saúde em Portugal.* http://cybersaude.wordpress.com/2006/11/15/faltam-estruturas-para-tratar-hiperactividade-e-defice-de-atencao-em-portugal/.

Cabral, Pedro. 2006. "Attention Deficit Disorders: Are We Barking Up the Wrong Tree?" *European Journal of Paediatric Neurology* 10: 66–77.

Caldas de Almeida, José, António Leuschner, Henrique Duarte, Isabel Paixão, João Sennfelt, Maria J. Heitor, and Miguel Xavier. 2007. *Proposta de Plano de Acção para a Reestruturação e Desenvolvimento dos Serviços de Saúde Mental em Portugal 2007–2016.* Lisbon: CNRSSM—Comissão Nacional para a Reestruturação dos Serviços de Saúde Mental, Ministério da Saúde. http://www.portaldasaude.pt/NR/rdonlyres/AC8E136F-50E4-44F0-817F-879187BD2915/0/relatorioplanoaccaoservicossaudemental.pdf.

Caldas de Almeida, José Miguel, Miguel Xavier, Graça Cardoso, Manuel Gonçalves Pereira, Ricardo Gusmão, Bernardo Corrêa, Joaquim Gago, Miguel Talina, and Joaquim Silva. 2013. *Estudo Epidemiológico Nacional de Saúde Mental, 1º Relatório.* Lisbon: Universidade Nova de Lisboa. http://www.fcm.unl.pt/main/alldoc/galeria_imagens/Relatorio_Estudo_Saude-Mental_2.pdf.

Carreira, Augusto. 2010. "Hiperatividade é a Perturbação Mais Diagnosticada." *Diário de Notícias*, May 18. http://www.dn.pt/inicio/portugal/interior.aspx?content_id=1572761&page=-1.

Cordinhã, Ana C., and José Boavida Fernandes. 2008. "A Criança Hiperactiva: Diagnóstico, Avaliação e Intervenção." *Revista Portuguesa de Clínica Geral* 24: 577–89.

Decreto-Lei N.º 3/2008. 2008. Ministério da Educação, Portugal. http://legislacao.min-edu.pt/np4/np3content/?newsId=1530&fileName=decreto_lei_3_2008.pdf.

Diário da República. 2009. Aviso N.º 3775/2009, vol. 33. 2ª Série. https://dre.pt/application/dir/pdf2s/2009/02/033000000/0662506628.pdf.

Edwards, Claire, Etaoine Howlett, Madeleine Akrich, and Vololona Rabeharisoa. 2014. "Attention Deficit Hyperactivity Disorder in France and Ireland: Parents' Groups' Scientific and Political Framing of an Unsettled Condition." *BioSocieties* 9: 153–72.

Ferreira, José Carlos. 2014. "Perspectiva Histórica da PHDA." In *Hiperatividade e Défice de Atenção*, edited by Ana Serrão Neto, 21–25. Lisbon: Verso de kappa.

Filipe, Angela M. 2014. "The Rise of Child Psychiatry in Portugal: An Intimate Social and Political History, 1915–1959." *Social History of Medicine* 27: 326–48. doi:10.1093/shm/hku006.

———. 2015. "Conceiving ADHD: Diagnosis and Practice in the Portuguese Clinic." PhD diss., King's College London.

———. 2016. "Making ADHD Evident: Data, Practices and Diagnostic Protocols in Portugal." *Medical Anthropology* 35: 390–403. doi:10.1080/01459740.2015.1101102.

Filipe, Angela M., Marta Roriz, Daniel Neves, Marisa Matias, and João A. Nunes. 2014. "Coletivos sociais na saúde: o ativismo em torno das doenças raras e do parto em Portugal." In *Saúde, Participação e Cidadania*, edited by Ana R. Matos and Mauro Serapioni, 175–94. Coimbra: CES-Almedina.

Filipe, Carlos. 2004. "A Perturbação de Hiperactividade Com Défice de Atenção No Adulto." *Revista Portuguesa de Clínica Geral* 20: 733–37.

Fonseca, António, Mário Simões, José Rebelo, Luís Borges, José Boavida Fernandes, Guiomar Oliveira, Susana Nogueira, Helena Porfírio, and Paula Temudo. 1998. "Hiperactividade na Comunidade e Hiperactividade em Meio Clínico: Semelhanças e Diferenças." *Psychologica* 19: 111–22.

Furtado, Cláudia. 2015. "Hiperatividade: Análise à Utilização de Medicamentos em Portugal Continental." *Boletim Infarmed Notícias* 54. Lisbon: Infarmed—Autoridade Nacional do Medicamento e Produtos de Saúde. http://www.infarmed.pt/portal/page /portal/INFARMED/PUBLICACOES/INFARMED_NOTICIAS/infarmed%20 not%EDcias%20N.%BA%2054%20-%20maio%202015_1.pdf.

Gomes Pedro, João. 2015. "Hiperatividade Está Mal Diagnosticada em Portugal." *Diário de Noticias*, March 23. http://www.dn.pt/inicio/portugal/interior.aspx?content_id =4469884&page=2.

Hespanha, Pedro. 2010. "A Reforma Psiquiátrica Em Portugal: Desafios e Impasses." In *Desinstitucionalização, Redes Sociais e Saúde Mental: Análise de Experiências da Reforma Psiquiátrica em Angola, Brasil e Portugal*, edited by Breno Fontes and Eliana da Fonte, 137–61. Recife: Editora Universitária da UFP.

Infarmed. 2009. "Informação Aos Profissionais de Saúde (Recomendações Relativas À Segurança Do Metilfenidato)." http://www.infarmed.pt/infarmedia/47/infarmedia .pdf.

International Narcotics Control Board (INCB). 2016. "Availability of Internationally Controlled Drugs: Ensuring Adequate Access for Medical and Scientific Purposes." New York: INCB, United Nations (E/INCB/2015/1/Supp.1), http://www.incb.org/doc uments/Publications/Annual Reports/AR2015/English/Supplement-AR15_availabil ity_English.pdf.

Jornal i. 2012. "Vendas de Medicamentos Para Concentração Aumentaram 78% em Cinco Anos." *iOnline*, May 4. http://www.ionline.pt/artigos/portugal/vendas-medicamentos -concentracao-aumentaram-78-cinco-anos.

Jutel, Annemarie, and Sarah Nettleton. 2011. "Towards a Sociology of Diagnosis: Reflections and Opportunities." *Social Science & Medicine* 73: 793–800. doi:10.1016/j .socscimed.2011.07.014.

Kooij, Sandra, and M. H. Franken. 2010. "Entrevista de Diagnóstico de PHDA em Adultos (DIVA) 2.0." DIVA Foundation, Portuguese translation supported by CADIn—Centro de Apoio ao Desenvolvimento Infantil. http://www.divacenter.eu/Content/VertalingPDFs/DIVA_2_Portugees_FORM.pdf.

Lakoff, Andrew. 2000. "Adaptive Will: The Evolution of Attention Deficit Disorder." *Journal of the History of the Behavioral Sciences* 36: 149–69.

———. 2004. "The Anxieties of Globalization: Antidepressant Sales and Economic Crisis in Argentina." *Social Studies of Science* 34: 247–69.

Legido-Quigley, Helena, Marina Karanikolos, Sonio Hernandez-Plaza, Cláudia de Freitas, Luís Bernardo, Beatriz Padilla, Rita Sá Machado, Karla Diaz-Ordaz, David Stuckler, and Martin McKee. 2016. "Effects of the Financial Crisis and Troika Austerity Measures on Health and Health Care Access in Portugal." *Health Policy* 120: 833–39.

Lopes, Ana, Alexandra Paul, Núria Madureira, and José Boavida Fernandes. 2007. "Perturbação de Hiperactividade e Défice de Atenção na Infância e Adolescência: Problemas Associados." *Saúde Infantil* 29: 19–28.

Maia, Catarina, Micaela Guardiano, Victor Viana, J. Paulo Almeida, and Maria Júlia Guimarães. 2011. "Auto-Conceito em Crianças com Hiperactividade e Défice de Atenção." *Acta Médica Portuguesa* 24: 493–502.

Marques, Cristina, and Teresa Cepeda. 2009. *Recomendações para a Prática Clínica da Saúde Mental Infantil e Juvenil nos Cuidados de Saúde Primários.* Lisbon: CNSM—Coordenação Nacional para a Saúde Mental. http://www.acs.min-saude.pt/pt/saudemental.

Marques, Cristina, Marco Torrado, Adriano Natário, and Maria José Proença. 2006. *Rede de Referenciação Hospitalar de Psiquiatria da Infância e da Adolescência. Documento técnico de suporte.* Lisbon: CNSM—Coordenação Nacional para a Saúde Mental/ ACCS—Administração Central do Sistema de Saúde. http://www.acss.min-saude.pt/Portals/0/DOCUMENTO%20T%C3%89CNICO%20DE%20SUPORTE_RRH_PSIQ%20IA_VERS%C3%83O_%2023%20NOV.pdf.

Mol, Annemarie. 2002. *The Body Multiple: Ontology in Medical Practice.* Durham, NC: Duke University Press.

Mota, Henrique C. 1999. "Bichos carpinteiros normalizados." *ASIC—Revista de Saúde Infantil*: 69–70.

National Institute for Health and Clinical Excellence (NICE). 2008. *Attention Deficit Hyperactivity Disorder: Diagnosis and Management of ADHD in Children, Young People and Adults.* Manchester: National Institute for Health and Clinical Excellence. www.nice.org.uk/nicemedia/pdf/ADHDFullGuideline.pdf.

National Institute of Mental Health (NIMH). 2012. *Attention Deficit Hyperactivity Disorder (ADHD).* Booklet 12-3572. Bethesda, MD: National Institute of Mental Health. http://www.nimh.nih.gov/health/publications/attention-deficit-hyperactivity-disorder/adhd_booklet_cl508.pdf.

Neto, Ana Serrão, ed. 2014. *Hiperatividade e Défice de Atenção.* Lisbon: Verso de kappa.

Observatório Português dos Sistemas de Saúde (OPSS). 2013. *Relatório de Primavera 2013: Duas Faces Da Saúde.* Coimbra: Observatório Português dos Sistemas de Saúde.

Oliveira, Guiomar, Frederico Duque, Cristina Duarte, Fernanda Melo, Luisa Teles, Mafalda Brito, Maria Carmo Vale, Maria Júlia Guimarães, and Rosa Gouveia. 2012.

"Pediatria do neurodesenvolvimento. Levantamento nacional de recursos e necessidades." *Acta Pediátrica Portuguesa* 43: 1–17.

Padilhão, Carla, Margarida Marques, and Cristina Marques. 2009. "Perturbações do Comportamento e Perturbação de Hiperactividade xom Défice de Atenção: Diagnóstico e Intervenção nos Cuidados de Saúde Primários." *Revista Portuguesa de Clínica Geral* 25: 592–99.

Pais, Sofia Castanheira, Isabel Menezes, and João Arriscado Nunes. 2016. "Saúde e Escola: Reflexões em Torno da Medicalização da Educação." *Cadernos de Saúdo Pública* 32: e00166215.

Palha, Miguel. 2012. "Pediatra Denuncia Ruptura de Stock de Medicamento Para a Concentração." *Público*, May 3. http://www.publico.pt/n1544535.

Parens, Erik, and Josephine Johnston. 2009. "Facts, Values, and Attention-Deficit Hyperactivity Disorder (ADHD): An Update on the Controversies." *Child and Adolescent Psychiatry and Mental Health* 3. doi:10.1186/1753-2000-3-1.

Petrina, Stephen. 2006. "The Medicalization of Education: A Historiographic Synthesis." *History of Education Quarterly* 46: 503–31.

Pimentel, Maria J., Salomé Vieira-Santos, Vanessa Santos, and Maria C. Vale. 2011. "Mothers of Children with Attention Deficit/Hyperactivity Disorder: Relationship among Parenting Stress, Parental Practices and Child Behaviour." *Attention Deficit and Hyperactivity Disorders* 3: 61–68.

Pinto Costa, Rui. 2009. *O Poder Médico No Estado Novo, (1945–1974)*. Porto: Universidade do Porto Editora.

Porfírio, Helena, José Boavida Fernandes, and Luís Borges. 1998. "Intervenção Psicofarmacológica na Perturbação por Défice de Atenção com Hiperactividade." *Psychologica* 19: 201–7.

Provedor da Justiça. 2008. *Subsídio por Frequência de Estabelecimento de Educação Especial*. http://www.provedor-jus.pt/?action=5&idc=67&idi=1116.

Rebelo, José. 1986. "Para Uma Delimitação Da Noção de Criança Hiperactiva." *Revista Portuguesa de Pedagogia* 20: 203–18.

Rodrigues, Ana Nascimento. 2007. "Escalas Revistas de Conners: Formas Reduzidas para Pais e Professores." In *Avaliação Psicológica. Instrumentos Validados para a População Portuguesa*, edited by Mário Simões, Carla Machado, Miguel Gonçalves, and Leandro Almeida, 203–26. Coimbra: Quarteto Editora.

Rodrigues, Ana, and Nuno Antunes. 2014. *Mais Forte Do Que Eu! Hiperactividade e Défice de Atenção: Causas, Consequências e Soluções*. Lisbon: Lua de Papel.

Rosenberg, Charles. 2006. "Contested Boundaries: Psychiatry, Disease, and Diagnosis." *Perspectives in Biology and Medicine* 49: 407–24. doi:0.1353/pbm.2006.0046.

Santos, Boaventura de Sousa. 1985. "Estado e sociedade na semiperiferia do sistema mundial: O caso português." *Análise Social* 21: 869–901.

Santos, Maria J., and Maria F. Gaspar. 2015. "Projeto Contra Desigualdades Sociais No Pré-Escolar Obtém Apoio Internacional." Educare.pt. http://www.educare.pt/noticias/noticia/ver/?id=37245&langid=1.

Sardica, José. 2008. *Twentieth Century Portugal: A Historical Overview*. Lisbon: Universidade Católica Editora.

Simões, Mário, Miguel Gonçalves, and Leandro Almeida, eds. 1999. *Testes e Provas Psi-cológicas em Portugal.* Braga: Sistemas Humanos e Organizacionais/Associação dos Psicólogos Portugueses.

Singh, Ilina. 2002. "Bad Boys, Good Mothers, and the 'Miracle' of Ritalin." *Science in Context* 15: 577–603.

Singh, Ilina, Angela M. Filipe, Imre Bard, Meredith Bergey, and Lauren Baker. 2013. "Globalization and Cognitive Enhancement: Emerging Social and Ethical Challenges for ADHD Clinicians." *Current Psychiatry Reports* 15: 385. doi:10.1007/s11920-013-0385-0.

Soeiro, José. 2015. "Toma o Comprimido e Cala-Te?" *Jornal Expresso*, May 29. http://expresso.sapo.pt/blogues/jose-soeiro/2015-05-29-Toma-o-comprimido-e-cala-te-.

8

Transformations in the Irish ADHD Disorder Regime—from a Disorder "You Have to Fight to Get" to One "You Have to Wait to Get"

Claire Edwards
Órla O'Donovan

Under the headline "Hyperactivity Still Regarded as New Phenomenon Here," an article published in *The Irish Times* in 1998 reported on a conference held at a teacher training college at which a keynote speaker asserted that "many people [in Ireland] are only hearing about ADHD [attention deficit–hyperactivity disorder]" (McLoughlin 1998). Also reported in the article was the establishment of the first Irish ADHD service, run by a clinical psychologist in a children's hospital, and the emergence of a network of ADHD support groups around the country. That same year, a discussion took place in the upper house of the Irish parliament involving the minister for health and children at which the lack of popular and professional recognition of the disorder and the concomitant lack of treatment services were highlighted. Relying on their own personal resources, at the time many Irish parents who suspected their children had ADHD were making costly diagnostic and treatment odysseys abroad. A decade later, ADHD had been transformed from a largely institutionally unrecognized disorder to being a "matter of fact" and recognized as the primary reason for children attending the state-run Children and Adolescent Mental Health Services (CAMHS). Widely held up as a prototypical "contested illness" and what Joe Dumit (2006: 577) referred to as an illness "you have to fight to get," in this chapter we show how in Ireland the fight to get childhood ADHD has been won.

ADHD is now officially recognized as "the most common behavioural disorder among children" (Health Service Executive 2015). We argue that in the Irish context, childhood ADHD has changed from being a disorder "you have to fight to get" to being one "you have to wait to get" since lack of professional recognition has been replaced by public health care waiting lists as the main obstacle to diagnosis.

Guided by Bruno Latour's (2004) model of the social critic as one who assembles rather than debunks, we explore the participants or ingredients—human and nonhuman—gathered around the *thing* ADHD that made it exist and maintain its existence specifically in the Irish context. This mix includes medical professionals, scientists, teachers, politicians, the pharmaceutical industry, ADHD treatments, drug regulation authorities, US ADHD organizations, and more. In our discussion, particular attention is given to Irish-based ADHD organizations and their "evidence-based activism" in the assemblage that gathered to state the fact of ADHD and constitute the Irish ADHD "disorder regime."

Both conceptually and empirically, our discussion draws on the European Union–funded research project European Patient Organisations in Knowledge Society (EPOKS). This study investigated patients' organizations' knowledge production activities across four conditions (ADHD, Alzheimer's disease, rare diseases, and childbirth) and four national contexts (Ireland, the United Kingdom, France, and Portugal). "Evidence-based activism" is the term we use to refer to the diverse epistemic activities of these patients' organizations and to capture the many forms of knowledge they mobilize (Rabeharisoa, Moreira, and Akrich 2014). The term highlights both the articulation between knowledge and politics and the work entailed in that articulation. Further features of this distinct form of health activism are the articulation of experiential and credentialed knowledge and the formation of alliances between patients' organizations and medical and scientific specialists. Documentary analysis of texts published by and about the organizations significantly informed our research, but fieldwork was also undertaken and included interviews with leading members and personnel, as well as attendance at conferences they organized.

In the first phase of this project, which began in early 2009, we traced the histories of a number of organizations. Primarily on the basis of documentary-archival analysis, we systematically tracked the organizations' historical trajectories along a number of dimensions (e.g., cause, constituency, and web of relations). Using a common framework, for each organization we sought to identify main historical turning points and characterize public positionings.

Questions posed included: When and why was the organization established? As what kind of organization has it self-identified (e.g., self-help, advocacy, or "war on disease")? What are the main changes it has sought to bring about? Who are its allies (and opponents)?

The second phase of EPOKS focused on developing detailed analyses of recent knowledge-related activities of the organizations. Again, we used a common framework for each of the case study organizations and asked how its knowledge-related activities could best be characterized. Is its propensity to embrace or to challenge biomedical knowledge? What is the content of the knowledge it produces and/or circulates? What is the nature and scope of its target audiences? What tools does it use for staging, legitimizing, and circulating knowledge? Does it participate in research projects at the European level? Case study reports were prepared for all of the organizations studied in EPOKS; these reports formed the basis of extended cross-national and cross-condition analysis and the identification of overarching themes and conclusions. Here we draw on the case study report on the Irish National Council of ADHD Support Groups (INCADDS) and a series of EPOKS publications (Edwards and Howlett 2013; O'Donovan, Moreira, and Howlett 2013; Edwards et al. 2014; Rabeharisoa, Moreira, and Akrich 2014; Rabeharisoa and O'Donovan 2014).

Conceptually, we also draw on Maren Klawiter's (2004) work on breast cancer activism. Following Michel Foucault's (1987) identification of the task of the genealogist as the analysis of "regimes of practices," she offers the concept of the "disease regime" as a way of conceptualizing the structural shaping of illness experiences. Pointing to another kind of assemblage, she defines a disease regime as being composed of "the institutionalized practices, authoritative discourses, social relations, collective identities, emotional vocabularies, visual images, public policies and regulatory actions through which diseases are socially constituted and experienced" (Klawiter 2004: 851). In contrast to many Foucauldian analyses of the regimes of practices of public health and medicine that adopt a totalizing view of power, Klawiter illustrates how disease regimes change over time and, in the case of the transformation of the US breast cancer regime between the late 1970s and late 1990s, the significant role played by the breast cancer movement in that process. Adapting Klawiter's concept, in this chapter we consider the emergence of the current Irish ADHD disorder regime.

We begin by considering the fight for recognition of childhood ADHD, a fight that intensified in the late 1990s. This was the period referred to as the "Celtic Tiger" years (the mid-1990s–2008), during which the Irish economy recorded record growth rates and during which certain public services expanded, including educational services for children with disabilities. Second, now that the existence of ADHD is officially recognized, we outline what it is recognized as being in institutionalized discourses. In the context of the crash in the Irish economy in 2008, together with inbuilt inequalities in the Irish health care system that result in public patients waiting longer than private patients to access many specialist consultations, we discuss how childhood ADHD has become a disorder you have to wait to get. Third, we consider how, following a successful "stating of the fact" of ADHD, ADHD activism remains a dynamic field in which organizations continue to redefine the very thing around which they are mobilized.

The Fight to Get Childhood ADHD in Ireland

The narrative of ADHD in Ireland is one in which over a relatively short period of time—some 10 years—the disorder shifted from being relatively unknown to being a key focus of the work of child and adolescent psychiatric services. This coincided with the Celtic Tiger boom years and the hailing of Ireland as "a crowning glory of neoliberalism"; between 1993 and 2000, the gross national product grew by an average of 9% (Finn 2011: 7). Particularly significant to this discussion, the decade between the 1990s and 2000s also witnessed an expansion of some public services such as educational supports for children with "special needs." For example, the Special Needs Assistance Scheme in Irish schools expanded from employing 2,988 Special Needs Assistants in 2001 to employing 10,442 in 2008 (Department of Education and Skills 2011: 23). This period also saw the introduction of significant disability legislation such as the Disability Act of 2005, which entitled parents who felt their child may have a disability to a professional assessment of their child's health and educational needs. Here, we consider the various players and the shifting public policies, social relations, and institutional practices and knowledge that led to a successful "stating of the fact" of ADHD. Mentions of ADHD first emerged in the Irish media in the 1980s, and that decade too saw the formation in Dublin of the first ADHD organization, then known as the Hyperactive Children's Support Group Ireland. However, it was from the mid-1990s that the disorder became more prominent and debated in both governmental and popular discourse; according to a 1995 article in *The Irish Times*, ADHD was a "hidden handicap" that psychiatrists had, up until that point, been unwilling to diagnose (Thompson 1995).

Facing Down "Bad Parenting": The Emergence of ADHD Activism

Linked to international sociotechnical networks, organizations consisting of parents of children with the disorder played a central role in shaping the emerging ADHD disorder regime and shifting the dynamic of unwilling diagnosis that had characterized Irish child psychiatry. An initial focus of these organizations when they were established was to destabilize existing professional knowledge of the disorder, develop a new collective illness identity, and transform the social relations of the disorder. There was a mushrooming of groups in the 1990s, and in 1999 an umbrella body for these organizations, the Irish National Council of AD/HD Support Groups (INCADDS), was formed. Today there are some 22 local ADHD organizations in existence. When we interviewed them, group members expressed how, in the early years, they felt castigated by the medical profession (and psychiatrists in particular) as "bad parents" and had a desperate need for information and support about how to deal with their children's behavior. Exemplifying this mission, a document describing the history of the Cork group, HADD Cork (Hyperactive Attention Deficit Disorders Cork), identified awareness-raising and mutual support as central to the group's cause: "Our aims and objectives at that time were to raise awareness about this treatable 'chronic' condition among parents and professionals, to care and share and to utilise our knowledge especially when we felt so isolated, living and dealing with a condition so very few know about in this country" (Lordan 2001: 2).

The emergence of HADD Cork, like so many of these groups, reflected a local activism in which the provision of self-help and mutual support was central. Through face-to-face support groups and telephone helplines, groups emerged as spaces for the sharing of experiential knowledge about ADHD in the face of a disbelieving public and a medical profession unwilling to validate the disorder. However, their activities extended far beyond the provision of mutual support. In the same way that Klawiter (2004: 851) notes how social movements "can have an impact on an individual's illness experience by transforming her perceptions of, and relationship to, practices of the regime," so the organizations provided sites of knowledge circulation in which parents, and indirectly their children, were socialized into being parents of a child with, or sufferer of, ADHD identities. This socialization was grounded in shifting the understanding of ADHD from a disorder of poor parenting to one of (in part, at least) neurobiology.

The awareness-raising missions of these ADHD organizations in the 1990s were framed as a struggle for recognition of a disorder that was widely known elsewhere but not yet recognized in Ireland. For example, the public notice about the meeting that led to the establishment of the group in the midwest of Ireland stated, "This disorder was first widely-recognised some 10 years ago in the US. It is not yet generally known about in Ireland."[1] The idea that Ireland was lagging behind other countries in recognizing ADHD as a medical condition of "brain dysfunction [that] relates to the left lobe of the brain and that a sufferer cannot take responsibility for his or her actions" was voiced in the national parliament by a politician member of ADD Midwest (Government of Ireland 1998). She stated that even though "ADHD has been treated for over 30 years in most parts of the world, it is still a relatively new phenomenon in Ireland" (Government of Ireland 1998). The organizations therefore contributed to the production of "development rankings" or ideas about how "advanced" or "backward" various countries were with respect to the recognition, authorization, and provision for the disorder. The diffusion of knowledge and practices from the United States and the United Kingdom was particularly significant for the groups, not least in a context in which many families traveled to the United Kingdom to obtain a diagnosis for their children in the absence of sympathetic practitioners in Ireland. Describing the difference between the United Kingdom and Ireland, in the late 1990s a UK pediatrician who had provided a source of diagnosis for Irish families stated that "Irish parents are coming to the centre because it has a different way of understanding these things. It's not just about parenting and your environment; while these are important, ADHD is about a brain that has a different way of functioning" (Holmquist 1998).

The Development of Credentialized Networks

Drawing on the expertise of professionals and establishing collaborative relationships between patients and credentialed experts are key aspects of evidence-based activism. This was evident in the early years of Irish ADHD activism, a feature of which was the forging of alliances with certain key sympathetic professionals, including a small number of health professionals from the United States. The INCADDS website is dedicated to a US clinical psychologist, Deirdre Killelea, who is identified as having made a significant contribution to the establishment of the national organization, but who died in 2005. Prior to moving to Ireland in 1994, she had worked in a treatment center for children with ADHD in the United States; she was also the mother of a child diagnosed with ADHD, thus positioning her as a credentialed and experienced authority on the disorder (Purcell 1998). Similarly, HADD Ireland for a number of years counted David Carey, a US educational psychologist based in Dublin, as one of its advisors.

Another key ally of INCADDS and its member groups has been Michael Fitzgerald, the first professor of child psychiatry in Ireland. Described by members of INCADDS as "our savior," he was, in the past, one of the few Irish psychiatrists willing to diagnose ADHD, and was described by a psychologist in our study as the "one recognised psychiatric expert in the country . . . and would be a referral source for hundreds and hundreds of people."[2] Presented with an award in 2012 from INCADDS to mark "his dedication and support over the years to all those living with ADD" (ADD Midwest Support Group 2015), he has contributed considerably to the promotion of ADHD within the domain of child psychiatry, and in the 1990s, was vocal about the lack of awareness of the disorder. Fitzgerald has been extremely prolific in his scientific publications about the disorder and has pushed the research agenda on the links between genetics and ADHD.

Prior to the 1990s, it seems Fitzgerald was largely a lone voice in child psychiatry, and parents reported how, in the 1980s and even through the early 2000s, they encountered a lack of understanding about ADHD in the face of a disorder regime that viewed their children as "brats" and that engendered a culture of parental blame. When we interviewed Fitzgerald, he attributed this "blame culture" to the hegemony of John Bowlby's (1982) attachment theory in Irish psychiatry and psychology: "It was John Bowlby—mothers were responsible for everything—it was, inverted commas, the bad mother caused all psychological problems so what child psychiatrists and child psychologists did was they just bashed the mothers. It's your fault that you have a child with ADHD. That went on well into the 90s and, for some people, into the 21st century as well."[3] But Fitzgerald's willingness to prescribe medication for ADHD also sparked controversy in the media. In a 1995 newspaper article, he stated that "there was an unwillingness to prescribe medication to children in the past but this is one area where it is helpful and parents who are at their wits end are extremely grateful when they see the changes in their child once on Ritalin" (Thompson 1995). These views were contested by developmental psychologists, who urged caution in associating ADHD with brain dysfunction. Indeed, battles over definitions between professionals from various fields appeared with regularity during the late 1990s and early 2000s, with one prominent media psychologist, Tony Humphreys, describing the labeling of children with disorders such as ADHD as "sins against children" (O'Neill 2006) and questioning the existence of ADHD itself as a biological entity.

For parents, then, stating the fact of ADHD involved contesting such arguments and establishing the materiality of ADHD in the biology of the brain, as part of an understanding of the disorder as complex and multidimensional. Neurobiological understandings increasingly became embedded in public policy discourses about the disorder from the late 1990s, following the discussion of ADHD in the Irish parliament initiated by a senator and member of ADD Midwest. That parliamentary discussion led to the establishment of a working group on the disorder, under the Joint Committee on Health and Children, to explore the prevalence and provision of services for children with ADHD. The report of the working group, *Report on Attention Deficit Disorder in Ireland* (*RADDI*), published in 1999, was a significant coup for the ADHD organizations, and drew on interviews with professionals, including Fitzgerald, as well as parents of children with the disorder. The report stated that "there is genetic and neurobiological evidence that ADD/H[4] has a biological basis" (Joint Committee on Health and Children 1999: 2) and that "new research by scientists at Trinity College Dublin . . . has confirmed that sufferers from ADHD have a genetic abnormality causing the condition" (10). A report published by the Working Group on Child and Adolescent Psychiatric Services (WGCAPS), set up a year later by the Department of Health and Children and made up predominantly of child psychiatrists and psychologists, was rather more circumspect, noting that even though ADHD "is a clinical diagnosis, there is no blood or x-ray type test available to confirm it. Assessment therefore means considering whether there are alternative causes of inattentive, impulsive and/or restless behaviour" (Department of Health and Children 2001: 5).

Enumerating ADHD and Its Treatment in "Official" Discourse

Both these reports provided official recognition of ADHD as a matter of fact and were some of the first attempts to quantify its prevalence in Ireland. The WGCAPS, established with a broad remit to examine the state of child psychiatry services in Ireland and services for children with ADHD specifically, estimated the prevalence to be between 1% and 5% of school-age children; extrapolating from this, it argued that "500 school aged children per 200,000 population will suffer from ADHD/HKD at any one time and 50 new cases of children will present for treatment each year" (Department of Health and Children 2001: 6).[5] It noted that with increased awareness of the disorder, the number of children referred to child and adolescent psychiatry teams would increase substantially. The *RADDI* report, in contrast, asserted that "ADD/H affects approximately 5–10% of the general population based on the criteria published in the *Diagnostic and Statistical Manual of Mental Disorders* of the American Psychiatric Association (DSM)" (Joint Committee on Health and Children 1999: 2), but also noted that there was a serious underdiagnosis of the disorder. This politics of numbers (Alonso and Starr 1987)—particularly of those undiagnosed—became, and remains, a key trope of parents' organizing.[6] For example, during an ADHD awareness week in 2010, hosted by the ADHD organizations, the media widely reported that there were 60,000 children with ADHD in Ireland, many of whom were undiagnosed. When confusion emerged around this figure, a child psychiatrist, Fiona McNicholas, explained: "I don't think there are 60,000 children *diagnosed* with ADHD. There's about 60,000 children under the age of 15 who you might expect to have ADHD based on a 5% prevalence rate" (Drivetime 2010).

Crucially, both working group reports also addressed the deficit in services for children with the disorder and set out some benchmarks for how ADHD should be treated. Parents' activism in Ireland emerged in a context of limited access to publicly funded child psychiatry services, and despite a couple of specialist ADHD centers being established in hospitals during the 1990s (in particular, one at Our Lady's Hospital for Sick Children, Crumlin, which was established in 1998 and funded by parents' groups), these were only available in Dublin (Joint Committee on Health and Children 1999: 23). During the interviews we conducted with support groups, a number of the interviewees emphasized that access to specialist services, especially diagnostic and support services, quickly emerged as priorities for the support groups. As stated on the INCADDS website, for example:

> It is the core mission of INCADDS to ensure that the difficulties for sufferers of AD/HD are minimised by the development and promotion of early diagnosis; the promotion of appropriate and comprehensive person-centred treatment; and by raising awareness of the disorder so that its sufferers will be better understood. In addition, INCADDS wants to ensure that the families of sufferers of AD/HD are adequately supported so that they in turn can support their children and relatives. (INCADDS 2015)

The two working group reports also provided official endorsement of parents' concerns about the lack of diagnostic and treatment options. The *RADDI* report noted "that quite a large number of children wait five to eleven years for a diagnosis of ADD/H after parental identification of problems" (Joint Committee on Health and Children 1999: 3), and in Ireland's two-tier health system, acknowledged that many families resorted to paying privately for a diagnosis. In recommending multidisciplinary teams as the best model for treating ADHD, the WGCAPS report suggested that the state required some 25 new consultant-led CAMHS teams, as well as the enhancement of many existing teams that were not fully staffed, at a total cost of £39 million.

While discussion of the need for greater ADHD services was relatively settled, what constitutes appropriate treatment remains controversial. ADHD organizations have, since their inception, argued for multimodal approaches to the treatment of ADHD, and this was acknowledged in both reports. The WGCAPS, for example, stated that components of treatment may include education of the child and his family, as well as teachers, family therapy, and pharmacotherapy. In relation to medication, it noted that "in most cases, a stimulant is the first choice medication e.g. Ritalin (Methylphenidate) or Dexedrine (Dexamphetamine)" (Department of Health and Children 2001: 7). Perhaps more controversially, the *RADDI* report, while also stating the need for multimodal treatment, recommended the regulatory action that the Irish Medicines Board "need[s] to approve a far greater number of medicines that are not available at present . . . Medications have been unequivocally shown to reduce core symptoms of hyperactivity, impulsivity and inattentiveness" (Joint Committee on Health and Children 1999: 4). Such statements did not reflect the concerns that many parents expressed in interviews around decisions to medicate their children, or the controversies that rage around ADHD medications to this day. Methylphenidate (Ritalin) was first licensed in Ireland in 1980, but as with the numbers of children with ADHD, there are no accurate figures available on children being prescribed the drug from this time. What is apparent is that there has been a significant upward trajectory in rates of prescribing; figures from the Health Service Executive suggest that there was a 62% increase in drugs being prescribed for ADHD between 2007 and 2012 (from 32,701 prescriptions in 2007 to 52,988 in 2012), with Ritalin accounting for the largest proportion of these prescriptions (from 24,423 in 2007 to 37,154 in 2012) (Byrne 2013). For some, this dynamic reflects an epistemic shift in psychiatry in Ireland and a change in its institutionalized practices. One psychiatrist told us:

When I was training to be a psychiatrist a long time ago and I did my child psychiatry, at that time, my colleagues in child psychiatry were very proud of the fact that they very rarely prescribed any medication . . . Now the situation has dramatically changed and child psychiatrists, very many of them, not everyone, but I would think probably the majority prescribe quite a lot . . . the whole orientation of child psychiatry has become a lot more biomedical and its understanding of problems and its responses to problems has become a lot more biomedical.[7]

This shift, which we discuss in the following section, is in part due to the successful stating of the fact of ADHD and is evident in the contemporary Irish ADHD disorder regime. Indeed, this success saw the aforementioned psychologist Tony Humphreys publicly castigated by the minister for health and children and the Psychological Society of Ireland in 2012 for suggesting that conditions such as autism and ADHD did not exist (Rogers 2012).

Recognized as What? The Current Irish ADHD Disorder Regime

Having considered the contributions of ADHD organizations toward making the *thing* ADHD exist in Ireland, we now turn to addressing the authoritative understandings of what that thing is, or dimensions of the Irish ADHD disorder regime. As we will show, although the existence of ADHD is now widely accepted in Ireland, uncertainties about how it should be diagnosed and treated remain. The problem is recognized, but its solutions continue to be disputed. Furthermore, we argue that for those without the private resources to bypass waiting lists to access publicly funded health care services, ADHD has become a disorder you have to wait to get.

Enunciating ADHD Today: State Discourses and Uncertainties

The Irish government's 2006 mental health policy, *A Vision for Change*, made provision for CAMHS, staffed by community and hospital-based multidisciplinary teams, for young people up to the age of 18 years. Published in 2008, the first CAMHS annual report notes that the most frequently occurring "primary presentations" (29% of cases) were "hyperkinetic disorders/problems," a category that included "ADHD and other attentional disorders" (Health Service Executive 2008: 17). Illustrating a shift in the institutionalized nomenclature, the 2013 CAMHS annual report records that the "ADHD/hyperkinetic category (31.6%)

again was the most frequently assigned primary presentation," and that "ADHD and other attentional disorders (31.6%) were the most frequently assigned primary presentation overall and in each of the regions" (Health Service Executive 2013: 7). Categorizing ADHD as a psychiatric disorder, the 2013 annual report notes the outcomes of a study to determine the prevalence of psychiatric disorders in the Irish adolescent population; this study showed that 3.7% met the criteria for ADHD. This authoritative discourse of ADHD also recognizes it as a gendered disorder in which the "male to female ratio for ADHD or other attentional disorders is 4:1" (Health Service Executive 2013: 36). According to the 2013 CAMHS data, boys made up 75% of children in the 5- to 9-years-old age group who used the service, and ADHD and other attentional disorders accounted for 44% of primary presentations in boys in that age group. In contrast, girls made up 25% of the 5- to 9-year-olds seen by the service, and of those, 34% had ADHD and other attentional disorders. The 2013 CAMHS annual report also notes that as a consequence of the emergence of ADHD as "the largest diagnostic category attending community CAMHS teams, dedicated ADHD clinics have developed to meet this demand" (Health Service Executive 2013: 60). In other words, within the mental health services, ADHD is now recognized as a gendered psychiatric disorder, the high prevalence of which has created the need for dedicated clinics.

Within the educational realm, official definitions of special educational needs categorize ADHD as an "emotional disturbance and/or behaviour problem" (National Council for Special Education 2014: 21). Similar to the emergence of ADHD as the largest diagnostic category within the child and adolescent mental health services, the largest category of students deemed to have special educational needs are those with "emotional/behavioural disturbance" (National Council for Special Education 2010: 2).

Despite the dramatic increase in the diagnosis of ADHD in Irish children, the institutionalized practices and authoritative discourses that contribute to the constitution of the disorder regime acknowledge a series of uncertainties surrounding the condition. Adapted from a British National Health Service source, the information about ADHD provided on the Irish Health Service Executive's website reflects a series of ongoing uncertainties that are attributed to lack of research, or what Hess (2009) referred to as "undone science." Among these are uncertainties about (1) adult ADHD diagnostic practices "because there is no definitive set of age-appropriate symptoms," (2) the symptoms since it "is not fully understood whether these problems are an extreme form of normal behaviour, or part of a separate range of behaviour," (3) its etiology since the "exact cause of attention deficit hyperactivity disorder (ADHD) is not fully understood," and (4) its treatment since, for example, in regard to the widely prescribed drug Ritalin it is noted that "it is not completely clear how it works" (Health Service Executive 2015). Notwithstanding these uncertainties, the Health Service Executive's information presents ADHD as a disorder caused by a combination of genetic causes, brain function and anatomy, and environmental factors, including exposure to toxins such as tobacco smoke during pregnancy. (The latter suggests that ADHD groups have not been entirely successful in their efforts to rid understandings of the disorder from notions of maternal blame.)

Treating ADHD in an Era of Welfare Restraint

The Health Service Executive's website also prescribes a diagnostic route for parents who suspect their child may have ADHD, beginning with a consultation with a medical general practitioner who may provide a referral to specialists such as psychiatrists, pediatricians, or the multidisciplinary CAMHS teams mentioned above. At odds with the official recognition of the ongoing uncertainties surrounding the disorder, assurance is provided that these specialists "can make an accurate diagnosis after a detailed assessment," including a physical examination, several tests, a series of interviews with the child and other significant people, and adherence to a set of strict diagnostic criteria (Health Service Executive 2015). The institutionalized treatment practices specified in the Health Service Executive's information about ADHD reflect the kind of multimodal understanding of the disorder promoted by ADHD organizations, often in the face of professionals' tendency to reduce the disorder to their specific domains of knowledge and competency. These treatments are a combination of medication (the psychostimulants methylphenidate and dexamfetamine and the selective noradrenaline uptake inhibitor atomoxetine) and therapies such as psychotherapy, behavior therapy, and cognitive-behavioral therapy, in addition to dietary changes and parent training programs.

The establishment of ADHD as a disorder that can be responsive to pharmaceutical treatment is also evident in Irish drug reimbursement policy and practices. Data provided to us by the Health Service Executive's Primary Care Reimbursement Services indicate that methylphenidate (Ritalin) is the most frequently prescribed of the three ADHD medicines, at least to those eligible for public reimbursement for their medicines. These data also provide evidence of gradual year-by-year increases in public expenditure on the reimbursement of drugs used in the treatment of ADHD. For example, in 2010, public expenditure on methylphenidate, atomoxetine, and dexamfetamine amounted to €2.5 million, and by 2013 this had increased to €2.8 million.[8] Following a complaint to the public service ombudsman made by the mother of a child with ADHD, since 2014 ADHD has been officially recognized as constituting a mental illness that entitles people up to 16 years of age who have the diagnosis to a Long Term Illness Card and access to medications free of charge. This will further contribute to increases in public expenditure on ADHD medications.

The treatment of ADHD in Ireland can perhaps best be described as being shaped by an eclecticism in which medication plays a dominant role. There are no official data regarding the total numbers of children with ADHD receiving particular treatments, or indeed on the types of treatments being offered. There is, however, a fragmented, yet burgeoning research scene exploring the efficacy of different treatments for ADHD; this ranges from small-scale research focused on brain training and neurofeedback to randomized, controlled trials seeking to evaluate early-years parenting programs for families of children with the condition (McGilloway et al. 2013). This disparate assemblage of research and therapeutic actions reflects the view that ADHD must be tackled through a multimodal approach in which psychosocial interventions often go hand in hand with psychostimulant medication.

For professionals working in the Irish mental health services, borrowing from international practices and guidelines in relation to treatment appears to be commonplace. As one child psychiatrist who treats ADHD noted in an interview, "You know we've got the UK NICE guidelines, we've got the American academy guidelines, we don't need to create our own Irish guidelines, we'd be wasting loads of time and they're going to be no different to any of the others, and most practitioners would follow the guidelines."[9] Despite these guidelines, the apparent consensus on the need for multimodal approaches to treat ADHD has not precluded a specifically Irish moral debate and contestation between different professionals and parents about the efficacy and availability of different treatments. For example, a guide entitled *The A-Zee of ADHD*, which was published by one of the main ADHD organizations, HADD Ireland, described the pitfalls of treatment in Ireland: "Professionals tend to specialize in one or a few related areas, and so treating ADHD will often require a few different practitioners and services . . . Some clinics have a multi-disciplinary team, but most don't. Even if they do there might be something they don't offer" (Carr-Fanning 2011).

Since the widespread recognition of the disorder in Ireland, ADHD organizations have highlighted the poor availability of child and adolescent psychiatry in the public sector, the significant geographical variations in service availability, and the high costs of seeking private treatment (Edwards and Howlett 2013). Banner headlines in the Irish media such as "More Than 2,500 Children Waiting for HSE [Health Services Executive] Mental Health Services," combined with reports of great increases in demand for the services (such as 11% between 2012 and 2013), reiterate the organizations' concerns (Hennessy 2014). Both the major increase in referrals to the CAMHS and the enforced "austerity" measures from the European Union and International Monetary Fund, introduced since the crash in the Irish economy in 2008, have contributed to making childhood ADHD a disorder "you have to wait to get." Delays in accessing services are not, however, new to Irish public health care. Ireland has one of the highest levels of private health insurance in the Organisation for Economic Co-operation and Development member countries, which has come to operate primarily as a supplementary form of health care coverage offering subscribers a means of bypassing public waiting lists (McDonnell and O'Donovan 2009). In the past, before the existence of ADHD was recognized in Ireland, parents who could afford to do so traveled abroad for the diagnosis and treatment of ADHD in their children. Currently, those who can afford to do so access private child psychiatric services in Ireland, whereas those without the means to do so wait.

Furthermore, parents have expressed concerns that the primary (and often only) publicly funded treatment option available for them is medication. As one parent stated in an interview: "the problem isn't necessarily always getting a diagnosis and getting treatment, the problem is all you might get is a diagnosis and a prescription and that's where it finishes."[10] For parents, the biomedical "fix" for ADHD via medication is a source of constant concern, not least in a context of regularly appearing alarmist headlines such as "Thousands of Children on ADHD Drugs" (Hough 2011b), "Concern at ADHD Medication Rates" (Hough 2011a), and "Trained Parents Could Help Avoid Medication of Children with ADHD" (Ring 2013). In our research, parents repeatedly expressed how the decision to medicate is not taken lightly. It is largely for this reason that a key focus of ADHD organizations' activism since "stating the fact" of ADHD has been to push the boundaries of ADHD treatment beyond medication. Indeed, investigating alternative treatments in an arena of scarce resources, along with expanding the boundaries of ADHD patienthood, have become two key matters of concern for ADHD groups since the relative settling of ADHD as a neurobiological disorder. This in turn is reorienting the dynamics of the ADHD disorder regime as new actors are brought in as sufferers and as offering new forms of treatment.

Patient Activism since "Stating the Fact" of ADHD

Klawiter (2004) argues that social movements have the potential to change illness experiences, not just by shifting patient subjectivities and the positioning of the sufferer in relation to regime practices (such as formalized modes of treatment and the health care or pharmaceutical industry), but also by changing regime practices themselves. We have suggested that, in Ireland, ADHD organizations have contributed to successfully shifting the vocabulary of, and subjectivities associated with, ADHD from those that speak of "brats," "bad behavior," and "poor parenting," to "neurobiology," "brain chemicals," and biomedical legitimacy, such that formalized health care systems and child and adolescent psychiatry (as the dominant treating profession) have overwhelmingly come to accept ADHD as a valid disorder. However, the ADHD disorder regime is dynamic; in a circularity of activism, groups' redefinition of the condition, and the subsequent consequences of this for institutionalized practices, leads them to rearticulate their cause(s). This is visible both in terms of campaigns around treatment of the disorder and in groups' redefinition of sufferer subjectivities.

In the first of these, disputes that remain around access to treatment beyond the biomedical are increasingly leading organizations to intervene in terms of investigating alternative treatments to medication. Reflecting their role as contributors to the production of knowledge about the ADHD disorder, ADHD organizations have acted as conduits for the recruitment of research participants, and in some cases, have commissioned their own research into specific interventions as a response to a lack of choice in public health service provision (Edwards and Howlett 2013). Constrained by limited options in the public health service, they have sought to open up the field of practice around ADHD by investigating interventions such as family therapy programs and neurofeedback as additional forms of treatment (Edwards and Howlett 2013). One group, ADD Midwest, based in Limerick, for example, raised money to fund psychotherapists to run sessions with both parents and their children over a two-year period; the group also used this money to fund an evaluation of the project, which was carried out by the local university. Similarly, another group built linkages with a local university's psychology department to run a trial of a neurofeedback intervention with a small number of children.

ADHD organizations have also initiated and run particular interventions such as group therapy for young adults and brought international experts to Ireland to speak about novel therapeutic approaches. For example, one of the main organizations, HADD Ireland, based in Dublin, has been critical of the lack of parenting courses focused on the specificities of parenting an "ADHD child." This organization offers its own parenting program, ParentsPlus, which it describes as being specially adapted for parents of children with ADHD. As its website also states of the workshops: "They are also facilitated by an experienced representative from HADD, who either has ADHD themselves and/or is a parent of a child or adult with ADHD" (HADD Ireland 2015b). This embodied knowledge of the condition exemplifies the lay expertise that has come to shape the field of ADHD, such that treatment strategies around the disorder have increasingly articulated credentialed and lay knowledges, as parents look beyond biomedical interventions.

Extending ADHD Patient Identities

Interventions can be read as an attempt by parents to further expand the current contours of knowledge around ADHD held by credentialed experts (in particular, in child and adolescent psychiatry). In doing so, the field of action that is the treatment of ADHD has come to encompass a broader range of health professionals, including neuroscientists, psychologists, psychotherapists, and social scientists—to name but a few—and a greater multiplicity of forms of knowledge (Rabeharisoa, Moreira, and Akrich 2014: 114). This expansion of the domain of ADHD is also happening in terms of the patient identities ascribed to persons with ADHD. Groups still cite awareness-raising of the disorder as one of their missions, as exemplified by a recent talk entitled "ADHD Is Real." (This talk, hosted by HADD Ireland, was by a clinical psychologist and an assistant clinical professor of psychiatry at Yale University, Thomas E. Brown) (HADD Ireland 2015a). However, today awareness-raising is shifting from children with the condition to adults with the condition. The groups have been relatively successful in their attempts to get ADHD recognized as an established disorder within mainstream child and adolescent psychiatry. Today, the battleground for recognition is adult psychiatry since groups describe the condition as one that often goes unrecognized or undiagnosed in adults with debilitating effects, including potential for substance misuse, educational underattainment, and difficulties in the workplace. For example, in 2013, a seminar organized by INCADDS entitled "An Educational Programme for the Rapid Recognition of ADHD in Adults" was advertised as providing a diagnostic toolkit to medical and other professionals;

presentations at the seminar emphasized the benefits of ADHD medicines for adults with the disorder but also considered other treatments, including cognitive-behavioral therapy, neurofeedback, and the increasingly popular practice of mindfulness. This boundary expansion in terms of ADHD has become apparent in the membership of certain groups and the embodied politics of illness that they represent. Thus, the key organizers of the groups are as likely to be adults with the disorder themselves as they are to be parents of children with the condition.

Such a shift is associated with a move to assert a more positive ADHD identity. For example, the chairperson of HADD Ireland identifies herself as someone with ADHD, and HADD Ireland regularly organizes events where celebrity figures who have ADHD talk about how the disorder has affected them, including the positive attributes it brings. Advertising a talk by one such celebrity as part of ADHD Awareness Week in 2013, for example, the group's website states, "Celebrated Chef Rozanne Stevens & recently diagnosed adult with ADHD talks about how getting a diagnosis really helped her. She talks about adapting her strengths and downplaying her weaknesses, finding her passion in life and how to channel her creative energy" (HADD Ireland 2015c). A headline in one national daily newspaper, *The Irish Independent*, is also evidence of this continuing shift in public discourse: "From Jamie Oliver to Richard Branson: ADHD isn't Just for Kids" (*The Irish Independent* 2012). Such discourse may not be a feature of all ADHD organizations in Ireland, but it is a growing trend that builds on the notion of neurodiversity to express this positive identity—a term that embraces and celebrates human difference in brain functioning and highlights the ways in which society needs to adapt itself to the neurodiverse person, rather than the other way around (Armstrong 2010).

SHIFTING SCALES OF ACTIVISM

Another changing dynamic of ADHD organizing in Ireland relates to the scale at which organizations are targeting their activism. Although many groups emerged at a local level in order to provide direct support to children and their families, they are increasingly scaling up their activism to the European level (Edwards 2014). Two organizations, INCADDS and HADD Ireland, are members of the European ADHD umbrella organization, ADHD Europe, which was formed in 2008 and seeks to "advance the rights of, and advocate on every level throughout Europe for people affected by AD/HD and co-morbid conditions in order to help them reach their full potential" (ADHD Europe 2015). These groups in particular have deployed European-level actions (such as ADHD Europe's annual awareness-raising weeks) to leverage local and national support for their cause in what Della Porta and Caiani (2007: 3) refer to as "boomerang effects."

Involvement at the European scale has brought the organizations into new coalitions with certain professionals and politicians. For example, the chairperson of HADD Ireland was a contributor to a European Expert White Paper on ADHD entitled "ADHD: Making the Invisible Visible," written by three experts (including Irish child psychiatrist Michael Fitzgerald) and supported by Irish Member of the European Parliament Nessa Childers, chair of the European Parliament Interest Group on Mental Health, Wellbeing and Brain Disorders. Through such actions, groups are clearly trying to position themselves as "insiders" in the European political process (Rabeharisoa and O'Donovan 2014).

However, these new coalitions have also led to contention and criticism in terms of the allies and allegiances of ADHD organizations. The Expert White Paper, along with another European initiative designed to create information about the disorder (and in which another Irish-based psychiatrist, Fiona McNicholas, has been involved), known as the ADHD Institute, were both funded by the pharmaceutical company Shire. In a recent post on the website *Mad in America* (which hosts writers who are critical of psychiatric modes of care and practice), blogger Maria Bradshaw takes issue with Shire's funding of the expert paper, which she describes as little more than a "content marketing tool designed not to inform but persuade" (Bradshaw 2014). She highlights the funding received from Shire by multiple members of the expert group, including members of ADHD organizations (and representatives from Irish ADHD organizations that were part of the group and contributed to the paper). Criticizing Childers for associating herself with the company, Bradshaw writes: "I am not questioning the commitment Ms. Childers has to improving the lives of children . . . What I am questioning is her vigilance in ensuring she is not being used by Shire Pharmaceuticals to promote drug sales rather than promote child well-being." These disputes echo those that have been a feature of US-based ADHD activism (Conrad 2007) and raise questions about the pharmaceutical industry becoming an increasingly powerful, if sometimes hidden, participant in maintaining the existence of ADHD.

Conclusion

In this chapter, we have considered some of the participants gathered around the *thing* ADHD who made it exist and maintain its existence specifically in the Irish context. Furthermore, we have demonstrated how the experience of ADHD has been shaped "by culturally, spatially, and historically specific regimes of practices" (Klawiter 2004: 846) that make up the Irish ADHD disorder regime. In particular, we have explored the contribution of ADHD organizations to stating the fact of ADHD and to the fight to get it recognized as a bona fide disorder that psychiatrists are willing to diagnose—a fight that intensified and was won between the late 1990s and 2000s. In that short period of time, ADHD was transformed from being a contested disorder that most Irish psychiatrists were unwilling to diagnose to being the disorder most frequently diagnosed in children attending CAMHS. In addition, in the institutionalized discourses and practices of the Irish educational and mental health services, ADHD was transformed from being a disorder associated with bad parenting to one understood as being complex and multidimensional, which materialized in the brain. A crucial aspect of the evidence-based activism of the ADHD organizations that contributed to these transformations was their allying with sympathetic experts who shared the same understanding of the disorder and their articulation of experiential with credentialed knowledge (Rabeharisoa, Moreira, and Akrich 2014). Although allying with these psychiatrists and psychologists, many of whom had been practicing outside the orthodoxies of their own professions, a marked feature of this activism has been their insistence on a multimodal approach to the treatment of the disorder that extends beyond the expertise of any single profession.

Our story of ADHD and ADHD activism in Ireland also highlights the importance of the cross-national diffusion of practices and ideas about the disorder. The initial years of ADHD activism were shaped by influences from the United States and the United Kingdom; latterly, the European context has become more important for the groups in terms of achieving leverage in Ireland. It is also a story of ongoing struggles. Having won the fight to get childhood ADHD recognized, ADHD organizations have been confronted by inequalities in the two-tier Irish health care system, specifically waiting lists to access publicly funded mental health services. Other more recent struggles and shifts in their cause, such as the fight to get adult ADHD recognized and the associated redefinition of the disorder and the identities of concerned people, point to the ongoing co-production of ADHD in Ireland and these organizations' evidence-based activism. It is an activism that, as we suggest, is likely to contribute not just to a boundary expansion in the contours of the disorder, but also to growing sites of contestation as a greater number of "experts" from different backgrounds (psychology, psychiatry, pharmacology, neuroscience, and social science, to name

but a few) jostle for position in the search for a "solution" to the dilemmas generated by ADHD and the creation of new needs for professional intervention.

NOTES

1. Notice of meeting held on March 15, 1997, supplied by ADD Midwest.

2. Interview conducted with a psychologist, November 8, 2010.

3. Interview conducted with Michael Fitzgerald, May 25, 2010.

4. Variations in how state bodies and ADHD organizations enunciated the disorder—
including ADD, ADD/H, ADHD/HKD, and AD/HD—reflected, and indeed still reflect, the
absence of a fully stabilized vocabulary for the condition. Reasons for the groups' choice
of acronym are rarely explicitly stated, but variations appear, in some cases, to be dependent on whether the organization draws on the *DSM-IV* (*Diagnostic and Statistical Manual
of Mental Disorders* of the American Psychiatric Association) classification, which uses
ADHD, or the *ICD-10* (*International Classification of Diseases*) classification, which uses hyperactivity kinetic disorder, or a combination of both.

5. It is not clear exactly what diagnostic criteria the report drew on, but it explains in
a footnote that "ADHD is the DSM-IV . . . Hyperactivity kinetic disorder is the ICD 10
classification" (Department of Health and Children 2001: 5).

6. As explained by Alonso and Starr (1987: 3) the "politics of numbers" is a term that
refers to the political judgment that is "implicit in the choice of what to measure, how to
measure it, how often to measure it, and how to present and interpret the results."

7. Interview with a psychiatrist, conducted March 22, 2012.

8. Figures requested and obtained via personal communication with Health Service
Executive.

9. Interview with a child and adolescent psychiatrist, conducted November 8, 2010.

10. Interview conducted with a parent and member of an ADHD organization, July 13,
2010.

REFERENCES

ADD Midwest Support Group. 2015. "Presentation to Prof. Michael Fitzgerald from
    INCADDS." http://addmidwestsupport.com/2012/10/08/16/.
ADHD Europe. 2015. "Welcome to ADHD Europe." http://www.adhdeurope.eu/.
Alonso, William, and Paul Starr, eds. 1987. *The Politics of Numbers.* New York: Russell Sage.
Armstrong, Thomas. 2010. *Neurodiversity: Discovering the Extraordinary Gifts of Autism,
    ADHD, Dyslexia and Other Brain Differences.* Cambridge, MA: Da Capo.
Bowlby, John. 1982. "Attachment and Loss: Retrospect and Prospect." *American Journal
    of Orthopsychiatry* 52 (4): 664–78.
Bradshaw, Maria. 2014. "Shire Pharmaceuticals and the MEP—a Case Study in Manipu-
    lation?" *Mad in America* (blog), February 17. http://www.madinamerica.com/2014/02
    /38836/.

Byrne, Luke. 2013. "Prescriptions for ADHD Drugs Soar by More Than 60pc." *The Herald*, September 14. http://www.herald.ie/news/prescriptions-for-adhd-drugs-soar-by-more-than-60pc-29579137.html.

Carr-Fanning, Kate. 2011. *The A to Zee of ADHD.* Dublin: HADD Family Support Group. http://www.hadd.ie/publications/z-adhd.

Conrad, Peter. 2007. *The Medicalization of Society.* Baltimore: Johns Hopkins University Press.

Della Porta, Donatella, and Manuela Caiani. 2007. "Europeanization from Below: Social Movements and Europe." *Mobilization: An International Quarterly* 12 (1): 1–20.

Department of Education and Skills. 2011. *The Special Needs Assistant Scheme: A Value for Money Review of Expenditure on the Special Needs Assistance Scheme 2007/8–2010.* Dublin: Department of Education and Skills. https://www.education.ie/en/Publications/Value-For-Money-Reviews/pub_sna_vfm_june_2011.pdf.

Department of Health and Children. 2001. *Working Group on Child and Adolescent Psychiatric Services: First Report.* Dublin: Department of Health and Children.

Drivetime. 2010. Radió Teilifís Éireann (RTÉ) Radio 1, September 20.

Dumit, Joe. 2006. "Illnesses You Have to Fight to Get: Facts as Forces in Uncertain, Emergent Illnesses." *Social Science & Medicine* 62 (3): 577–90.

Edwards, Claire. 2014. "Spatialising the Contentious Politics of ADHD: Networks and Scalar Strategies in Health Social Movement Activism." *Health and Place* 29: 52–59. doi:10.1016/j.healthplace.2014.05.005.

Edwards, Claire, and Etaoine Howlett. 2013. "Putting Knowledge to Trial: 'ADHD Parents' and the Evaluation of Alternative Therapeutic Regimes." *Social Science & Medicine* 81: 34–41. doi:10.1016/j.socscimed.2013.01.015.

Edwards, Claire, Etaoine Howlett, Madeleine Akrich, and Vololona Rabeharisoa. 2014. "Attention Deficit Hyperactivity Disorder in France and Ireland: Parents' Groups' Scientific and Political Framing of an Unsettled Condition." *BioSocieties* 9: 159–72. doi:10.1057/biosoc.2014.3.

Finn, Daniel. 2011. "Ireland on the Turn? Political and Economic Consequences of the Crash." *New Left Review* 67: 5–39.

Foucault, Michel. 1987. "Questions of Method: An Interview with Michel Foucault." In *After Philosophy: End or Transformation,* edited by Kenneth Baynes, James Bohman, and Thomas McCarthy, 100–117. Boston: MIT.

Government of Ireland. 1998. *Parliamentary Debates—Seanad Éireann,* October 14. http://debates.oireachtas.ie/seanad/1998/10/14/00010.asp.

HADD Ireland. 2015a. "'ADHD IS REAL.' Talk by Prof. Thomas E. Brown." http://www.hadd.ie/article/adhd-real-talk-prof-thomas-e-brown.

———. 2015b. "Parenting Courses." http://www.hadd.ie/resources/parenting-courses-0.

———. 2015c. "Rozanne Stevens, Celebrated Chef on How ADHD Works for Her." http://www.hadd.ie/article/rozanne-stevens-celebrated-chef-how-adhd-works-for-her.

Health Service Executive. 2008. *Child and Adolescent Mental Health Services: First Annual Report.* http://www.hse.ie/eng/services/Publications/Mentalhealth/camhsrpts/camhs2008.html.

———. 2013. *Child and Adolescent Mental Health Services Annual Report 2012–13.* http://www.hse.ie/eng/services/Publications/Mentalhealth/camhsrpts/CAMHS12-13.html.

———. 2015. "Health A–Z." *ADHD.* http://www.hse.ie/portal/eng/health/az/A/ADHD/.

Hennessy, Michelle. 2014. "More Than 2,500 Children Waiting for HSE Mental Health Services." *thejournal.ie,* February 13. http://www.thejournal.ie/children-waiting-list-mental-health-1313982-Feb2014/.

Hess, David J. 2009. "The Potential and Limitations of Civil Society Research: Getting Undone Science Done." *Sociological Inquiry* 79 (3): 306–27. doi:10.1111/j.1475-682X.2009.00292.x.

Holmquist, Kathryn. 1998. "Ain't Misbehavin'." *The Irish Times,* February 23.

Hough, Jennifer. 2011a. "Concern at ADHD Medication Rates." *Irish Examiner,* March 28. http://www.irishexaminer.com/ireland/health/concern-at-adhd-medication-rates-149575.html.

———. 2011b. "Thousands of Children on ADHD Drugs." *Irish Examiner,* March 28. http://www.irishexaminer.com/ireland/health/thousands-of-children-on-adhd-drugs-149539.html.

The Irish Independent. 2012. "From Jamie Oliver to Richard Branson: ADHD Isn't 'Just for Kids.'" October 12. http://www.independent.ie/lifestyle/health/from-jamie-oliver-to-richard-branson-adhd-isnt-just-for-kids-28892712.html.

Irish National Council of ADHD Support Groups (INCADDS). 2015. "About INCADDS." http://www.incadds.ie/about-us.html.

Joint Committee on Health and Children. 1999. *Report on Attention Deficit Disorder in Ireland.* Dublin: Joint Committee on Health and Children.

Klawiter, Maren. 2004. "Breast Cancer in Two Regimes: The Impact of Social Movements on Illness Experience." *Sociology of Health & Illness* 26 (6): 845–74.

Latour, Bruno. 2004. "Why Has Critique Run Out of Steam? From Matters of Fact to Matters of Concern." *Critical Inquiry* 30: 225–48.

Lordan, Mags. 2001. "Cork HADD The History." *Working for You: Newsletter of Hyperactivity Attention Deficit Disorder Cork Support Group* 1: 2.

McDonnell, Orla, and Órla O'Donovan. 2009. "Private Health Insurance as a Technology of Solidarity? The Myth of 'Community' in Irish Healthcare Policy." *Irish Journal of Sociology* 17 (2): 6–23.

McGilloway, Sinead, Grainne Ni Mhaille, Yvonne Leckey, Paul Kelly, and M. Bracken. 2013. *Proving the Power of Positive Engagement: The Effectiveness of Psychosocial Behavioural Training Interventions for Children with Symptoms of ADHD: A Randomised Controlled Trial Evaluation of the Incredible Years Basic Parent Training and Small Group Dina Programme.* Dublin: Archways.

McLoughlin, Brian. 1998. "Hyperactivity Still Regarded as New Phenomenon Here, Conference Told." *The Irish Times,* October 5.

National Council for Special Education. 2010. *NCSE Statistics on Resource Allocations: August 2010.* Dublin: National Council for Special Education.

———. 2014. *Children with Special Educational Needs: Information Booklet for Parents.* Dublin: National Council for Special Education.

O'Donovan, Órla, Tiago Moreira, and Etaoine Howlett. 2013. "Tracking Transformations in Health Movement Organisations: Alzheimer's Disease Organisations and Their Changing 'Cause Regimes.'" *Social Movement Studies* 12 (3): 316–34. doi:10.1080/14742837.2013.777330.

O'Neill, Luke. 2006. "Labels Are 'Sins against Children'—Psychologist." *The Irish Times*, June 20.

Purcell, T. 1998. "Provision Made for Children with ADD." *Irish Examiner*, October 5.

Rabeharisoa, Vololona, Tiago Moreira, and Madeleine Akrich. 2014. "Evidence-Based Activism: Patients', Users', and Activists' Groups in Knowledge Society." *BioSocieties* 9: 111–28. doi:10.1057/biosoc.2014.2.

Rabeharisoa, Vololona, and Órla O'Donovan. 2014. "From Europeanisation to European Construction." *European Societies* 16 (5): 717–41.

Ring, Evelyn. 2013. "Trained Parents Could Help Avoid Medication of Children with ADHD." *Irish Examiner*, November 22. http://www.irishexaminer.com/ireland/train ed-parents-could-help-avoid-medication-of-children-with-adhd-250428.html.

Rogers, Stephen. 2012. "Comments 'Likely to Cause Upset.'" *Irish Examiner*, February 10. http://www.irishexaminer.com/ireland/comments-likely-to-cause-upset-183321.html.

Thompson, Sylvia. 1995. "The Hidden Handicap." *The Irish Times*, October 31.

9

The Journey of ADHD in Argentina

From the Increase in Methylphenidate Use to Tensions among Health Professionals

Silvia A. Faraone
Eugenia Bianchi

This chapter focuses on the rise of attention deficit–hyperactivity disorder (ADHD) as a childhood behavioral disorder in Argentina. In this country, diverse health and education professionals (with diverse theoretical and therapeutic positions) are intensely debating issues regarding the diagnosis and treatment of this condition.

The Argentine case is of particular interest owing to, among other factors, the coexistence of psychoanalytical and biological psychiatric approaches in the practices of health professionals and the cultural and political influence of psychoanalysis in the country. The current conflict in approaches to the diagnosis and treatment of ADHD is between the more psychoanalytical approach and the more biology- and psychiatry-oriented one. Psychoanalysis-related professional groups are resistant to what they call tendencies toward the medicalization and pathologization of children. Psychoanalysts postulate that the iatrogenic effect provoked by stimulants and the use of the American Psychiatric Association's (APA) *Diagnostic and Statistical Manual of Mental Disorders (DSM)* for diagnosing mental pathologies in children violate the Ley Nacional de Salud Mental 26.657 and the UN Convention on the Rights of the Child, which Argentina ratified and adopted through the *Convención sobre los derechos de niños* (Ley 23.849) in the 1990s.

The Ley Nacional de Salud Mental, which was passed by Congress in 2010, empowered professional groups that stand against the pathologization of childhood because it devoted central attention to the concept of mental suffering; in doing so, it confronted medical-pharmaceutical hegemony. The UN Convention on the Rights of the Child (adopted by the General Assembly of the United Nations and ratified by Argentina in 1990) led to the inclusion of these rights in the Argentine Constitution, which guaranteed children the right to receive health-related assistance and to be kept safe and sound, protected from cruelty, negligence, and injustice.[1]

To explore the conflicting approaches to the diagnosis and treatment of ADHD in children in Argentina, we present the results of three studies carried out by the authors between 2007 and 2012. We include data from national and international specialized literature and newspaper articles. We also evaluate statistical data from the Confederación Farmacéutica Argentina (or COFA, a professional association of colleges) and the Administración Nacional de Medicamentos, Alimentos y Tecnología Médica (or ANMAT, the national agency that regulates, certifies, and monitors drugs, foods, and medical devices). In addition, we include data from 63 in-depth individual interviews and 2 in-depth group interviews with health professionals. Some further interviews were carried out with key informants such as renowned child psychiatrists and pediatricians, chief pharmacists, and pharmaceutical sales representatives. In addition, scientific and academic publications on ADHD from Argentine authors were analyzed, along with psychiatric manuals used to assist in diagnosis and treatment. These manuals were chosen because of their widespread use in Argentina and the frequency with which professionals referred to them.

Drawing on this nationwide research, this chapter provides information on the increasing sales of methylphenidate since the 1990s and, more recently, the growing distribution of these sales in the country. We also describe the ways in which the conflicting views and tensions among professionals have influenced diagnostic and therapeutic decisions. These decisions are intertwined with children's-rights perspectives, state-orientated demands, and professionals' critical views on their own practices. Even though it is not possible to delineate a single map of the alignment of the various disciplines and organizations, this chapter anticipates some future areas of conflict and resistance.

Medicalization and Biomedicalization

According to the canonical definition, "medicalization" is the process by which previously nonmedical problems become defined and treated as medical problems (Conrad 2013: 196). Today, medicalization is characterized by issues that go beyond those of the pioneering studies a half century ago that dealt with the influence of doctors and law reformers as well as medical and scientific discoveries. Studies carried out during the 1970s from a medicalization perspective identified physicians, social movements, and interest groups, as well as organizational or inter-professional activities, as the core forces of these processes. Since then, medicine has undergone significant changes through which other forces have come to contribute substantially to the current medicalization process.

In the twenty-first century, the three key actors that guide medicalization worldwide are biotechnology, consumers, and managed care (Conrad 2007: 133). As Conrad examined in a 2007 analysis, many of the key studies of medicalization were completed more than a decade or even two decades ago; however, some changes in medicalization have occurred in the context of important changes in medicine such as the widespread corporatization of health care, the rise of managed care, the increasing importance of the biotechnological industry (especially the pharmaceutical and genomics industries), and the growing influence of consumers and consumer organizations (Conrad 2007: 16). Although actors involved in this global trend are similar, they differ in their emphasis, as indicated by the fact that important zones of medicalization are moving from a medical-professional predominance to a market predominance (Conrad 2005: 10).

Other authors have incorporated these transformations and reconfigured topics in medicalization as part of "biomedicalization" (Clarke et al. 2003: 162). Following Michel Foucault's theory of "biopower" and Paul Rabinow's concept of "biosociality," these authors emphasize that biomedicalization is focused on health as a moral mandate, and it is characterized by the internalization of control, vigilance, and personal transformation. Biomedicalization has acquired a wider scope than medicalization, but both concepts still exist and coexist, and they share a similar focus on actors, strategies, technologies, frameworks, and practices.

The Argentine health sector has undergone a silent reform since the 1990s (Iriart, Faraone, and Waitzkin 2000: 62). Deep transformations have occurred without a declared global project and without explicit objectives from the government or multilateral credit organizations. It is within this framework of micro- and macro-politics, within contradictory developments, that the medicalization and biomedicalization processes in Argentina constitute a paradigmatic case for the context of Latin America. Underlying this framework are the social security sector in Argentina (*obras sociales*), which handles a high percentage of the overall public expenditures, and the unions, which directly run many of the institutions that offer services in this sector. These institutions play a central role in the development of medical social care in Argentina, and the reform of the system that comprises them may be analyzed in parallel to the incidence of multilateral credit agencies on health investment for Latin American countries (in Argentina, especially the World Bank and the International Monetary Fund, or IMF) and their allied administrations (Iriart, Faraone, and Waitzkin 2000: 61).

An Introduction to the Argentine Panorama

In Argentina, the analysis of the interplay of various perspectives of ADHD has a special significance. The recent extension of the phenomenon, the shortage of comprehensive studies, and the coexistence of pediatric medicine with biological psychiatry, neurology, cognitive behavioral psychology, the neurosciences, and psychoanalysis in professionals' training and practices create a particular and interesting view of the problem.

Psychoanalysis has an important role, too. It has been part of the field of mental health in Argentina since the 1960s (Dagfal 2009: 299) and has gradually gained considerable influence in the education and practice of institutions and providers who care for persons with physical and mental health problems. However, since the mid-1990s, there have been two coexisting realities. On the one hand, there has been an ever-growing emergence of many new so-called alternative therapies such as mental control, transcendental meditation, and self-help techniques (Visacovsky 2001: 41). On the other hand, there has been a growing influence of all branches within the neurosciences, so that psychoanalytical primacy has given way to biological hegemony in the conception and treatment of mental suffering.

Outside these advances and growing influences, the position that psychoanalysis has occupied within Argentina is unique as compared with its role in other Latin American and European countries. In Argentina, psychoanalysis has numerous staunch supporters among professionals, and through them, it has had an effect on clinical practice. In cities such as Buenos Aires, São Paulo, and Rio de Janeiro, psychoanalysis exceeds clinical practice in terms of mental health care, and its influence has spread in the urban culture (e.g., in the language, as Visacovsky's observations reveal in the following paragraph). Professionals in the academic, research, and clinical practice worlds in these cities have contributed to sets of regulations for the country that favor certain actions in mental health issues.

The dissemination of psychoanalysis in Argentine society was also analyzed by Visacovsky (2001: 31). He describes the quantity and impact of institutions such as the pioneering Asociación Psicoanalítica Argentina, which was founded in 1942 and associated with the International Psychoanalytical Association (IPA). He also mentions the Asociación Psicoanalítica de Buenos Aires, or APdeBA, which split from the APA and was founded in 1977. Today, there are more than 100 psychoanalytical institutions, most of them of Lacanian scope. Among these, there is the Buenos Aires's Escuela Freudiana de Buenos Aires, or EFBA, founded in 1974, and the Escuela de la Orientación Lacaniana, or EOL, founded in 1992.

Visacovsky (2001: 31) also describes the profusion of psychoanalytical concepts in everyday language, even if the terms do not retain their specialized meaning. He suggests that psychoanalysis can be considered a worldview or a culture that has an authorized public voice, opining on the most varied issues in the mass media.

The problems in Argentina differ from those in other countries such as Uruguay (Miguez 2010: 326). In Argentina, ADHD is identified mainly among persons in the middle and upper classes (mostly urban) who have access to education and health benefits. Whereas prescription of methylphenidate has a function of "domination and control" in Uruguay (as Miguez has documented), in Argentina it is used mainly for reinsertion and performance enhancement in high-exigency education modalities, with personalized treatment strategies (which are characteristic of the types of education expected in these social classes).

The controversy regarding ADHD in Argentina derives from the problems created by the reintroduction of methylphenidate in the market in the 1990s (its withdrawal during the 1970s will be expanded on in a later section) and the increase in ADHD diagnoses given the extension of the use of the *DSM* and its broader categories. These problems were presented by teachers and parents in a series of congresses, conferences, and symposiums intended for health professionals. They were also expressed in several books (Joselevich offered a compilation in 2003, re-edited in 2005; and Janin wrote another one in 2004, re-edited in 2007) and in specialized journals such as *Terremotos y Soñadores* (*Earthquakes and Dreamers*), which began to be published in 2000.

A wide variety of Argentine authors have deepened the analysis of the problematics of ADHD. They have created dense academic works from various perspectives, including psychoanalysis clinical theories (Untoiglich 2011: 10), neoliberal politics in mental health (Barcala 2011: 220), and teaching conceptions (Dueñas 2011a: 145). Various books have also been published from the perspective of health and mental health. Moyano Walker (2004), Stiglitz (2006), Benasayag (2007), Janin (2007), Dueñas (2011b), Joselevich (2005), and Benasayag and Dueñas (2011) compiled health professional works from backgrounds such as medicine (pediatrics, neurology, and psychiatry), educational psychopedagogy, psychology, psychoanalysis, and journalism. However, in Argentina few studies approach ADHD from the perspective of the social sciences.

Argentina: An Emblematic Case

We now consider ADHD as a representative case for the debates on medicalization and biomedicalization—particularly in the use of psychopharmaceutical agents for the treatment of children. We offer some results of our investigation that map out the actual situation in Argentina.

When It Comes to Diagnosis: Actors and Struggles

Key historical moments mark peak levels of ADHD diagnosis in Argentina, and it is possible to systematize them. Initially, there was a marked growth and consolidation of the disease in the 1990s, with two significant events. First, a series of political, economic, social, and cultural transformations in Argentina (Barcala 2010: 70) translated into the implementation of a government program with a neoliberal bias. In addition, the fourth edition of the *DSM* (APA 1994) was published in the United States, and there was consequent global penetration of its use. In it, ADHD is typified for the first time. From 2001 on, in parallel with the deep social and political crisis in Argentina, there was a verifiable increase in psychopharmaceutical sales (Lakoff 2004: 248) (this will be described in detail later in the chapter). Various interviews show how groups and institutions, with their corresponding written publications and meetings (both scientific and professional), began to think about the problematic effects that psychopharmaceuticals have on children.

During interviews in the course of our fieldwork, we documented a variety of positions related to the existence and status of ADHD diagnosis and treatment (Arizaga and Faraone 2008: 177). Most of the professionals we interviewed (especially pediatricians and neurologists belonging to health services) expressed their agreement on the existence of the clinical features or psychiatric classification of ADHD. However, they admitted a significant diagnostic imprecision and certain confusion due to diagnostic masking (resulting from other pathologies or problematic situations, such as social or family issues such as violence or abuse) (Bianchi 2012: 1034). They also noted high comorbidity (allowing for the observation of simultaneous pathologies such as child psychosis, Asperger's syndrome, or other disorders, while ADHD appears as a main diagnosis) (Bianchi 2012: 1034).

Moreover, these professionals asserted that ADHD is an old-fashioned diagnosis, based on outdated classifications in older versions of the *DSM* or old denominations such as "minimal cerebral dysfunction" (Strother 1973: 6), and they insisted that the changes in its iterations throughout the years were only at the denomination level, while its essence was maintained. This perspective focuses on the recognition of ADHD as a real disorder and one that is widely recognized as such (Mayes, Bagwell, and Erkulwater 2008: 157).

However, in Argentina, and linked to the field of psychoanalysis, ADHD has aroused criticism and refutations of a varied nature, practically from the time of its configuration in the *DSM-III-R* (APA 1987) as a behavioral disorder in childhood. Apart from the creation of a critical battlefront on the existence of ADHD, the most resounding polemic involves the very existence of the diagnosis as a clinical entity. These perspectives, mainly ascribed by the educational community, emphasize the subjectivity involved in treating each child with her unique symptoms or personality characteristics. Certain ideals of the era are critically questioned (i.e., "performance," "success," and "consumption") as the main conditions of the production of subjectivity in the care of children and their families. In our interviews with teachers, this problem was illustrated as the case in point of a student who had lunch in the middle of a class because he had to attend meetings with so many professionals (psychopedagogists, neurologists, and psychologists) that he was completely overwhelmed by the whole situation and no longer cared about anything (fieldwork interview with a group of teachers from a private school of high exigency in the northern area of Greater Buenos Aires, socioeconomic status [SES] middle to high, from Arizaga and Faraone 2008: 130).

Approaches and Treatments: A Troubled Journey

An emerging result from the interviews is the differentiation of diagnoses, depending on which health subsector the professionals work in. Mental health professionals who specialize in children and work in the state public subsector often receive referrals to take care of more complex cases than those with ADHD. These professionals postulated that certain lower socioeconomic populations were being underdiagnosed, and they associated this underdiagnosis with the presence of other social and cultural problems in childhood and adolescence. In more vulnerable and marginalized sectors, both inattention and hyperactivity in children are often referred to as "behavioral problems" or as a "characteristic of the child's personality." From the interviews with teachers, we verified that "there are no expectations or learning possibilities attributed to these children, except that they do not disturb the classroom, and pass the primary school subject examinations" (Arizaga and Faraone 2008: 268).

As these professionals pointed out, most children diagnosed with ADHD are cared for by health care providers belonging to the social security subsector or the private subsector (through prepaid plans). According to data from the Instituto Nacional de Estadísticas y Censos (INDEC), in Argentina only 7% of the population has prepaid medical insurance, 45% of the population receives health care services through their social security coverage, and 48% of the population has coverage from the state public sector (INDEC 2013).

A possible interpretation is to associate diagnoses with the various social classes at the different stratification levels of the health care system, according to social status and the expectations of the population who have access to it. However, another important indicator of the process in Argentina is the differentiation in discounts on prescribed medication and benefits according to the health care subsector the patient belongs to. The drug kit distributed by the Argentine state to public health care providers through the program called REMEDIAR (i.e., the public subsector in which health care is accessible free of charge) does not include methylphenidate. However, it does include drugs of a varied nature in keeping with its aim of "contributing to prevent the worsening of health conditions of the poorest families in the country, guaranteeing timely access to adequate treatment and medicines for at least 90% of their 'prevalent pathologies'" (AGN 2011). This makes access difficult for persons in these sectors who are generally of low or middle-low socioeconomic levels. Under the *obras sociales*, 40% of the cost of methylphenidate is covered, whereas some provincial medical insurance policies such as those in Tierra del Fuego, one of the jurisdictions selected in this research given its high sales margin, cover up to 70%.

So, the progression of the problem in Argentina is particular for its focus mainly on children who are not characterized by social vulnerability or social exclusion, or by deprivation of rights or health care access. Instead, these children are described by health professionals as being from educated middle- and upper-class families who regularly go to consultations with health professionals. The extension of medicalization and biomedicalization to this population illustrates the multiplicity of forms of social control for childhood sectors that were not reached by other earlier historical mechanisms. This multiplicity is focused on what Donzelot defined as the "tutelary complex" (Donzelot 1998: 99) and what Rose termed "technologies of government" (Rose 1999: 131) that are aimed at working-class families and children by means of moralizing, coercive, and persuasive mechanisms (Rose 1999: 132).

Nevertheless, health care systems and medication coverage have been and remain central to the debates concerning ADHD in Argentina. On the one hand, existing movements led by patients and families, some specialists, and even the pharmaceutical industry strive to have medical social security cover 100% of methylphenidate costs—as is the case for children who receive state coverage. One strategy to achieve this end is to have ADHD included as a disability (Superintendencia de Servicios de Salud 2015). On the other hand, other social actors, among them multidisciplinary professional associations, confront this situation by establishing a strong polemic against the prescription of psychiatric medication for children. Thus, a diverse range of positions supports both the appropriateness of psychopharmacological therapy and its inadequacy.

One of the results of our investigation relates to the polemics concerning the psychoactive medication used in ADHD treatment. In one of the provinces studied (included in the core section of low methylphenidate sales), cases of neuroleptics and antidepressant prescriptions were documented for the treatment of ADHD. For instance, in the provinces of Tierra del Fuego and Corrientes, besides methylphenidate, the use of anxiolytics such as clonazepam (the most common brand of which is Rivotril) or neuroleptics (such as risperidone in Dropicine or Risperin) was documented. These drugs are intended to reduce or control anxiety levels, and doctors remarked that some antidepressants are used for the same purpose since all types of psychoactive drugs of this kind are used "for everything" (as a pediatrician said). Only one of the key informants interviewed referred to the lack of rigorous longitudinal scientific studies involving children in relation to these psychopharmaceuticals.

Pharmacological Therapy for ADHD

As already mentioned, our analysis of the interviews during fieldwork reveals a trend in the increase in ADHD diagnoses in Argentina in recent decades. In addition, our review of statistical documents reveals an increase in the dispensation of methamphetamines as a response to the symptomatic framework of ADHD.

Nosological categories and psychopharmaceutical therapy today appear to be joint aspects that should be considered together. In some specific cases, both dimensions are articulated in different ways. Several authors worked on various aspects of the relationship between the diagnosis of depression and the use of antidepressant medication—depression constituted an example of reformulated nosology through psychopharmaceutical advances. Similarly, Ehrenberg pointed out that biological psychiatry is not so strict with respect to the correlation between biochemical alterations in the nervous system resulting from antidepressants and their therapeutic effects, and therefore the biochemical heterogeneity of forms of depression is not constrained within all antidepressant medication options (Ehrenberg 2000: 177). Caponi emphasized that antidepressants have a preponderant position in the rationale behind the characterization of the depression diagnosis (Caponi 2009: 334). Finally, Shorter remarked that systems for classifying diseases do not tell us which patients will respond to which drugs (Shorter 2009: 5). In the case of ADHD, the link between psychopharmaceuticals and nosology is different. Even when new psychopharmaceutical agents such as atomoxetine (which entered Argentina in 2004) were incorporated, changes in nosological criteria were not primarily led by the introduction of these new drugs.

In our fieldwork analysis, methylphenidate emerged as the first drug of choice in the treatment of ADHD, and methylphenidate is the drug with the highest sales in Argentina for the treatment of this condition (fig. 9.1). The ratio of national sales between methylphenidate and atomoxetine is 3.5 to 1, as figure 9.2 illustrates.

Therefore, in the case of ADHD, it is possible to assert that methylphenidate itself has undergone a process of modifications in terms of forms of administration (ER, or extended release; MR, or modified release; OROS, or osmotic release oral system; SODA, or spheroidal oral drug absorption system; and the transdermal patch, among others) by virtue of its association with nosology. This emphasizes the fact that the depression model, despite being frequently chosen by researchers, does not bear out the explanatory possibilities of medicalization processes in the twenty-first century. Although other drugs such as atomoxetine have been used, research on them is not as significant as it is for new antidepressant drugs, and nosological criteria are not driven by the introduction of

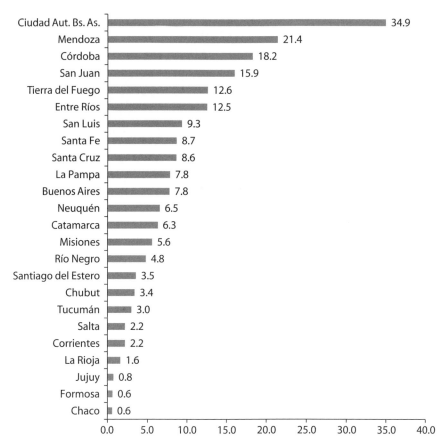

Fig. 9.1. Dispensed units of methylphenidate per 1,000 children aged 5–19, by province, 2006. *Source*: COFA

new drugs. In this way, the association with nosology has been sustained and continuous—predominantly by the administration of the same psychopharmaceutical, methylphenidate—and what changed throughout time was its form of administration, in order to adjust the intake to the requirements of the child's daily life.

Methylphenidate Behavior

Not many statistics on the prescription and consumption of psychostimulants have been published in Argentina. However, as our fieldwork interviews revealed, different professionals, medical associations, and journal articles have referred to the continuous increase of methylphenidate sales.

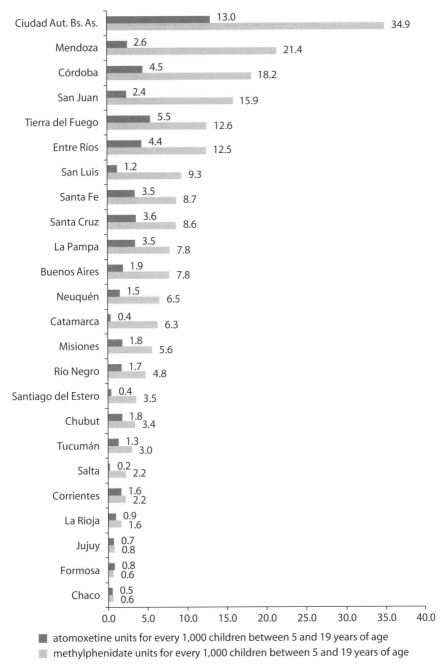

Province	atomoxetine	methylphenidate
Ciudad Aut. Bs. As.	13.0	34.9
Mendoza	2.6	21.4
Córdoba	4.5	18.2
San Juan	2.4	15.9
Tierra del Fuego	5.5	12.6
Entre Ríos	4.4	12.5
San Luis	1.2	9.3
Santa Fe	3.5	8.7
Santa Cruz	3.6	8.6
La Pampa	3.5	7.8
Buenos Aires	1.9	7.8
Neuquén	1.5	6.5
Catamarca	0.4	6.3
Misiones	1.8	5.6
Río Negro	1.7	4.8
Santiago del Estero	0.4	3.5
Chubut	1.8	3.4
Tucumán	1.3	3.0
Salta	0.2	2.2
Corrientes	1.6	2.2
La Rioja	0.9	1.6
Jujuy	0.7	0.8
Formosa	0.8	0.6
Chaco	0.5	0.6

■ atomoxetine units for every 1,000 children between 5 and 19 years of age
▨ methylphenidate units for every 1,000 children between 5 and 19 years of age

Fig. 9.2. Dispensed units of methylphenidate and atomoxetine per 1,000 children aged 5–19, by province, 2006. Source: COFA

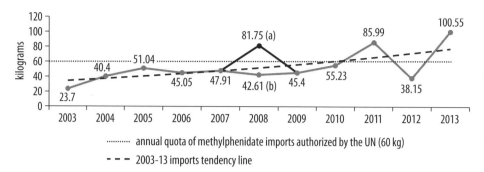

Fig. 9.3. Methylphenidate annual imports in Argentina (kg). *Sources:* Carbajal 2007; Arizaga and Faraone 2008; Maniowicz 2011; pers. comm. with ANMAT, 2014

Information provided by the Argentine Administración Nacional de Medicamentos, Alimentos y Tecnología Médica (ANMAT), from the Departamento de Psicotrópicos y Estupefacientes, identifies 2004 as the year in which the quantity of active ingredients imported into the country began its escalation from 23.7 kilograms in the previous period to 40.4 kilograms, in an upward trend that has been consolidated ever since (as figure 9.3 illustrates). The Departamento de Psicotrópicos y Estupefacientes does not have records about atomoxetine (which is classified as an antidepressant) because the drug is not included in its psychotropic lists. Atomoxetine is commercialized and sold in Argentina by 2 laboratories in 10 formulations and 5 different concentrations.

As can be deduced from the previous analysis, the prescription and consumption of methylphenidate is a crucial element in the current configuration of ADHD in Argentina. This psychostimulant had not been marketed in the country for several decades when its use became popular among university students in the 1970s. It was commercialized as metamphetamine racemate and was used to optimize academic performance. Due to the death of some women who were using it in order to lose weight, the Sociedad Argentina de Cardiología warned against its effects in the adult population and it was withdrawn from the pharmacological market all across the country. Later, as we pointed out, it was reintroduced for sale in the 1990s, this time as methylphenidate and in response to a demand from parents and physicians (see Carbajal 2007: 238, though the author does not specify from which interest groups this demand came) who were interested in accessing the drug without having to manage purchases from the United States. At present, sales require the submission of an official prescription issued by the Ministerio de Salud, and physicians must have acquired this prescription form previously with the subsequent authorization of the Ministerio de Salud. Prescriptions are handled in triplicate and under a filing procedure by ANMAT. Since reintroduction of the drug in the 1990s, methylphenidate has been exclusively prescribed for the treatment of ADHD, and the trend of the annual importation quota for its commercialization is markedly upward (as fig. 9.3 illustrates). This tendency is consistent with the global trend, as expressed by the International Narcotics Control Board (INCB) in its 1995 and 2006 reports.

The reintroduction of the drug can be seen as the expression of the establishment of a new relationship among parents, professionals of diverse specialties, and pharmaceutical laboratories, centered around the acquisition of a fundamental supply of certain therapeutics. The reintroduction of methylphenidate in Argentina (with the exclusive prescription for ADHD treatment) opens the possibility of the emergence and proliferation of a diagnosis that includes the use of this drug as the first-choice treatment. This reintroduction also gave way to "possibility conditions" (in the Foucauldian sense) involving a whole series of discourses and practices in specific child health field sectors and pressure groups that offered—and still offer today—strong resistance, formulating and proposing diagnostic and therapeutic modalities that are not centered on the drug. Presently, methylphenidate is produced in Argentina by 5 laboratories in 17 formulations and 8 different concentrations, and it is distributed in fast-acting and extended-release forms.

Despite the limitations and difficulties related to obtaining data on methylphenidate, we reconstructed the series of its importation for the years 2003–13 from various sources that ANMAT uses as data providers. The 2003–4 series was taken from Carbajal (2007: 239); for the 2005–8 series, we used Arizaga and Faraone's research (2008: 81); for the 2008–10 period, we obtained data from Maniowicz (2011); and for the 2011–13 period, we requested data directly from ANMAT.

Figure 9.3 records discrepancies in the values in 2008: Arizaga and Faraone referred to values over 80 kilograms (81.75, see [a]), and Maniowicz referred to a lower value (42.61, see [b]). These differences are significant because the quota that Argentina agreed to with the United Nations is established at 60 kilograms/year. However, as a tendency, all sources appear to indicate a sustained increase in the importation of methylphenidate.

In this polemic scenario of strong public debates around the consumption of psychotropic medication, an important milestone was the publishing, in 2005, of the "Consenso de expertos del área de la salud sobre el llamado Trastorno por Déficit de Atención con o sin Hiperactividad" ("Health Area Experts Consensus on Attention Deficit Disorder with or without Hyperactivity"), a statement signed by approximately 200 renowned professionals of various specialties on the issue (it has more than 1,100 signatures). It was addressed to the Argentine Ministerio de Salud and submitted to it through the executive power, including a formal information request on ADHD diagnosis. The document criticized the spread of the ADHD diagnosis and the psychopharmaceutical prescription for its treatment, and it highlighted some side effects of methylphenidate. It also proposed that only expert professionals in the field assess children, that medication be a last resort only, that the child's family and social context be taken into account, and that the broadcasting of information about ADHD in the mass media be restricted, given the controversies among professionals on the very existence of the symptomatic frame (Forum Infancias 2015). The document was reviewed by Congreso Nacional, the Argentine Cámara de Diputados Nacional in 2006, and the Comisión de Acción Social y Salud Pública, de Educación y de Familia, Mujer, Niñez y Adolescencia. Moreover, in 2007, ANMAT ordered the laboratories that sell both of the main psychopharmaceuticals used in ADHD treatment (methylphenidate and atomoxetine) to improve their package leaflets so that they included warnings, precautions, and associated contraindications (ANMAT 2007).

Strategies of the Pharmaceutical Industry and the Biomedical Technologies

As already pointed out, the pharmaceutical industry has a central role in the medicalization and biomedicalization of childhood processes. Conrad (2007: 133), Moynihan and Cassels (2007: 19), Cabral Barros (2008: 580), and Iriart (2008: 1623) note that the pharmaceutical industry and biotechnology are the main actors in the new configuration, in which psychoactive medication is integrated as a fundamental piece in the institutionalization of pharmacologization in the first years of a child's life. Conrad analyzes the global picture in his 2004 study: consumers become the target for market expansion, with physicians largely remaining as gatekeepers prescribing treatment. In private medical markets, due to limits in types of permitted promotion (e.g., for off-label uses), corporations offer promotions indirectly to providers or consumers (e.g., on the Internet). Thus, consumers are the prime driver for demand—generally without insurance support—and must pay directly for medical products or services. Then, physicians are necessary facilitators for treatment and sometimes promoters (i.e., entrepreneurs) of the product (e.g., cosmetic surgery) as well.

Contributing to this scenario, the pharmaceutical industry has occupied new niches as it puts forward other ways of advertising to the general public, such as indirect promotion to providers via off-label use or to consumers on the Internet (Conrad and Leiter 2004: 168). This global trend, which is no stranger to Argentina, has erupted in recent decades as a radical transformation from the concept of health users to the idea of health consumers. Broadly speaking, this notion can be analyzed through Michel Foucault's considerations on the spread of the *homo œconomicus* model, typical of American neoliberalism, into all forms of behavior. In Foucault's words, *homo œconomicus* is "someone who is eminently governable" (Foucault 2004: 270). The adoption of this model results in the concealment of the social dimension of these processes because it turns claims and demands on health rights into health services acquisition issues and places access to medication and treatment in the place of a free choice (Conrad and Leiter 2004: 169).

In our analysis of pharmaceutical industry sale strategies in Argentina, we observed a mixture of a physician-oriented marketing model (in which the physician is the main target) and a direct-to-consumer–oriented one (family and school included). In the analysis of the former, especially within the medical field, our research revealed a close monitoring by the pharmaceutical industry of what and when doctors prescribe, through important marketing companies (Jara 2007: 197) and the growing use of sales representatives. In the analysis of the latter, an essential component is the uneven relation between pharmaceutical companies and family and patient associations.

With regard to the physician-oriented marketing model, in Argentina the main market research companies are International Market Survey and Close Up. For the latter, Lakoff (2004: 258) has analyzed how data are registered per doctor, product, and prescribed quantity according to the copies of microfilmed prescriptions obtained from big pharmaceutical brands in the city of Buenos Aires. Within this model, pundits play another important role in pharmaceutical marketing strategies: pharmaceutical sales representatives detect and value physicians according to their role within their specialty, and those physicians are then promoted as part of the "expert" category. As experts, they spread their latest findings on diseases and possible pharmaceutical therapies in journals, scientific sessions of all kinds (lectures, meetings, conferences, etc.), and guidelines for consent based on evidence. These experts generally belong to prestigious private institutions in the city of Buenos Aires and elsewhere in the country.

With regard to the consumer-oriented marketing model (and in a parallel fashion), some family and patient associations have gradually gained stature as new relevant actors. In the case of ADHD, one of the most important associations in the United States is Children and Adults with Attention Deficit/Hyperactivity Disorder (CHADD). Conrad (2007: 139) and Moynihan and Cassels (2007: 73) agree that these groups, whose speakers support pharmaceutical research and treatment, are in some cases funded by pharmaceutical companies. As Conrad and Bergey (2014: 36) pointed out, the pharmaceutical industry is expanding its marketing strategies to nonmedical professions. These authors have found these groups mainly in the educational field and named them "sickness and treatment brokers" or "disease spotters": they constitute a main element in the circuit of referrals and treatment for ADHD since teachers contribute to its diagnostic evaluation by filling out forms and the like.

In Argentina, the alliance between industry and parents and patients is still in an emerging phase and lacks the development acquired in the United States and some European countries. Our fieldwork in Argentina revealed the existence of collaboration among teachers and educational psychologists in the diagnosis and early detection of ADHD (Faraone et al. 2010: 494). This takes shape in two different ways. First, pharmaceutical sales representatives—with or through medical specialists—go to schools or carry out informational talks in educational psychology offices (these encounters are referred to as *mesas de ayuda* [help desks]). The second involves teacher-oriented information in the form of handbooks, manuals, and briefs that include statistical data, general advice for profile detection, and detailed information on psychopharmaceuticals.

These modalities (both help desks and the use of these publications) are not allowed in Argentina because, as already mentioned, they constitute a violation of the Ley Nacional de Salud Mental passed in 2010 (INFOLEG 2010). Apart from this, according to national legislation on control of technical and economic norms on medicines through Ley 16.463 of 1964, all forms of publicity on prescribed medicines are forbidden in Argentina (INFOLEG 1964). We were able to document some other modalities of pharmaceutical publicity and marketing aimed at the education community in Argentina, including the distribution of merchandising in the form of school stationery at Buenos Aires institutions (in both the city and the province) with logos, images, and slogans of both the laboratory and the specific drugs. We also found the dissemination of academic articles on ADHD in specialized magazines for teachers and psychopedagogists.

In conclusion, both marketing models can be observed in Argentina: the physician-oriented model and the consumer-oriented model. Within the latter, four modalities can be found in relation to educational institutions: the use of help desks, the distribution of merchandising inside schools, the publishing of booklets on ADHD-related information addressed to teachers, and the dissemination of academic articles on ADHD in specialized magazines for teachers and psychopedagogists.

Mental Health Law and Classification Manuals

As mentioned before, the process of the nosological redefinition of ADHD is central in Argentina, especially since the global spread of the use of the *DSM-III* (APA 1980) because it reveals an increase in the diagnosis and psychopharmacological treatment of ADHD and suggests close relationships among classification manuals, diagnostic constructions, and the pharmaceutical industry (Bianchi 2012: 1029). It seems that the *DSM* has a core role in the problematics of ADHD in Argentina. References to other manuals were marginal in our interviews. For example, the *ICD-10*, which is published by the World Health Organization (WHO), was seldom mentioned even though it was obligatory for diagnosis and statistics on public health in the country. Mentions of the *Classification française de troubles mentaux de l'enfant et de l'adolescent* (CFTMEA) were even rarer.

The repetition of definitions, references, and allusions to the *DSM* as the almost exclusive source of conceptualization for ADHD during our fieldwork interviews shows the preeminence of this manual over other available references (Stagnaro 2006: 339). This manual is referred to as the primary instrument for practice or as the basis of a theoretical framework. However, it is not exempt from tensions since it has become the source of doubts, debates, and questions. These polemic expressions link to the concept of a mental disorder that has defenders and detractors and the questioning about whether it is a valid concept with which to approach childhood problems.

In the case of ADHD in Argentina, the criticisms of the *DSM* are also currently related to the Ley Nacional de Salud Mental. In its first article, the aim of this law is defined as "the enjoyment of human rights of those people with mental suffering" (INFOLEG 2010). This definition often leads to intense debates in legislative chambers because the concept of "mental suffering" displaces, on the one hand, the concept of a "mental disorder" and, on the other hand, medical-pharmaceutical hegemony. In relation to this concept, the law emphatically expresses the need for an interdisciplinary approach to populations with "mental suffering" and reserves the use of drugs exclusively for therapeutic ends, never as a punishment or for the benefit of a third party. These two assertions are deliberate; they explicitly depict the permanent struggle among the professional sectors involved in the field of mental health. In the case of ADHD, the law strengthens groups that, as we have pointed out, are positioned against the pathologization of childhood.

Conclusion

In Argentina, the pharmacologization of childhood that derives from the use of methylphenidate for ADHD treatment has caused and still causes many controversies. The panorama that is outlined is extremely complex and involves multiple actors (from fields such as health, education, economics, and politics) and their related frameworks. This panorama also presupposes the deployment of legislation, norms, classifications, and technologies, with no unitary or lateral effects to the process. ADHD appears as the meeting point for all these fields and actors. It is an arena in which they intersect, and far from developing it in harmony, they fill it with tensions and debates. At the same time, it is an arena in which strong articulations take place.

Although the *DSM-5* (APA 2013) was published in Spanish in 2014, even before its publication we have documented various scientific meetings, conferences, and gatherings of a different nature offered to professionals in Argentina in order to guarantee that the manual will prevail. In light of the actors involved in the problem, we do not dismiss the fact that the emergence of the *DSM-5* will reignite the conflicts with associations that have already established deep disagreement with the manual.

Another aspect worth mentioning is the distinctive configuration of ADHD's problematics in Argentina. Three matters emerge as relevant. First, there is the focus on rights (in the Ley Nacional de Salud Mental, with its human rights perspective, and the UN Convention on the Rights of the Child, which Argentina ratified and links to its legislation in general and the law mentioned in particular) and the stance taken by some professionals who contest the validity of a pharmaceutical-centered treatment of ADHD and the pathologization of childhood. Second, actions from diverse psychoanalytic-related therapeutical-clinical perspectives and from different professional associations tend to halt the advances of the pharmaceutical industry and of the classification of the *DSM*. Third, there is the target of diagnosis and treatment for ADHD: children of middle-class families. In this sense, the high costs of methylphenidate and its exclusion from health care coverage end up constituting an obstacle to a bigger expansion. However, within the middle-class sectors, certain familial and pedagogical expectations are reconfigured as health services for consumers' demands and are accompanied by personalized treatments.

Yet another aspect of legislative matters is the verification of active normatives that can be a frame for controlling the expansion of the sales of psychopharmaceuticals for use in children. By and large, as Conrad and Bergey describe (2014: 36), countries that impose strong legal constraints on the use of stimulants represent an obstacle for the penetration of pharmaceutical companies' marketing strategies; conversely, countries that impose laxer constraints result in more accessible markets. This is the case in Argentir.a. Moreover, as we have described, it has coincided in recent years with the opening up of pharmacological industries' marketing strategies, which have directed their efforts toward consumers and familial organizations and toward educational communities. Even if these actions are forbidden by legislation proper, within their gaps specific actions consolidate therapeutic strategies in which the prescription of psychostimulants is a first choice for treatment.

NOTES

We would like to thank Isabel Ballesteros for her helpful analysis of the data and Andrés Faraone and Diana Rossi for their invaluable revision of the text in English. We are also particularly grateful to Natalia Barry, who was in charge of the revised version for the printed edition.

1. Local psychiatric associations, particularly the *Asociación de Psiquiatras Argentinos*, or APSA, vigorously resisted the Ley Nacional de Salud Mental. The law's first article guarantees full enjoyment of human rights for people with mental suffering. When the bill was proposed in Congress, this definition provoked intense debate for two reasons. First, the concept of "mental suffering" displaces the notion of "mental disorder" used by biological psychiatry. The eighth article of the law promotes the creation of interdisciplinary teams that should include psychologists, psychiatrists, social workers, nurses, occupational therapists, and professionals from other disciplines to care for patients. Second, the law confronts medical-pharmaceutical hegemony by stating that medications must only be prescribed for therapeutic purposes to people undergoing mental suffering; they should never replace therapeutic accompaniment or special care. Moreover, the 12th article of the law also establishes that psychopharmaceutical treatments must be used in the frame of interdisciplinary approaches. Finally, the UN Convention on the Rights of the Child and the local law based on it guarantee human health care rights to all children in Argentine territory. This questions the very nature of pathologization as a valid claim for treatment. Thus, on a regulatory level, this was another

element that helped some sectors resist the increase of the ADHD diagnosis and the rise in psychopharmaceutical use related to it. As will be seen in the analysis, from both exclusively medical perspectives and regulatory approaches, Argentina has traced a unique path regionally and worldwide.

REFERENCES

American Psychiatric Association (APA). 1980. *Diagnostic and Statistical Manual of Mental Disorders (DSM-III)*. 3rd ed. Washington, DC: American Psychiatric Association.

———. 1987. *Diagnostic and Statistical Manual of Mental Disorders (DSM-III-R)*. 3rd ed., revised. Washington, DC: American Psychiatric Association.

———. 1994. *Diagnostic and Statistical Manual of Mental Disorders (DSM-IV)*. 4th ed. Washington, DC: American Psychiatric Association.

———. 2013. *Diagnostic and Statistical Manual of Mental Disorders (DSM-5)*. 5th ed. Washington, DC: American Psychiatric Association.

Arizaga, M. Cecilia, and Silvia Faraone. 2008. "La medicalización de la infancia. Niños, escuela y psicotrópicos. Informe Final." Observatorio Argentino de Drogas. SEDRONAR. Instituto de Investigaciones Gino Germani, Facultad de Ciencias Sociales, Universidad de Buenos Aires. December. http://www.observatorio.gov.ar/media/k2/attachments /LaZMedicalizacinZdeZlaZInfancia.ZNiosZEscuelaZyZPsicotrpicos.ZA0Z2008 .-.pdf >

Auditoría General de la Nación (AGN). 2011. "Programa REMEDIAR. Ministerio de Salud de la Nación. Auditoría de Gestión." http://www.agn.gov.ar/files/informes/f_007 _11_04_02.pdf.

Barcala, Alejandra. 2010. "Estado, infancia y salud mental: Impacto de las legislaciones en las políticas y en las prácticas de los actores sociales estatales en la década del 90." PhD diss., Buenos Aires University.

———. 2011. "El impacto de las políticas neoliberales en el ámbito de la salud mental." In *Invención de enfermedades. Traiciones a la salud y a la educación*, edited by León Benasayag and Gabriela Dueñas, 219–32. Buenos Aires: Noveduc.

Benasayag, León, ed. 2007. *ADDH. Niños con déficit de atención e hiperactividad. ¿Una patología de mercado? Una mirada alternativa con enfoque multidisciplinario*. Buenos Aires: Noveduc.

Benasayag, León, and Gabriela Dueñas, eds. 2011. *Invención de enfermedades. Traiciones a la salud y a la educación*. Buenos Aires: Noveduc.

Bianchi, Eugenia. 2012. "Problematizando la noción de trastorno en el TDAH e influencia del manual DSM." *Revista Latinoamericana de Niñez y Juventud* 10: 1021–38.

Cabral Barros, J. Augusto. 2008. "Nuevas tendencias de la medicalización." *Ciência & Saúde Coletiva* 13: 579–87. http://www.redalyc.org/pdf/630/63009704.pdf.

Caponi, Sandra. 2009. "Un análisis epistemológico del diagnóstico de depresión." *Interface-Comunicação, Saúde, Educação* 13 (29): 327–38. http://www.scielo.br/pdf/icse /v13n29/v13n29a07.pdf.

Carbajal, Mariana. 2006. "La supuesta enfermedad del chico inquieto y las pildoritas mágicas." *Página 12*. *El país*, October 17. http://www.pagina12.com.ar/diario/elpais /subnotas/74605-24184-2006-10-17.html.

———. 2007. "ADD y ADHD, una mirada desde el periodismo." In *ADDH. Niños con déficit de atención e hiperactividad. ¿Una patología de mercado? Una mirada alternativa con enfoque multidisciplinario*, edited by León Benasayag, 237–44. Buenos Aires: Noveduc.

Clarke, Adele E., Janet K. Shim, Laura Mamo, Jennifer R. Fosket, and Jennifer Fishman. 2003. "Biomedicalization: Technoscientific Transformations of Health, Illness, and U.S. Biomedicine." *American Sociological Review* 68: 161–94. http://www.jstor.org /action/showPublisher?publisherCode=asa.

Confederación Farmacéutica Argentina (COFA). 2012. "Quiénes somos." http://www .cofa.org.ar/?p=29.

Conrad, Peter. 2013. "Medicalization: Changing Contours, Characteristics, and Contexts." In *Medical Sociology on the Move*, edited by William C. Cockerham, 195–214. Dordrecht: Springer.

———. 2007. *The Medicalization of Society: On the Transformation of Human Conditions into Treatable Disorders*. Baltimore: Johns Hopkins University Press.

———. 2005. "The Shifting Engines of Medicalization." *Journal of Health and Social Behavior* 46 (1): 3–14.

Conrad, Peter, and Meredith Bergey. 2014. "The Impending Globalization of ADHD: Notes on the Expansion and Growth of a Medicalized Disorder." *Social Science & Medicine* 122: 31–43.

Conrad, Peter, and Valerie Leiter. 2004. "Medicalization, Markets and Consumers." *Journal of Health and Social Behavior* 45: 158–76. http://hsb.sagepub.com/.

Convención sobre los derechos de niños. Argentina. 1990. "Ley No. 23 849." http://www .refworld.org/docid/4b0d3cee2.html.

Dagfal, Alejandro. 2009. *Entre París y Buenos Aires. La invención del psicólogo (1942–1966)*. Buenos Aires: Paidós.

Donzelot, Jacques. 1998. *La policía de las familias*. Valencia: Pre-textos.

Dueñas, Gabriela. 2011a. "Cuestionando prácticas desubjetivantes en salud y educación." In *Invención de enfermedades. Traiciones a la salud y a la educación*, edited by León Benasayag and Gabriela Dueñas, 145–66. Buenos Aires: Noveduc.

———. 2011b. *La patologización de la infancia. ¿Niños o síndromes?* Buenos Aires: Noveduc.

Ehrenberg, Alain. 2000. *La fatiga de ser uno mismo: Depresión y sociedad*. Buenos Aires: Nueva Visión.

Faraone, Silvia, Alejandra Barcala, Flavia Torricelli, Eugenia Bianchi, and Cecilia Tamburrino. 2010. "Discurso médico y estrategias de marketing de la industria farmacéutica en los procesos de medicación de la infancia en Argentina." *Interface-Comunicação, Saúde, Educação* 34: 485–97. http://www.redalyc.org/articulo.oa?id=180115835020.

Forum Infancias. 2015. "Consenso de expertos del área de la salud sobre el llamado 'Trastorno por Déficit de Atención con o sin Hiperactividad.'" Comité Ejecutivo. http://foruminfancias.com.ar/consenso/.

Foucault, Michel. 2004. *The Birth of Biopolitics*. London: Palgrave Macmillan.

Información Legislativa (INFOLEG). 1964. "Ley de Medicamentos. Importación y Exportación." Ley 16.463. Información Legislativa, Centro de Documentación e Información. Ministerio de Economía y Finanzas Públicas. http://www.infoleg.gob.ar /infolegInternet/anexos/20000-24999/20414/norma.htm.

———. 2010. "Ley Nacional de Salud Mental." Salud Pública, Ley 26.657. Información Legislativa, Centro de Documentación e Información. Ministerio de Economía y Finanzas Públicas. http://www.infoleg.gob.ar/infolegInternet/anexos/175000-179999 /175977/norma.htm.

Instituto Nacional de Estadísticas y Censos (INDEC). 2013. Censo 2010. "Resultados definitivos." http://www.censo2010.indec.gov.ar/index_cuadros_2.asp.

Iriart, Celia. 2008. "Capital financiero versus complejo médico-industrial: los desafíos de las agencias regulatórias." *Ciência & Saúde Coletiva* 13 (5): 1619–26. http://www .redalyc.org/articulo.oa?id=180125203020.

Iriart, Celia, Silvia Faraone, and Hugo Waitzkin. 2000. "Atención Gerenciada: La reforma silenciosa." *Nueva época. Salud Problema* 5 (9): 47–75.

Janin, Beatriz. 2007. *Niños desatentos e hiperactivos. ADD/ADHD. Reflexiones críticas acerca del trastorno por déficit de atención con o sin hiperactividad.* Buenos Aires: Noveduc.

Jara, Miguel. 2007. *Traficantes de salud: Cómo nos venden medicamentos peligrosos y juegan con la enfermedad.* Barcelona: Icaria-Antrazyt.

Joselevich, Estrella. 2005. *AD/HD. Qué es, qué hacer. Recomendaciones para padres y docentes.* Buenos Aires: Paidós.

Lakoff, Andrew. 2004. "The Anxieties of Globalization: Antidepressant Sales and Economic Crisis in Argentina." *Social Studies of Science* 34 (2): 247–69.

Maniowicz, Deborah. 2011. "Malos diagnósticos y sobremedicación." *Revista Veintitrés*, June 26. http://veintitres.elargentino.com/nota-2927-portada-titulo.html.

Mayes, Rick, Catherine Bagwell, and Jennifer Erkulwater. 2008. "ADHD and the Rise in Stimulant Use Among Children." *Harvard Review of Psychiatry* 16 (3): 151–66.

Miguez, María N. 2010. *La sujeción de los cuerpos dóciles: Medicación abusiva con psicofármacos en la niñez uruguaya.* Buenos Aires: Estudios Sociológicos Editora.

Moyano Walker, José M. 2004. *ADHD ¿Enfermos o singulares? Una mirada diferente sobre el síndrome de hiperactividad y déficit de atención.* Buenos Aires: Lumen.

Moynihan, Ray, and Alan Cassels. 2007. *Medicamentos que nos enferman e industrias farmacéuticas que nos convierten en pacientes.* Barcelona: Terapias Verdes.

Rabinow, Paul. 1988. "Polemics, Politics, and Problematizations: An Interview with Michel Foucault." In *The Essential Works of Foucault 1954–1988*, vol. 1, *Ethics, Subjectivity and Truth*, edited by Paul Rabinow, 111–19. New York: The New Press.

Rose, Nikolas. 1999. *Governing the Soul: The Shaping of the Private Self.* London: Free Association Books.

Shorter, Edward. 2009. *Before Prozac: The Troubled History of Mood Disorders in Psychiatry.* Oxford: Oxford University Press.

Stagnaro, Juan C. 2006. "Los nombres de la locura: Nosografías psiquiátricas contemporáneas." *Vertex Revista Argentina de Psiquiatría* 17 (69): 337–39. http://www.editorial polemos.com.ar/docs/vertex/vertex69.pdf.

Stiglitz, Gustavo. 2006. *DDA, ADD, ADHD, como ustedes quieran: El mal real y la construcción social.* Buenos Aires: Grama.

Strother, Charles R. 1973. "Minimal Cerebral Dysfunction: A Historical Overview." *Annals of the New York Academy of Sciences* 1 (205): 6–17.

Superintendencia de Servicios de Salud. 2015. "Buscador de genéricos con cobertura del 70%." *Consultas. Buscador de genéricos.* http://www.sssalud.gov.ar/index/index.php ?cat=consultas&opc=busgene.

Untoiglich, Gisela. 2011. *Versiones actuales del sufrimiento infantil: Una investigación psicoanalítica acerca de la desatención y la hiperactividad.* Buenos Aires: Noveduc.

Visacovsky, Sergio E. 2001. *El Lanús: Memoria, política y psicoanálisis en la Argentina (1956–1992).* Buenos Aires: Alianza.

10

Academic and Professional Tensions and Debates around ADHD in Brazil

Francisco Ortega
Rafaela Zorzanelli
Valéria Portugal Gonçalves

The diagnosis of attention deficit–hyperactivity disorder (ADHD) was shrouded in controversy before the current term was defined in the fourth edition of the *Diagnostic and Statistical Manual of Mental Disorders (DSM-IV)* of the American Psychiatric Association (APA) (APA 1994). The classification of ADHD by the APA raised doubts in professional and academic communities about whether it constituted a real disease or simply emerged as a social construct in response to a supposed demand for the medicalization of child and adolescent behaviors. In the absence of clear boundaries for the pathology, the main claim put forward by those who argue that such a condition does not exist is that its main symptoms (attention deficit, hyperactivity, and impulsivity) fall within the range of behaviors expected in childhood and adolescence.

In Brazil, only physicians can diagnose ADHD and provide pharmacotherapy for it. Pharmacological treatments are frequently combined with psychosocial treatments such as behavioral therapy and lifestyle changes, which are facilitated mostly by psychologists, teachers and other educational professionals, and parents. Still, it is difficult to ascertain whether and when both types of interventions are being provided in each particular case. ADHD is diagnosed in Brazil on the basis of the *ICD-10* (WHO 2008), which is the main disease classification system in use in the country. The *DSM* is used only for research purposes.

After decades of debate, the issues have been hotly contested and several documents have been published defending various positions; the controversy, however, remains. In Brazil, the debate is polarized around movements that reject the legitimacy of research into the diagnosis of ADHD and its psychopharmacological treatment, and those that support the description and classification of ADHD based on the countless scientific studies published on the topic (Fórum 2011; Mattos, Rohde, and Polanczyk 2012; ABP 2014; ABRASME 2014).

In this chapter, we provide an overview of the various discourses that circulate in Brazil about ADHD. First, we present the findings of the main research groups involved in both investigating the prevalence of ADHD and in making psychological tests for its diagnosis—either cultural adaptations of existing tests or new versions. Next, we introduce data from the Brazilian sanitation regulatory agency Agência Nacional de Vigilância Sanitária (ANVISA) about the control of methylphenidate prescription and the construction of a medical discourse about ADHD in the country. ANVISA is responsible for monitoring drug prices and medical devices, for inspecting tobacco products, and for controlling technical support in the granting of patents by the Instituto Nacional de Propriedade Industrial (INPI). It also exercises control over the production and marketing of products and services that are subject to sanitary surveillance, and it controls ports, airports, and borders. It is linked to both the Brazilian Ministério de Saúde and the Brazilian Ministério de Relações Exteriores. Finally, we present some controversies and opposing discourses about ADHD from Brazil's professional and academic fields, the stances taken by the movements involved in the debate about ADHD's medicalization, and the competing discourses about ADHD in the country.

Epidemiological Data on ADHD in Brazil

The literature on ADHD reports a wide range of prevalence estimates for the disorder. For example, the prevalence in Colombia is estimated to be 20.4% (Pineda et al. 1999; Cornejo et al. 2005); in Spain it is 3.1% to 6.8% (Pino and Mojarro-Praxedes 2001; Catalá-López et al. 2012); in the United Kingdom it is 2% to 5% (Polanczyk et al. 2007; Polanczyk and Jensen 2008); and various studies in Australia indicate a range from 2.4% to 9.9% (Gomez et al. 1999).

Various epidemiological studies in Brazil have found a 3.6% to 5% prevalence of ADHD among school-age children (Barbosa and Gouveia 1993). With the use of *DSM-IV* criteria, one study found a prevalence of 5.8% in a sample of teenagers (Rohde, Biederman, and Busnello 1999). Another study, which evaluated students at four public schools in southeastern Brazil, found a prevalence of 13% (Fontana et al. 2007); yet in the same region of the country, a different study found a prevalence of 17.1% (Vasconcelos et al. 2003). Internationally, it has been noted that studies that use the *DSM-IV* tend to find a higher prevalence than those that use previous versions of the manual (Baumgaertel, Wolraich, and Deitrich 1995).

According to Freire and Pondé (2005), one of the reasons for the discrepancies between the results is that the *DSM-IV* focuses on the symptoms observed, while disregarding criteria such as impairment, onset, duration, and severity of symptoms. Their study involved 763 children attending a public school in Salvador,[1] in the state of Bahia in northeastern Brazil. They found that 12 children (8%) had a high probability of having ADHD. In a different study conducted in the same state, on an island called Ilha da Maré, involving a predominantly Afro-Brazilian population, Goodman et al. (2005) found a prevalence of ADHD of 0.9% among children.

Using the *DSM-IV*, Guardiola, Fuchs, and Rotta (2000) found an 18% prevalence of ADHD among 35,521 first-grade students who were 6 to 14 years of age in elementary school in the city of Porto Alegre. Of those students, 64.7% were in state public schools, 11.9% in municipal schools, and 23.4% in private schools. A proportional random sample of 484 children was selected for the study. This was higher than a similar study in the United States, which found a prevalence of 15.9% among elementary school children (5 to 12 years of age) (Nolan, Gadow, and Joyce 2001). Guardiola, Fuchs, and Rotta (2000) attributed the high prevalence estimates in their studies (18%) to the fact that the diagnostic classifications in the US manuals are not precise enough for the disorder to be identified and should therefore be supplemented by neuropsychological evaluations.

Azevêdo et al. (2010) conducted a study of the prevalence of ADHD in a Brazilian indigenous population from the Karaja ethnic group living in isolated settlements in the Amazon. Children and adolescents ages 7 to 16 years from five Karaja settlements were examined. The proportion of children and adolescents ages 7 to 16 years with emotional and behavioral problems compatible with ADHD was found to be 24.5%: 21.9% for boys and 28.6% for girls. The authors suggested that the prevalence of ADHD could have been overestimated because the sample was restricted to children and adolescents whose parents believed they had behavioral problems.

One meta-analysis of the global prevalence of ADHD that was conducted by Brazilian researchers sought to find an explanation for the size of the variation in the prevalence estimates found in different studies of the disorder (Polanczyk et al. 2007). They found that the reason lay in the different methodologies used, adding that if the methodological differences were taken into consideration, an estimated 5% of the global population of school-age children would fit the diagnostic criteria for ADHD (Polanczyk et al. 2007). However, Singh et al. (2013) argue that viewing the quest for standardized diagnostic methods for ADHD as a strictly methodological problem in itself presupposes that a universally valid diagnosis is possible, thereby failing to take into account the ethical dimensions of the relative harms and benefits of globalization.

We could not find any Brazilian study examining changes in prevalence of ADHD diagnosis over time. Variations in prevalence are largely interpreted as resulting from the type of sample examined (from school or community settings), the different instruments and diagnostic criteria used, and, above all, the person providing the information during diagnostic evaluation—parents, children, adolescents, or teachers (Rohde et al. 1998; Vasconcelos et al. 2003).

The widely varying prevalence of ADHD reported in the literature prompts some questions. Attributing such variations to methodological differences presupposes that reaching a global consensus on the diagnostic criteria of the disorder would suffice for definitive answers to be given about the existence of the disease. In other words, the diagnostic criteria, the methods used to make these diagnoses, and the characteristics of the disorder—which are themselves compatible with normal behaviors in children's daily lives—will each in their own way cause differences in the observed prevalence estimates reported in studies.

These variations demonstrate how fluid and unclear the boundaries of ADHD are—as, indeed, are those of other contemporary psychiatric conditions (Rosenberg 2002, 2006). It is not without reason, then, that the apparent variations in ADHD prevalence are being addressed by the Brazilian research community, contributing to debates about the high numbers of diagnoses in people who may not have the disorder, as well as the underdiagnosis of people who may have it.

There is a significant lack of data concerning the historical context of the emergence of ADHD in Brazil as well as its incorporation within medical practices and lay discourses (Rohde et al. 1998; Caliman 2009; Itaborahy and Ortega 2013). Brazilian publications do not specifically address the historical aspects of the emergence of the disorder in the country. We do not find this information in the published material, which frequently reports on the emergence of ADHD in the US context. If one wants to trace the emergence, uses, and misuses of the ADHD diagnosis in Brazil, one is left with only a few pieces of unpublished material (mainly master's theses and PhD dissertations) that examine some elements of this history.

Consumption and Prescription of Methylphenidate in Brazil

Methylphenidate is the most widely consumed stimulant in Brazil and around the world. In 1998, the drug was authorized in Brazil for the treatment of ADHD.[2] Now it is commercialized under the trade names Ritalin and Concerta. Although in the 1950s the use of methylphenidate did not have a precise indication, as of the 1990s its therapeutic value started to be based on the possibility of treating ADHD in an international context (Conrad 1975, 2007; Shorter 2009). In addition, its increased consumption and reliability started to be used to underpin the legitimization of the diagnosis (Dupanloup 2004; Singh 2007). It is believed that an increasingly direct association between methylphenidate consumption and ADHD has been responsible for the increased production and use of this psychostimulant around the world since the 1990s. According to UN data, the world production of methylphenidate increased 1,200% between 1990 and 2006 (INCB 2008), whereas total global consumption of the substance rose from 21.8 tons in 2002 to 35.8 tons in 2006 (INCB 2008). Its increased consumption worldwide continued between 2005 and 2009, rising 30% in the period to reach a total production of 40 tons (INCB 2010b).

In 2005, Brazil's methylphenidate production reached 167 kilograms, supplemented by imports of 133 kilograms. By 2009, its production had dropped to 111 kilograms, but imports had risen to 919 kilograms (INCB 2010a). In 2011, domestic output fell to just 81 kilograms, and imports also dropped to 210 kilograms (INCB 2013). More recent data are unavailable because Brazil, like other major producers (Germany, Austria, Canada, the United States, France, Japan, the Netherlands, and Pakistan), failed to report statistics on psychotropic substances from 2012 to the International Narcotics Control Board (INCB) in time for its 2013 publication (INCB 2013)—this fault has caused concern at the board, as expressed in its latest annual reports (INCB 2012, 2013).

The use of psychopharmacological medications, including methylphenidate, is attracting increasing attention in Brazil. Since the early 2000s, reports about the pharmaco-epidemiological distribution in Brazil of controlled substances such as amphetamines and other appetite inhibitors and methylphenidate have been one of ANVISA's priority targets.

Before 2007, there was no electronic system for regulating controlled medications in Brazil (ANVISA 2010). Records of purchases and sales by drugstores had to be checked by local inspectors. A study from the early 2000s already noted the high level of erroneous and missing data on the forms that recorded sales of controlled psychotropic drugs (Noto et al. 2002). ANVISA did not have access to these local data. Since the introduction of the Sistema Nacional de Gerenciamento de Prescrição Controlada (SNGPC), handwritten records have been phased out, enabling the easy extraction of consolidated electronic data. Prior to this switch, consumption was calculated by summing the volumes produced and the volumes imported, and then subtracting the volumes exported. The data resulting from this operation were sent to the INCB. With the current system, the volumes are recorded when sales are made. This means that variations in the buying habits of users and sales of drugs can be broken down per state. The data from ANVISA for 2009 are from the initial stage of implementation of the SNGPC system, when only private pharmacies and drug stores had joined (ANVISA 2010). By 2011, the system had a nationwide footprint for prescriptions dispensed in private pharmacies, so the data were taken to be an acceptable approximation of consumption of some controlled substances in Brazil (SNGPC 2012).

According to ANVISA, the consumption of methylphenidate in Brazil in 2009 ranged from 5 million milligrams in January to 20 million milligrams in October. This is probably because children and adolescents who are on vacation from school may take less medication. We can therefore infer that the consumption data supplied by the SNGPC system that year corresponded with the consumption of the substances and products subject to special control acquired from private-sector establishments (ANVISA 2010). In the last three-year period analyzed, with the new information system fully functioning, annual consumption of 156,623,848 milligrams was recorded in 2009, 266,092,536 milligrams in 2010, and 413,383,916 milligrams in 2011 (SNGPC 2012).

Some of the legal measures for controlling the sale and use of methylphenidate have been criticized by Brazilian physicians who argue that the notification procedure for its prescription is excessive and disproportionate to the risks it poses to users (Carlini et al. 2003). Since 1998, the Ministério de Saúde has required methylphenidate prescription to be notified in the same way as opiates; this differs from the WHO classification, in which the latter are handled differently. To acquire his first prescription pad, a physician must submit an application using a registration form bearing his signature, which must be formally witnessed by a notary public. Subsequent prescription pads may only be obtained in the presence of an official from ANVISA, who checks, one by one, that all the pages are stamped by the physician (Ministério da Saúde 1998). Carlini et al. (2003) reported that 72% of the physicians who prescribed methylphenidate believed this notification process intimidated their patients and their patients' relatives, making them think their condition was more serious than it was. Meanwhile, 86% said that these regulatory requirements increase bureaucratic procedures and discourage the storage of methylphenidate by the pharmacies, making it harder for patients to find. Finally, 70% opined that the notification process was a cause of embarrassment for those who bought the drug.

While national and international agencies demonstrate concern over the increased consumption of methylphenidate and seek better ways to control its sale, Gomes et al. (2007) are convinced that the biggest problem is how little is known about the disorder and its treatment, among professionals and laypersons alike. They reached this conclusion after analyzing information gathered from health and education professionals and laypersons from 61 municipalities in rural areas and 39 municipalities in metropolitan areas from every region of Brazil (Gomes et al. 2007). Main prescribers are general practitioners, cardiologists, and occupational health doctors (SNGPC 2012).

In an effort to support the hypothesis that ADHD is undertreated in Brazil, the researchers Paulo Mattos, Luis Augusto Rohde, and Guilherme Polanczyk published a letter in 2012 to the editors of the official journal of the Associação Brasileira de Psiquiatria (www.abp.org.br) in which they demonstrated that by the number of methylphenidate pills sold in 2010 (40,585,870, according to IMS Health 2012), they could estimate that this drug was used by only 184,481 individuals that year. The authors stressed that this number represented just 16.9% to 19.2% of the people diagnosed with ADHD in Brazil, if a conservative prevalence of 0.9% was considered (Goodman et al. 2005) rather than the estimate published in a meta-analysis (5.3% among children and adolescents and 2.5% among adults) (Polanczyk et al. 2007). The criteria they used to make this calculation were continuous treatment over a 1-year period (1 pill taken 22 days a month for 10 months), assuming breaks in its use during school vacations and weekends. With this calculation, they aimed to show the country's scientific community that even if lower prevalence estimates were used instead of the expected prevalence, it could still be concluded that more than 80% of individuals with the disorder were not receiving medication-based treatment (Mattos, Rohde, and Polanczyk 2012).

On the other side of the debate are persons for whom the sudden rise in the number of people diagnosed with ADHD and the significant increase in the consumption of methylphenidate over the world are motives for questioning what role the drug industry has in encouraging the potentially abusive prescription of methylphenidate and even legitimizing ADHD as a neurological disease. In Brazil, this movement is organized by the Fórum sobre Medicalização da Educação e da Sociedade (www.medicalizacao.org.br), whose members include researchers, medical professionals, psychologists, and educators. The forum is led by Maria Aparecida Moysés, a pediatrician and researcher who stated in an interview with the press that "methylphenidate has the same mechanism of action and the same adverse reactions as cocaine and amphetamines" and that precisely the effect expected in restless children is one of the effects of its toxicity: zombie-like behavior that makes individuals more docile. Hence its name, "the drug of obedience." She goes on to question the existence of "a neurological disease that only alters behavior and learning" (Moysés 2011).

As we can see, not all of the professionals involved in treating ADHD in Brazil agree that medicating is the best method. As we will see further on, many Brazilian professionals, mainly in the fields of education, psychology, and psychoanalysis, believe it is necessary to adopt a broader perspective to engage with learning difficulties, restlessness, and inattention. In Brazil, ADHD is largely considered a neurodevelopmental disorder, although most of the non-physician professionals dealing with it come from the field of education. These professionals adopt a multidisciplinary and psychosocial approach, leaving the prescription of methylphenidate for the most severe cases.

Medical Discourse about ADHD, Professional Associations, and Patient Support Groups

Patient and family support groups can initiate social movements organized around a diagnosis with aims that vary from spreading knowledge and awareness about a disease to fighting for better treatments or more research for a cure (Nunes, Matias, and Filipe 2007). Some of them reject the prevailing scientific medical discourse about the disease, calling for recognition of their illnesses and their subjective meanings (Epstein 2008).

Although Brazil does not have the same tradition of patient support groups as the United States, it does have some associations for patients with diseases such as autism, ADHD, and obsessive-compulsive disorder and their family members. These associations have an important function in spreading knowledge about these diseases and fighting for better treatments and citizens' rights (Nunes 2014; Rios and Andrada 2015). In countries such as the United States, Canada,

Australia, and South Africa, some groups have organized into social movements that reject the scientific medical discourse about pathology and cure. Their struggle is not so much to ensure citizens' rights and social inclusion as to affirm the right to a different identity from the normative standard (Orsini 2009, 2012; Orsini and Smith 2010; Baker 2011; Silverman 2012).

In the case of ADHD, these groups have a peculiar composition, encompassing not just patients in their membership. The best-known national group is the Associação Brasileira do Déficit de Atenção (ABDA). Created in 1999, its members include not only people with ADHD and their relatives, but also professionals and researchers. It is a nonprofit entity that aims to spread knowledge about ADHD. Its website (www.tdah.org.br), which appears in a wide range of scientific periodicals and journals, receives an average of 200,000 visits every month. Also, the mixed membership of ABDA makes it a prime medium for communication between lay and professional audiences, as well as for spreading the biomedical discourse on ADHD in the country. The academic studies published on the website and in journals aim to legitimize ADHD as a biologically based disorder. The association is sponsored by Novartis and Shire Pharmaceuticals, and its members pay an annual membership fee. Through its website, the association divulges what ADHD is; its causes, diagnosis, and treatment; and ways of dealing with the disorder regarding pharmacological and lifestyle aspects, recommendations for family members and patients, and contact details for professionals working in the field. Professionals and researchers also use the ABDA website to post comments on articles on ADHD in the mainstream press, and they use the site as a means of communicating their opinions and positions on the validity or legitimacy of such articles.

Some of the most important centers for ADHD research in Brazil such as the Grupo de Estudos do Déficit de Atenção (GEDA) are linked with ABDA. This group is also linked to the Instituto de Psiquiatria of the Universidade Federal do Rio de Janeiro, which receives funding from Janssen-Cilag, the manufacturer of Concerta. Some of GEDA's members are speakers for Janssen-Cilag, Eli Lilly (the manufacturer of Strattera), Novartis, and GlaxoSmithKline. The group is responsible for much of the research published in the country on methylphenidate and ADHD, and some of its members sit on the ABDA scientific board.

Another example is the Programa de Transtornos de Déficit de Atenção/Hiperatividade (ProDAH; www.ufrgs.br/prodah), a research group inside the Faculdade de Medicina of the Universidade Federal do Rio Grande do Sul, in southern Brazil. ProDAH receives funding from the pharmaceutical companies Bristol-

Myers Squibb, Eli Lilly, Janssen-Cilag, and Novartis. Some of its members sit on the ABDA scientific board.

Santa Casa de Misericórdia do Rio de Janeiro is a philanthropic hospital funded by donations and public resources for some of the hospital services it provides for the population. It has specialized outpatient clinics providing free health care, including its infant psychiatry service. Some of its professionals are members of the ABDA scientific board and are speakers for the pharmaceutical companies Abbott, Astra-Zeneca, Janssen-Cilag, and Novartis.

Research is also conducted at the Ambulatório para Distúrbios Hiperativos e Déficit de Atenção (ADHDA) for children and adolescents and the Programa Déficit de Atenção e Hiperatividade em Adultos (PRODATH) for adults, both of which operate at the Hospital das Clínicas at the University of São Paulo, in the southeastern part of the country. Some of its members are speakers for Janssen-Cilag and Novartis and sit on the ABDA scientific board.

In yet another example, the alcohol and drug research unit (Unidade de Pesquisa em Álcool e Drogas, or UNIAD) at the Universidade Federal do São Paulo contributes a significant number of publications about methylphenidate. Some of its members are speakers for Janssen-Cilag.

The associations among the main research groups in Brazil that are engaged in building knowledge about ADHD, patient and family support groups, and drug companies constitute a significant production hub for the official discourse about the disorder. A study conducted by the Universidade do Estato do Rio de Janeiro's Instituto de Medicina Social identified partnerships and funding links between the main members of the research groups listed above. The authors analyzed 103 Brazilian publications about the uses of Ritalin that were published between 1998—the year in which the drug was authorized in Brazil—and 2008. Seventy-two of the publications were articles in the mainstream press (newspapers and magazines) and 31 were in psychiatry journals. Brazilian psychiatry periodicals indexed in the Scielo database were searched, as were high-circulation mainstream newspapers and magazines. The analysis provided inputs for the discussion of which points are highlighted in and which points are omitted from discourses about methylphenidate in Brazil, and their possible effects on clinical practice (Itaborahy and Ortega 2013). The authors reported that the *Jornal Brasileiro de Psiquiatria*, a leading periodical in the field, mostly published research by GEDA, often with advertising for Concerta. In the articles published in this journal, the authors declared a conflict of interest concerning the treatment of patients, but in other articles the funding received from drug companies was not explicitly stated. According to Itaborahy and Ortega, a supplement published by this journal in 2007 was funded entirely—from the articles to the advertisements—by a manufacturer of methylphenidate (Itaborahy and Ortega 2013).

The pharmaceutical companies' funding of research on ADHD should not automatically be seen as undermining its validity; after all, funding is needed to support the infrastructure required for complex investigation involving multiple research centers. In the case of epidemiological investigations of the disorder or surveys of the level of knowledge on the part of professionals and nonprofessionals in a country as large and culturally diverse as Brazil, the need for a more robust research infrastructure becomes even more critical. Nonetheless, in view of the potential power of drug companies to influence research findings when they are directly involved in funding research and researchers, it is worth considering the need to control, evaluate, and question such influences and the ethical implications arising from such sponsorship (Itaborahy and Ortega 2013).

Itaborahy and Ortega (2013) found that all of the scientific publications agreed that the use of methylphenidate was indispensable for the treatment of ADHD, whereas the lay reports included other approaches, mentioning social pressures and demands on the patient and noting that the patient's psychodynamic state contributes to an individual's altered attention, self-control, and capacity for concentration. The benefits of methylphenidate use were discussed in 74% of the scientific publications but in only 40% of the newspaper and magazine articles. Despite the different percentages, both types of publications agreed on the main benefits of the use of the substance, such as improving academic performance and remission of symptoms of ADHD. In addition, they stressed that the antidependency effect of methylphenidate could help prevent addiction disorders (e.g., alcohol and substance abuse). However, where they diverged was in the role of psychotherapy in treatment; the scientific publications held that the combined use of the medication and psychological therapies yielded worse results than the use of the drug alone, whereas the lay reports argued that patients with ADHD benefited from psychotherapy (Itaborahy and Ortega 2013).

Mental Health Care in Brazil

The Brazilian health care system was organized after the 1988 Constitution was enacted. The Constitution states that health is a social right and that the state has a duty to provide health services. Since the creation of the Sistema Único de Saúde (SUS) in 1990, there have been steady and continuous efforts toward universal health coverage and care. The SUS system is organized region-ally, with a decentralized network of health services formed by a complex set of public, private, and philanthropic providers, under coordinated management at each level of government and with strong community participation (Lobato and Burlandy 2000; Souza 2002). In spite of the advances in the past two decades, there are several challenges to consolidating SUS as a universal public system that can provide quality services to the entire Brazilian population. These concern difficulties in attaining universal coverage and the proliferation of private health care plans among the middle and upper classes; insufficient and inadequate health care financing; challenges pertaining to the health care model, which was designed for acute diseases and neglects chronic conditions; an inade-quacy of human resources; and the challenge of social participation (Biehl 2005; CONASS 2006).

SUS mental health policies have been shaped by the Brazilian psychiatric re-form movement, which was inspired by the Italian democratic psychiatry move-ment led by Franco Basaglia in Trieste and the Lacanian-inspired institutional psychotherapy program of La Borde in France (Barros 1994; Passos 2009). In Brazil, this movement was started in the early 1970s by a faction of mental health professionals and relatives of patients with mental illnesses. Brazilian mental health workers, together with trade unions and left-wing politicians, advanced the *luta anti-manicomial* (anti-asylum struggle) and criticized the psychiatry establishment's collaboration with the dictatorship. This movement developed within the context of the country's redemocratization and the social-political mobilization (Delgado 1992; Amarante 1995; Tenório 2002). Following guide-lines set up by the Caracas Declaration (1990), in recent decades psychiatric care in Brazil has moved from a hospital-oriented system to primary health care, pro-moting alternative community-centered treatment models. In 2001, the Lei da Reforma Psquiátrica (Federal Law 10.216), which guards the protection and rights of those with mental disorders and redirects the model of care in mental health, was approved (Csillag 2001). Brazilian mental health policy originates from this law. It encourages the programmed reduction of admission to psychiat-ric wards for extended periods of time, promoting the idea that psychiatric ad-mission, when necessary, should take place in general hospitals and should last for only short periods of time. Apart from that, it promotes the deinstitutional-ization of patients who have been admitted for long periods of time in psychiatric wards and actions that advance psychosocial inclusion through work, culture, and leisure (Ministério da Saúde 2002, 2005).

The Centros de Atenção Psicossocial (CAPS) are specialized mental health services that provide outpatient care or partial hospitalization as day or night treatment. The CAPS system has become the basis of the Brazilian psychiatric reform, and mental health care is centralized at the CAPS level. CAPS are responsible for treating severe mental disorders and, if possible, for averting inpatient admissions (psychiatric hospitals or psychiatric wards in general hospitals). They are also responsible for articulating the link with primary care units to coordinate psychiatric care in a defined catchment area (WHO-AIMS 2007; Mateus et al. 2008). The CAPS system opposes framing mental health policies according to specific diseases and organizing specialized services for various diagnoses. Therefore, the notion of a "citizen burdened by mental suffering" should replace various psychiatric labels, regardless of whether the individuals are labeled "schizophrenic," "autistic," or "alcoholic." The Centros de Atenção Psicossocial Infantil (CAPSi) are strategic elements of mental public health attention for children and adolescents with persistent and severe mental disorders. They are organized in a network that extends beyond the health field and interacts with community resources in order to promote the social inclusion of children and adolescents. The interdisciplinary team at CAPSi may also count on the partnership of families, society, schools, and other sectors. Diagnoses in CAPSi are based on the principle of the *clínica ampliada* (amplified clinic), which conceives them as an ongoing process. Diagnoses should be made and reevaluated throughout the evaluation and treatment process, and the diverse elements of the care strategy (psychotherapy, rehabilitation, and medication) should always focus on the singularity of the child and her history, family, relationships, and everyday life (Couto 2004, 2012; Couto et al. 2008).

Debate about the Medicalization of ADHD in Brazil

The already mentioned marked increase in the use of methylphenidate, both internationally and in Brazil, in recent years is viewed with circumspection by some mental health professionals and educators in Brazil. This, alongside the strong involvement of the drug industry in research into ADHD and methylphenidate in Brazil, has prompted some researchers to question the findings of studies on the disorder and the validity of its diagnosis and medication-based treatment.

A directive issued by the Secretaria Municipal de Saúde of Sao Paulo—Brazil's most highly populated city in the southeast of the country and home to its leading industrial hub—has heightened feelings around a new agenda of topics in recent months. Its text (Portaria No. 986/2014 2014) intends to regulate the prescription of methylphenidate in the municipality, stating that users suspected of having ADHD should be sent to CAPSi. Wherever such services do not exist, patients should be referred to treatment units combined with therapeutic interventions of a psychosocial and educative nature from the public service (Portaria No. 986/2014 2014). The teams of CAPSi are responsible for treating all severe mental health cases in their catchment areas and for referring others to outpatient clinics and other health units in the system (Ministério da Saúde 2002).

The directive issued in São Paulo aligns with the national policy insofar as "from a clinical perspective, it is a complex task to distinguish cases of ADHD from parts of educational problems which derive from inadequate educational models for the children's social context, increasingly complex family issues, and a sociocultural context in which there is competition, the production of stigmas, and exclusion" (Portaria No. 986/2014 2014). The Associação Brasileira de Saúde Mental (ABRASME) (www.abrasme.org.br) has supported the regulation, regarding it as an exemplary measure that is in full agreement with the precepts of a broader understanding of the problem. ABRASME is an association that subscribes to the principles of the Brazilian psychiatric reform and aims to coordinate training, education, research centers, and mental health services to strengthen and expand dialogue with technical and scientific communities, government and nongovernmental organizations, and civil society (ABRASME 2010).

In the same period, the Associação Brasileira de Psiquiatria (ABP) published an open letter (entitled "Carta Aberta a População" ["Letter to the People"]) in which it declared its disapproval of the São Paulo directive. Ten regional medical, psychiatric, and neurology societies and associations signed the letter, as well as the Sociedade Brasileira de Neuropsicologia, the Sociedade Brasileira de Neurociência, and ABDA. An additional 60 medical professionals, psychiatrists, and psychologists with master's and doctoral degrees, working as university professors or chairing professional associations, signed the letter. In the document, the ABP claims that the measure introduced by the São Paulo Secretaria Municipal de Saúde "is restrictive, bureaucratizes respectful access to treatment, mainly by people at a social disadvantage, and positions itself against scientific systematization in a mystifying, disrespectful way" (ABP 2014). It continues: "it is an abusive barrier to access to pharmacological treatment by people with a low income, and places restrictions on the full exercise and autonomy of Brazilian medicine and science" (ABP 2014). The letter also argues that the *DSM* does not offer a defined etiology for ADHD, just as it does not for autism, depression, or schizophrenia, but that this has not prevented the development of effective therapeutic and diagnostic protocols for these conditions (ABP 2014).

Maria Aparecida Moysés, founder of the Fórum sobre Medicalização da Educação e da Sociedade was one of the researchers invited to contribute to the São Paulo directive that regulates the prescription of methylphenidate in the city (Portaria No. 986/2014 2014). The forum was created in 2010 in response to the public debate in the city of São Paulo about the programs created for dyslexia and later for ADHD. The focus of these programs was considered a step backward in overcoming the associated educational difficulties since, according to their critics, they reduced educational problems to a supposed individual pathology. The professionals involved in these discussions are mainly from the areas of health and education, and the Rio de Janeiro and São Paulo state councils for psychology are important spokespersons for the movement. Since it was created, the forum has set up partnerships with numerous groups from Brazil and other countries (Fórum 2013).

In 2011, the forum held a meeting with an Argentinean movement, Forumadd (www.forumadd.com.ar), a multidisciplinary group opposed to the pathologization and medicalization of childhood. As a result of this meeting, a document was drafted that establishes the initial framework for engaging professionals from both countries. In addition, it delineates the principles of the movement with the goal of raising the awareness of societies and entities throughout Latin America (Fórum 2011). The goals of the campaign against medicalization are the following: to speak out against the increasing use of psychotropic drugs among children and adolescents—especially methylphenidate; to support the position that learning difficulties and ADHD are not pathologies, or simply "do not exist," and that the identification of such disorders causes patients more harm than good; and to criticize government policies that address such disorders (Fórum 2011).

Clearly, the debate about medicalization in Brazil involves a variety of groups and associations with discourses that represent different and apparently contradictory interests. State governments are making policies that are guided by the principles of deinstitutionalization put forth by reformist psychiatrists in Italy (Rotelli, Leonardis, and Mauri 1990). These policies are supported by the Associação Brasileira de Saúde Mental. Another player on this side of the field is the Fórum sobre Medicalização de Educação e da Sociédade. In its discourse about how ADHD is constituted as a neurological pathology, the forum aligns itself with public mental health policies that propose a broader clinical approach that takes into consideration the psychosocial factors that trigger psychic suffering, rather than a pathology-oriented approach. On the other side of the field is the ABP, which has always resisted the idea of a broader approach that positions the physician as just one member of a multidisciplinary team. Generally speaking, the medical associations' position is that medical professionals must take the lead in ADHD's treatment, with psychologists or speech therapists taking a supporting role. (Other professionals, such as occupational therapists or social workers, are not even mentioned on the ABDA website or in the scientific research published by this sector.) The view these medical associations take seems to be that a multidisciplinary dynamic would reduce medicine's professional autonomy. Alongside these medical associations, we also identified some ADHD patient and family groups, research centers, and the main journals in the field of medical science. These stakeholders are the main components that formalize medical discourse about ADHD in Brazil.

Conclusion

Analysis of the academic and professional tensions and debates about ADHD in Brazil evinces how controversial the landscape surrounding this condition is. On the one hand, there is a strong group of defenders of the idea that the condition is underdiagnosed (Mattos, Rohde, and Polanczyk 2012) and that the general public, schools, and parents should be better informed about it. On the other hand, there is a force keen to warn about the overmedicalization of expected childhood behaviors, for which there is little tolerance in society. The latter is formed by physicians who differ from the overmedicalized position, and especially by professionals from the human sciences. Despite the considerable weight of the medical discourse in favor of communicating, popularizing, and spreading information (and diagnosing ADHD when applicable), it is impossible to ignore the polarization and power of these conflicting discourses. This is what springs to light in the gray literature—in the journals published by professional associations and in the open letters—where one group or another's responses and positions are presented, even if this positioning is not totally explicit. We could add that if there is one characteristic that marks the Brazilian landscape in its approach to ADHD, it is the controversy, the tension between these discourses, and the dispute between the groups over which one is telling the "truest" version of this clinical condition.

A final point deserves some attention. As Banzato and Zorzanelli (2014) noted, these polarized positions often spring from a shared assumption, whether they hold that disorders do correspond or should correspond in some future moment to natural types (entities that exist in nature, independent of the way humans have framed them), or that they are artificial (arbitrary human constructs). The touch-point of these two apparently mutually exclusive positions is the comparison of mental disorders with medical diseases, the physiopathological foundations of which are already known. The idea of a real disease is therefore its existence, given by its nature and its objectivity, qualities that should be ensured by the supposed natural, independent existence of human classifications. The debates around the diagnosis of ADHD in Brazil discussed in this chapter seem to incorporate this type of dilemma, which itself deserves much more space for debate than definitive solutions.

NOTES

1. Bahia showed that 763 was a reasonable sample calculation for this population.
2. This information was obtained only through personal correspondence with ANVISA, given the scarcity of historical studies about pharmaceuticals in Brazil.

REFERENCES

Agência Nacional de Vigilância Sanitária (ANVISA). 2010. "Relatório 2009—Sistema Nacional de Gerenciamento de Produtos Controlados (SNGPC)."

Amarante, Paulo. 1995. *Loucos pela vida: a trajetória da reforma psiquiátrica no Brasil.* Rio de Janeiro: SDE/ENSP.

American Psychiatric Association (APA). 1994. *Diagnostic and Statistical Manual of Mental Disorders (DSM-IV).* 4th ed. Washington, DC: American Psychiatric Association.

Associação Brasileira de Psiquiatria (ABP). 2014. "Carta Aberta a População." http://www.abp.org.br/portal/carta-aberta-a-populacao/.

Associação Brasileira de Saúde Mental (ABRASME). 2010. "Estatuto da associação brasileira de saúde mental," Assembleia Geral da ABRASME. http://www.abrasme.org.br/conteudo/view?ID_CONTEUDO=641.

———. 2014. "Transtorno de déficit de atenção e hiperatividade (ADHD) e a iniciativa exemplar da SMS de São Paulo." https://abrasmesp.wordpress.com/2014/07/23/nota-abrasme-transtorno-de-deficit-de-atencao-e-hiperatividade-tdah-e-a-iniciativa-exemplar-da-sms-de-sao-paulo/.

Azevêdo, Paulo, Verlaine Borges, Leonardo Caixeta, Laura Helena Silveira Andrade, and Isabel A. Bordin. 2010. "Attention Deficit/Hyperactivity Disorder Symptoms in Indigenous Children from the Brazilian Amazon." *Arquivos de Neuro-Psiquiatria* 68 (2010): 541–44.

Baker, Dana Lee. 2011. *The Politics of Neurodiversity: Why Public Policy Matters.* Boulder, CO: Lynne Rienner, 2011.

Banzato, Claudio, and Rafaela Zorzanelli. 2014. "Superando a falsa dicotomia entre natureza e construção social: O caso dos transtornos mentais." *Revista Latinoamericana de Psicopatologia Fundamental* 17 (2014): 110–13.

Barbosa, Genario A., and Valdiney V. Gouveia. 1993. "O fator hiperatividade do questionário de Conners: Validade conceitual e normas diagnósticas." *Temas* 23: 188–202.

Barros, Denise. 1994. *Jardins de Abel: Desconstrução do Manicômio de Trieste.* São Paulo: Editora da Universidade de São Paulo.

Baumgaertel, Anna, Mark L. Wolraich, and Mary Deitrich. 1995. "Comparison of Diagnostic Criteria for Attention Deficit Disorder in a German Elementary School Sample." *Journal of the American Academy of Child and Adolescent Psychiatry* 34 (1995): 629–38.

Biehl, João. 2005. *Vita: Life in a Zone of Social Abandonment.* Berkeley: University of California Press.

Caliman, Luciana Vieira. 2009. "A constituição sócio-médica do 'fato TDAH.' " *Psicologia & Sociedade* 21: 135–44.

Carlini, Elisaldo A., Solange A. Nappo, Vagner Nogueira, and Fernando G. M. Naylor. 2003. "Metilfenidato: influencia da notificação de receita A(cor amarela) sobre a prática de prescrição por médicos brasileiros." *Revista de Psiquiatria Clínica* 30: 11–20.

Catalá-López, Ferrán, Salvador Peiro, Manuel Ridao, Gabriel Sanfeliz-Gimeno, Ricard Genova-Maleras, and Miguel A. Catalá. 2012. "Prevalence of Attention Deficit Hyperactivity Disorder among Children and Adolescents in Spain: A Systematic Review and Meta-analysis of Epidemiological Studies." *BMC Psychiatry* 12: 168.

Conrad, Peter. 1995. "The Discovery of Hyperkinesis: Notes on the Medicalization of Deviant Behavior." *Social Problems* 23 (1): 12–21.

———. 2007. *The Medicalization of Society: On the Transformation of Human Conditions into Treatable Disorders.* Baltimore: Johns Hopkins University Press.

Conselho Nacional de Secretários de Saúde (CONASS). 2006. *SUS: avanços e desafios.* Brasilia: Conselho Nacional de Secretários de Saúde.

Cornejo, J. W., O. Osío, Y. Sánchez, J. Carrizosa, G. Sánchez, H. Grisales, H. Castillo-Parra, and J. Holguín. 2005. "Prevalencia del trastorno por déficit de atención-hiperactividad en niños y adolescentes colombianos." *Revue Neurologique* 40: 716–22.

Couto, Maria Cristina Ventura. 2004. "Por uma Política Pública de Saúde Mental para crianças e Adolescentes." In *A criança e a saúde mental: enlaces entre a clínica e a política*, edited by Tania Ferreira, 61–74. Belo Horizonte: Autêntica-FHC-FUMEC.

———. 2012. "Política de Saúde Mental para crianças e adolescentes: especificidades e desafios da experiência brasileira." PhD diss., Universidade do Estado do Rio de Janeiro.

Couto, Maria Cristina V., Cristiane S. Duarte, and Pedro G. Delgado. 2008. "A saúde Mental Infantil na Saúde Pública Brasileira: situação atual e desafios." *Revista Brasileira de Psiquiatria* 30: 390–98.

Csillag, Claudio. 2001. "Psychiatric Reform Law Comes into Effect in Brazil." *The Lancet* 357 (2001): 1346.

Delgado, Pedro Gabriel. 1992. *As razões da tutela: psiquiatria, justiça e cidadania do louco na Brasil*. Rio de Janeiro: TeCorá.

Dupanloup, Anne. 2004. "L'Hyperactivité infantile: analyse sociologique d'une controverse socio-médicale." PhD diss., University of Neuchâtel.

Epstein, Steven. 2008. "Patient Groups and Health Movements." In *The Handbook of Science and Technology Studies*, edited by Michael Lynch and Judy Wajcman, 499–539. Cambridge, MA: MIT.

Fontana, Rosiane da Silva, Márcio Moacyr de Vasconcelos, Jairo Werner Jr., Fernanda Veiga de Góes, and Edson Ferreira Liberal. 2007. "Prevalência de ADHD em quatro escolas públicas brasileiras." *Arquivos de Neuro-Psiquiatria* 65 (2007): 134–37.

Fórum sobre Medicalização da Educação e Sociédade. 2011. "Carta sobre medicalização da vida." Buenos Aires.

———. 2013. "Medicalização da Vida." *Jornal do Conselho Regional de Psicologia do Rio de Janeiro* 35: 8–9.

Freire, Antonio, Carlos Cruz, and Milena Pereira Pondé. 2007. "Estudo piloto da prevalência do transtorno de déficit de atenção e hiperatividade entre crianças escolares na cidade de Salvador, Bahia, Brasil." *Arquivos de Neuro-Psiquiatria* 63: 474–78.

Gomes, Marcelo, André Palmini, Fabio Barbirato, Luis Augusto Rohde, and Paulo Mattos. 2007. "Conhecimento sobre o transtorno do déficit de atenção/hiperatividade no Brasil." *Jornal Brasileiro de Psiquiatria* 56: 94–101.

Gomez, R., J. Harvey, C. Quick, I. Scharer, and G. Harris. 1999. "DSM-IV AD/HD: Confirmatory Factor Models, Prevalence, and Gender and Age Differences Based on Parent and Teacher Ratings of Australian Primary School Children." *Journal of Child Psychology and Psychiatry* 40: 265–74.

Goodman, Robert D. Neves dos Santos, A. P. Robatto Nunes, D. Pereira de Miranda B. Fleitlich-Bilyk, and N. Almeida Filho. 2005. "The Ilha de Maré Study: A Survey of Child Mental Health Problems in a Predominantly African-Brazilian Rural Community." *Social Psychiatry and Psychiatric Epidemiology* 40: 11–17.

Guardiola, Ana, Flavio D. Fuchs, and Newra T. Rotta. 2000. "Prevalence of Attention-Deficit Hyperactivity Disorders in Students: Comparison between DSM-IV and Neuropsychological Criteria." *Arquivos de Neuro-Psiquiatria* 58: 401–7.

International Narcotics Control Board (INCB). 2008. "Report of the International Narcotics Control Board for 2007." New York: United Nations.

———. 2010a. "Psychotropic Substances. Statistics for 2009. Assessments of Annual Medical and Scientific Requirements." New York: United Nations.

———. 2010b. "Report of the International Narcotics Control Board for 2009." New York: United Nations.

———. 2012. "Psychotropic Substances. Statistics for 2011. Assessments of Annual Medical and Scientific Requirements." New York: United Nations.

———. 2013. "Psychotropic Substances. Statistics for 2012. Assessments of Annual Medical and Scientific Requirements." New York: United Nations.

Itaborahy, Claudia, and Francisco Ortega. 2013. "O metilfenidato no Brasil: uma década de publicações." *Ciência e Saúde Coletiva* 18: 803–16.

Lobato, Lenaura, and Luciene Burlandy. 2000. "The Context and Process of Health Care Reform in Brazil." In *Reshaping Health Care in Latin America: A Comparative Analysis of Health Care Reform in Argentina, Brazil, and Mexico*, edited by Sonia Fleury, Susana Belmartino, and Enis Baris, 79–102. Ottawa, ON: IDRC Books.

Mateus, Mario D., Jair J. Mari, Pedro Gabriel G. Delgado, Naomar Almeida-Filho, Thomas Barrett, Jeronimo Gerolin, Samuel Goihman, Denise Razzouk, Jorge Rodriguez, Renata Weber, Sergio B. Andreoli, and Shekhar Saxena. 2008. "The Mental Health System in Brazil: Policies and Future Challenges." *International Journal of Mental Health Systems* 2: 12.

Mattos, Paulo, Luis Augusto Rohde, and Guilherme V. Polanczyk. 2012. "O ADHD é subtratado no país." Carta aos editores. *Revista Brasileira de Psiquiatria* 34: 513–16.

Ministério da Saúde. 1998. Portaria No. 344, May 12.

———. 2002. Portaria No. 336, February 19.

———. 2005. Secretaria de Atenção à Saúde. DAPE. Coordenação Geral de Saúde Mental. Reforma psiquiátrica e política de saúde mental no Brasil. Documento apresentado à Conferência Regional de Reforma dos Serviços de Saúde Mental: 15 anos depois de Caracas. OPAS. Brasília.

Moysés, Maria Aparecida. 2011. "A droga da obediência," Carta Fundamental. Interview, *Carta Capital*, February 20.

Nolan, Edith E., Kenneth D. Gadow, and Sprafkin Joyce. 2001. "Teacher Reports of DSM-IV ADHD, ODD, and CD Symptoms in Schoolchildren." *Journal of the American Academy of Child and Adolescent Psychiatry* 40: 241–49.

Noto, Ana Regina, Elisaldo de A. Carlinia, Patrícia C. Mastroianni, Vanete C. Alvesa, José Carlos F. Galduróz, Wagner Kuroiwa, Jussara Csizmar, Agrimeron Costa, Mariluci de A. Faria, Sônia Regina Hidalgo, Dirce de Assis, and Solange Aparecida Nappo. 2002. "Analysis of Prescription and Dispensation of Psychotropic Medications in Two Cities in the State of São Paulo, Brazil." *Revista Brasileira de Psiquiatria* 24: 68–73.

Nunes, Fernanda Cristina Ferreira. 2014. "Atuação política de grupos de pais de autistas no Rio de Janeiro: perspectivas para o campo da saúde." Master's thesis, Universidade do Estado de Rio de Janeiro.

Nunes, João Arriscado, Mariza Matias, and Ângela Marque Filipe. 2007. "As organizações de pacientes como atores emergentes no espaço da saúde: o caso de Portugal." *Revista Eletrônica de Comunicação, Informação & Inovação em Saúde* 1: 107–10. http://www.reciis.icict.fiocruz.br/index.php/reciis/article/view/894.

Orsini, Michael. 2009. "Contesting the Autistic Subject: Biological Citizenship and the Autism/Autistic Movement." In *Critical Interventions in the Ethics of Health Care*, edited by Stuart J. Murray and Dave Holmes, 115–30. London: Ashgate.

———. 2012. "Autism, Neurodiversity and the Welfare State: The Challenges of Accommodating Neurological Difference." *Canadian Journal of Political Science* 45: 805–27.

Orsini, Michael, and Miriam Smith. 2012. "Social Movements, Knowledge and Public Policy: The Case of Autism Activism in Canada and the US." *Critical Policy Studies* 4: 38–57.

Passos, Izabel C. F. 2009. *Reforma psiquiátrica: As experiências francesa e italiana*. Rio de Janeiro: Fiocruz.

Pineda, David Ardila, M. Rosselli, B. E. Arias, G. C. Henao, L. F. Gomez, S. E. Mejia, and M. L. Miranda. 1999. "Prevalence of Attention Deficit/Hyperactivity Disorder Symptoms in 4–17 Year Old Children in the General Population." *Journal of Abnormal Child Psychology* 27: 455–62.

Pino, Benjumea P., and Maria D. Mojarro-Praxedes. 2001. "Trastornos hipercinéticos: estudio epidemiológico en doble fase de una población sevillana." *Anales Psiquiatria* 17: 265–70.

Polanczyk, Guilherme, and Peter Jensen. 2008. "Epidemiological Considerations in Attention Deficit Hyperactivity Disorder: A Review and Update." *Child and Adolescent Psychiatric Clinics of North America* 17: 245–60.

Polanczyk, Guilherme, Mauricio Silva de Lima, Bernardo Lessa Horta, Joseph Biederman, and Luis Augusto Rohde. 2007. "The Worldwide Prevalence of ADAH: A Systematic Review and Metaregression Analysis." *American Journal of Psychiatry* 164: 942–48.

Portaria No. 986/2014. 2014. Secretaria Municipal de Saúde, Diário Oficial da Cidade de São Paulo. No. 109—Diário Oficial Municipal, June 12, p. 19.

Ribeiro, Marcelo, Luciane Ogata Perrenoud, Sérgio Duailibi, Lígia Bonacim Duailibi, Clarice Madruga, Ana Cecília Petta Roseli Marques, and Ronaldo Laranjeira. 2013. "The Brazilian Drug Policy Situation: The Public Health Approach Based on Research Undertaken in a Developing Country." *Public Health Reviews* 35: 1–32.

Rios, Clarice, and Barbara Costa Andrada. 2015. "The Changing Face of Autism in Brazil." *Culture, Medicine, and Psychology* 39 (2): 213–34.

Rohde, Luis Augusto, Genário Barbosa, Silzá Tramontina, and Guilherme Polanczy. 1998. "Transtorno de deficit de atenção/hiperatividade: revisando conhecimentos." *Revista ABP APAL* 20: 166–78.

Rohde, Luis Augusto, Joseph Biederman, and Ellis A. Busnello. 1999. "ADHD in a School Sample of Brazilian Adolescents: A Study of Prevalence, Comorbid Conditions and Impairments." *Journal of the American Academy of Child and Adolescent Psychiatry* 38: 716–22.

Rosenberg, Charles. 2002. "The Tyranny of Diagnosis: Specific Entities and Individual Experiences." *The Milbank Quarterly* 80: 237–60.

———. 2006. "Contested Boundaries: Psychiatry, Diseases and Diagnosis." *Perspectives in Biology and Medicine* 49: 407–24.

Rotelli, Franco, Ota Leonardis, and Diana Mauri. 1990. "Desinstitucionalização, uma outra via. A Reforma Psiquiátrica Italiana no Contexto da Europa Ocidental e dos 'Países Avançados.'" In *Desinstitucionalização*, edited by Maria Fernanda Nicácio, 27–59. São Paulo: Hucitec.

Shorter, Edward. 2009. *Before Prozac: The Troubled History of Mood Disorder in Psychiatry.* Oxford: Oxford University Press.

Silverman, Chloe. 2012. *Understanding Autism: Parents, Doctors, and the History of a Disorder.* Princeton, NJ: Princeton University Press.

Singh, Ilina. 2007. "Not Just Naughty: 50 Years of Stimulant Drug Advertising." In *Medicating Modern America: Prescription Drugs in History*, edited by Andrea Tone and Elizabeth Siegel Watkins, 131–55. New York: New York University Press.

Singh, Ilina, Angela M. Filipe, Imre Bard, Meredith Bergey, and Lauren Baker. 2013. "Globalization and Cognitive Enhancement." *Current Psychiatric Reports* 15: 385.

Sistema Nacional de Gestão de Prescrição Controlada (SNGPC). 2012. "Prescrição e consumo de metilfenidato no Brasil: Identificando riscos para o monitoramento e controle sanitário."

Souza, Renilson. 2002. *O Sistema Público de Saúde Brasileiro.* Brasília: Editora do Ministério da Saúde.

Tenório, Fernando. 2002. "A reforma psiquiátrica brasileira, da década de 1980 aos dias atuais: história e conceito." *História, Ciências, Saúde—Manguinhos* 9: 25–59.

Vasconcelos, Marcio M., Jairo Werner Jr., Ana Flávia de Araújo Malheiros, Daniel Fampa Negreiros Lima, Ítalo Souza Oliveira Santos, and Jane Bardawil Barbosa. 2003. "Prevalência do transtorno de déficit de atenção/hiperatividade numa escola pública primária." *Arquivos de Neuro-Psiquiatria* 61: 67–73.

World Health Organization (WHO). 2008. *International Classification of Diseases (ICD-10).* 10th ed. Geneva: World Health Organization.

World Health Organization (WHO)–Assessment Instrument for Mental Health Systems (AIMS). 2007. *Report on Mental Health System in Brazil.* Brasília: World Health Organization and Ministério da Saúde.

11

ADHD in the Italian Context

Children in the Midst of Social and Political Debates

Alessandra Frigerio
Lorenzo Montali

Compared to the United States, Australia, and the United Kingdom, attention–deficit hyperactivity disorder (ADHD) has been a recent issue for debate in Italy. Before the early 2000s, the ADHD diagnosis was still not recognized by many Italian child psychiatrists and psychologists, and it was mostly unknown to the general public. Moreover, no medication to treat ADHD was available in Italy's pharmaceutical market until 2007.

Things have since changed rapidly; today, ADHD is a recognized diagnosis among the majority of Italian child psychiatrists, psychologists, and social workers and it is a well-known disorder among laypeople. In this chapter, we frame the ADHD phenomenon within the Italian context, outlining the contingencies of its emergence and development, stakeholder activism raised around ADHD-related controversy and debate, social and school policies developed for ADHD, the condition's epidemiology, and the type of treatments available in Italy. Finally, we trace some cultural factors related to the discourses constructed and circulating around ADHD in Italy, and we discuss their influence on the subjective positioning of children with ADHD and the key adult stakeholders who interact with them.

Controversy and Debate: The Emergence of ADHD in Italy

The evolution of public discourse on ADHD in Italy is linked to the activity of associations and advocacy groups that are prominent voices in the Italian debate. Such groups produce and disseminate specific discourses and forms of knowledge about ADHD as well as attempt to influence social policies and legislation. On the one hand, the Associazione Italiana Disturbi Attenzione e Iperattività (AIDAI), which is composed of professionals such as child psychiatrists, psychologists, and pediatricians, and the Associazione Italiana Famiglie ADHD (AIFA) aim to promote the social acceptability of ADHD. They do so by creating supporting networks for parents, organizing trainings for teachers, countering critical perspectives (especially those based on psychodynamic and psychoanalytic approaches), and supporting the use of medication to treat ADHD. More specifically, the early 2000s saw the emergence of the project "Parents for Parents,"[1] which led to the formation of the parental association AIFA. On the association's website, parents state that this collective project started from the recognition of a diffuse absence of institutional responses to ADHD and the need to struggle against a scrutinizing and stigmatizing social context, which tended to blame parents for their children's behavior and did not recognize the validity of the ADHD diagnosis. In 2002, the association published a book, *Vorrei scappare in un deserto e gridare* (*I Would Like to Escape in a Desert and Shout*), which presented personal stories of many parents of children with ADHD; the book's aim was to sensitize public opinion with respect to parents' experiences and difficulties related to ADHD.

On the other hand, a number of associations and committees launched education and awareness campaigns criticizing the conceptualization of ADHD symptoms and the use of psychopharmacological treatments. Specifically, the organization Giù le mani dai bambini focused on the potential abuse of medication in childhood, and the campaign "Perché non accada anche in Italia" ("Let's Stop It from Happening in Italy") criticized the so-called pathologization and psychiatrization of human behavior and difficulties (Marzocchi, Re, and Cornoldi 2010).

The debate about the validity of the ADHD diagnostic category and the use of medication for its treatment was characterized by the stipulation of a number of statements of consensus, supporting different perspectives. In 2003, a consensus was written as the result of a national conference on ADHD (ISS 2003) held by a number of scientific and clinical experts on ADHD. The founder and representative of AIFA also participated in the conference. This consensus, entitled "Indicazioni e strategie terapeutiche per i bambini e gli adolescenti con disturbo da deficit attentivo e iperattività" ("Therapeutic Indications and Strategies for Children and Adolescents with ADHD"), was approved by a number of professional societies and organizations in the fields of pharmacology, psychopathology, and pediatrics. The consensus promoted the notion of ADHD as a chronic neurobiological disease and a specific approach to diagnosis and treating ADHD based on the revised fourth edition of the *Diagnostic and Statistical Manual of Mental Disorders* (*DSM-IV-R*) (APA 2000) and cognitive-behavioral intervention. The consensus also emphasized the use of pharmacological treatment, especially in cases in which intensive psychoeducational interventions are not available.

In response to these stances, criticisms came from a number of associations as well as from individual experts in the fields of psychology, education, and social science, whose opinions were frequently reported by the mass media addressing the topic of ADHD. In 2005, the association Giù le mani dai bambini promoted the definition of a consensus (Giù le mani dai bambini 2005) in the context of a broad campaign aimed at raising awareness about and preventing the risk of labeling children and giving them psychotropic medication. The consensus, entitled "Consensus internazionale: ADHD e abuso nella prescrizione di psicofarmaci ai minori" ("International Consensus: ADHD and Abuse in Prescription of Psychopharmacological Drugs to Minors"), was signed by more than 40 associations and institutions (such as parental associations, psychologists and psychotherapists' societies and institutes, cultural associations working with children, and associations promoting nonconventional medicine) and by a number of individuals (such as psychiatrists, psychotherapists, psychologists, sociologists, and psychoanalysts).

In the consensus, the nosography of ADHD is contested for its scientific inconsistency and for the implied strict pharmacological orientation toward intervention. The procedure to introduce methylphenidate to treat ADHD began with a petition directed to the minister of health at the time. The petition was proposed by the representatives of the "Parents for Parents" project and signed by a number of pediatricians and child psychiatrists. In 2007, methylphenidate, a psychostimulant that is recommended as a drug of first choice for ADHD, and atomoxetine, which is considered as a second choice (Germinario et al. 2013), were introduced to the Italian drug market by the Agenzia Italiana del Farmaco. Their commercialization inflamed debate; a number of official stances by experts (such as pediatricians, psychotherapists, and psychiatrists) and parliamentarians were collected in a document entitled "Allarme Reintroduzione Ritalin: Dichiarazione di Esperti e Parlamentari" ("Warning on Ritalin Reintroduction: Declarations by Experts and Parliamentarians") by the association Giù le mani dai bambini (Giù le mani dai bambini 2007). Moreover, awareness days were organized by experts and nonprofit associations to express approval or disapproval about the governmental decision.

As discussed above, the Italian debate on ADHD has been articulated around polarized positions. Today, the parental association AIFA claims that Italy is behind Anglophone countries, especially the United States, in terms of ADHD-related knowledge and practice. Parents declare their commitment to increase knowledge and acceptance around ADHD on their website, as well as in books and brochures published by the association. They also emphasize the importance of becoming "principle-centered," "executive," and "scientific parents" to manage the criticism toward ADHD and the related use of drugs (D'Errico and Aiello 2003: 28). In contrast, the committee Giù le mani dai bambini continues to organize events to discuss potential risks and side effects of the use of drugs for children diagnosed with ADHD and other psychopathologies. However, critical perspectives not ascribable to biomedical approaches, which address the importance of considering the social and relational aspects of ADHD, are mainly limited to minority communities of experts and journals with little influence on the Italian academic fields of psychology and psychiatry (Alegret 2012; Di Trani, Marinucci, and Tortolani 2012; Lambruschi and Bertaccini 2012; Leone 2012).

ADHD has entered the Italian public sphere and political arena, and the presence of social movements centered on ADHD diagnosis and treatments, such as AIFA and the association Giù le mani dai bambini, demonstrates that in contemporary society people are not passive subjects dependent on experts' judgments and advice; rather, they are increasingly active in the search for answers to common problems and questions (Beck 1992).

Social Policies and Legislation on ADHD

The first Italian guidelines for the diagnosis and treatment of ADHD were established by the Società Italiana di neuropsichiatria dell'infanzia e dell'adolescenza (SINPIA) in 2002 (SINPIA 2002), before methylphenidate and atomoxetine were introduced to the Italian drug market. The guidelines represented the first attempt in Italy to clinically define ADHD, establish a procedure to follow for its diagnosis, and articulate general principles for therapeutic intervention. Additional policy change began to occur in 2007 after years of debate (Bonati 2007; Costabile et al. 2007); significant political attention paid to the ADHD phenomenon led to the approval of a number of legislative measures.

First, the Agenzia Italiana del Farmaco decided in 2007 to authorize the use of drugs (i.e., methylphenidate and atomoxetine) for the treatment of ADHD. Moreover, a national protocol including guidelines was published in 2007 by the Istituto Superiore di Sanità (ISS), together with the Agenzia Italiana del Farmaco, to homogenize diagnostic procedures and give therapeutic directions (ISS 2007). Medication costs are covered by the national health system. A national ADHD register was created in conjunction with the publication of the national protocol (Panei et al. 2004; Bonati and Panei 2009). The register, instituted in 2007, was meant to include all Italian children and teenagers between 6 and 18 years of age who are diagnosed with ADHD and treated with methylphenidate or atomoxetine. The purpose of the register was to monitor and assess the clinical effects of the use of medications, including efficacy and adverse drug reactions (Knellwolf et al. 2006). According to the Italian legislation, children can receive pharmacological treatment for ADHD only if they are registered in the national register (Ruggero et al. 2012). In order to avoid improper use of medicines, the ADHD register allows the prescription of methylphenidate and atomoxetine only within a biannual therapeutic plan (Capuano et al. 2014).

The register is coordinated by the pharmacological department of the ISS and Agenzia Italiana del Farmaco, is supervised by a national panel of experts, and has to be administered by the ADHD regional reference centers that enroll the patients. ADHD regional reference centers are specialized centers for the diagnosis and treatment of ADHD; they were selected from the Unità Operative di Neuropsichiatria Infantile (UONPIA), the public child psychiatric services distributed throughout the Italian territory. The ADHD regional reference centers are UONPIA that were recognized by the regional health authorities as qualified centers for the diagnosis and treatment of ADHD.

According to a 2009 assessment of the implementation of the ADHD register (Bonati and Panei 2009), the practices related to the register varied depending on the specific reference center. Indeed, in 2009, two years after the creation of the register, one-third of the reference centers appeared not to have any patients under their care who were receiving pharmacological treatment, and 40% of all patients included in the register were from only three reference centers. Moreover, there was a gap between the population expected to need psychostimulants (about 45,000 people) and the number of patients enlisted in the register (1,050 people). The conclusion that could be drawn from these data is that the presence of an evidence-based tool, which the register is considered to be, is not sufficient to modify institutional medical practices. According to Bonati and Panei (2009), these differences might be due to limited human and financial resources available for the management of the register and to different therapeutic approaches and attitudes toward ADHD characterizing diverse geographic areas and cultural contexts. Overall, these aspects influence the register's level of compliance with the minister of health's established procedures. According to the ADHD register's newsletter from June 30, 2012 (ISS 2012), the number of registered patients in the 90 reference centers distributed throughout the Italian territory was 2,664. Medication was given to 2,239 patients—56.7% of whom were prescribed methylphenidate and 43.3% of whom were prescribed atomoxetine. The 2007 legislation also established that drugs can be prescribed only by the ADHD regional reference centers. The ADHD reference centers are responsible for defining a multimodal therapeutic plan, an appropriate combination of multiple methods of treatment such as medications, cognitive-behavioral therapy for children, parent training and educational interventions for teachers, and systematic follow-up to evaluate the security and efficacy of drugs.

Drugs to treat ADHD—methylphenidate and atomoxetine—are prescribed to 1.7% of the whole Italian population between the ages of 14 and 18 years, and the percentage of Italian children diagnosed with ADHD who are exposed to multimodal treatment—pharmacological treatment combined with other psychoeducational intervention—is between 7% and 17%, according to data collected in the years 2007–10 (Maschietto et al. 2012).

In 2011, the Registro ADHD della Regione Lombardia was activated to gather data about ADHD patients between 5 and 17 years of age and to guarantee homogeneous assessment and therapeutic plans for ADHD in the northern region of Lombardy, where there are 18 ADHD regional reference centers. A regional register is not yet activated in other areas of Italy. According to the data collected by the Registro ADHD della Regione Lombardia from 2012 to 2013 (Reale et al. 2014), 13% of patients with a diagnosis of ADHD received a prescription for multimodal treatment (a combination of pharmacological and psychological interventions), 2% received prescriptions for drugs alone, and 85% were prescribed psychological treatment only. The whole percentage of individuals pharmacologically treated was 15%. Among these patients, 83% were treated with methylphenidate, 7% with atomoxetine, and 10% with other drugs, especially risperidone. From 2011 to 2012, drug use decreased from 24% to 16% of patients

(Bonati and Reale 2013). Eighty-five percent of the patients received a prescription for a psychological type of intervention, involving mostly parent training (82%), child training (59%), and teacher training (33%). Patients with a combined type of ADHD received pharmacological treatment more frequently than patients with a predominantly inattentive or a predominantly hyperactive-impulsive type of ADHD. In contrast, patients with a predominantly inattentive ADHD type more frequently received psychological treatment alone.

ADHD is primarily diagnosed in Italy by child psychiatrists and in some cases by psychologists who work in public service or as private practitioners. Diagnosticians must conform to the 2007 national protocol to make the diagnosis, which is based on criteria from the American Psychiatric Association's (APA) *Diagnostic and Statistical Manual of Mental Disorders* (*DSM*), now in its fifth edition (APA 2013). The *International Classification of Diseases 10th edition* (*ICD-10*) (WHO 2010) is almost unused by Italian child psychiatrists and psychologists. The 2002 guidelines published by SINPIA explicitly stated that "it seems more appropriate to clinically assess children adopting the DSM-IV criteria instead of ICD-10 criteria, because the latter leaves children in a sort of 'nosographic limbo'" (SINPIA 2002: 9); in the guidelines' appendix, only the *DSM-IV* criteria are reported. In the 2003 consensus it is reported that "the diagnosis of ADHD must be based on the DSM-IV classification" (ISS 2003: 1). In the 2007 national protocol, the *ICD* is mentioned only to highlight its differences from the *DSM*. The diagnostic tools include semistructured interviews with parents (Kaufman et al. 2004) and rating scales for parents and teachers (Conners 2007). Cognitive and neuropsychological tests are suggested to define comorbidities, such as learning disabilities, and to provide a specific profile for each child (Marzocchi, Re, and Cornoldi 2010).

The Epidemiology of ADHD

In Italy, epidemiological studies have reported differing prevalence estimates for ADHD. Some studies conducted in the mid-1990s in three Italian central regions—Tuscany, Umbria, and Emilia—indicated a prevalence of around 3.6% in the population between 6 and 12 years of age (Gallucci et al. 1993; Camerini, Coccia, and Caffo 1996). Other studies conducted in the central area of Italy, specifically in the cities of Rome (region of Lazio) and Cesena (region of Emilia-Romagna) in the early 2000s, identified the prevalence of ADHD as ranging from 0.91% to 1.51% in children between 7 and 14 years of age (Ciotti 2003; Corbo et al. 2003; Sarno 2003). In contrast, a study conducted in 2002, in which a questionnaire was administered to 74 family pediatricians in a northern area of

Italy, the region of Friuli Venezia Giulia, suggested a prevalence of 0.43% (Besoli and Venier 2003).

According to the guidelines of SINPIA (SINPIA 2002), ADHD affects approximately 4% of children. Prevalence estimates from recent studies vary. A 2006 study estimated that ADHD affects 7.1% of children between 6 and 7 years of age (Mugnaini et al. 2006). In line with that, some researchers attested that the prevalence of ADHD in Italy is between 4% and 7% (Mazzotta et al. 2008). Didoni et al. (2011) estimated ADHD prevalence in the population (ages ranging from 6 to 17) to be 0.95%. Other recent surveys (Frigerio, Montali, and Marzocchi 2009; Maschietto, Re, and Cornoldi 2012) found that the prevalence of ADHD is between 1% and 2%. The ISS is more cautious with respect to the 2002 SINPIA guidelines and suggests that the prevalence of ADHD in the Italian population between 6 and 18 years of age is approximately 1% (Knellwolf et al. 2008). According to Maschietto, Re, and Cornoldi (2012), 1.2% is in line with previous epidemiological surveys conducted in Italy among the population between 6 and 18 years of age, but this rate is significantly lower (from two to four times lower) with respect to what is reported in the international scientific literature. The authors speculated that this difference may be due to a number of factors, including the criteria and procedures used to make the diagnosis, who is in charge of making the diagnosis in various countries, the willingness to prescribe drugs to children, and the availability of various therapeutic options. The wide variation between studies may be also due to other factors, such as the different diagnostic procedures adopted in different periods and areas, and the source of data used (e.g., data collected from schools or from pediatric private practices) (Costabile et al. 2007). Indeed, teacher-rated symptoms of ADHD tend to overestimate the prevalence of ADHD (Mugnaini et al. 2006) and to suggest that it is underdiagnosed in Italy (Frigerio, Montali, and Marzocchi 2014). The most recent survey on ADHD in Italy found a prevalence of 3% in the population between 5 and 15 years of age (Bianchini et al. 2013); data from the ADHD register set up in Lombardy indicate a prevalence of 3.51% in 5- to 17-year-old children and adolescents—a significantly lower percentage with respect to national data (Reale et al. 2014).

There are no studies on the prevalence of ADHD among adults in Italy. The ISS and the Istituto Mario Negri, a center for pharmacological research that collaborates with the ISS, also confirmed to us in an email exchange that there are no data on the prevalence of ADHD among adults (ISS, pers. comm.).

Among the children and adolescents (5 to 17 years of age) listed between 2007 and 2010 in the Italian ADHD register, 88.6% were male (Ruggiero et al. 2012).

According to data gathered by the ADHD register in Lombardy (Reale et al. 2014), in the period from 2012 to 2013, 85% of patients (ranging in age from 5 to 17 years) referred for assessment to the Lombardy ADHD reference centers were male and 15% were female. Among those children who after being assessed received a diagnosis of ADHD, 87% were male and 13% were female. Regarding differences across groups, data collected through the Lombardy ADHD register in the years 2012–13 suggest that the characteristics that are significantly associated with an ADHD diagnosis include the following: lower age at the time of diagnosis (5 to 11 years of age versus 12 to 17 years of age), being an only or an adopted child, a family history of ADHD, having an employed mother, delivery through natural childbirth, and a delay in language development (Reale et al. 2014).

Therapeutic Interventions for ADHD

According to the 2007 national protocol (ISS 2007), therapies for ADHD are divided into the following three types: psycho-behavioral, pharmacological, and multimodal. Psycho-behavioral therapies include intervention with children diagnosed with ADHD, parent training courses, and consultation with teachers. The type of treatment adopted for children is based on cognitive-behavioral psychology. Other approaches are increasingly used, such as the Summer Treatment Program (STP) (Pezzicca et al. 2011)—an intensive summer camp program aimed at developing pro-social behaviors in children, such as cooperation and communication skills, self-control strategies, and the ability to inhibit impulsivity. The activities proposed during the program are based on behavioral theory and meta-cognitive approaches. Recent research suggests that these programs may produce an improvement in the ability to use self-control strategies when specific tasks are proposed in the laboratory context, but they do not favor enhancement in everyday life (Pezzicca et al. 2011).

Parent training courses are frequently organized by hospitals, ADHD reference centers, and local divisions of the AIFA. They are organized as group sessions in which parents are instructed to analyze the children's problematic behaviors and receive specific instructions and behavioral strategies for children to use in different situations. Recently, a research team developed an integrated approach, called Cognitive Emotional Relational Groups (CERGs), to be applied for parent training (Paiano et al. 2012). This method integrates cognitive-behavioral psychology with attention to the emotional and relational aspects of children's behaviors. According to the 2007 national protocol published by the ISS and the Agenzia Italiana del Farmaco, teachers are sometimes included in the therapeutic program through a consultation, usually given by psychologists, in which they are instructed in procedures to modify a child's behavior and adapt their teaching approach to the specifics of a child with ADHD. With regard to school services, children who are diagnosed with ADHD do not have access to teaching aids unless they have major cognitive impairments or additional behavioral problems. There are no special classes for children diagnosed with ADHD. The Ministero dell'Instruzione, dell'Università e della Ricerca issued a ministerial circular for schools that provides some behavioral management strategies that can be used with children diagnosed with ADHD (MIUR 2010).

The national guidelines included in the national protocol suggest adopting a multimodal therapy—that is, a combination of cognitive-behavioral therapy for children, psychoeducational intervention with parents and schools, and pharmacological treatment. Despite the attempt to homogenize therapeutic interventions, there is much variability concerning the duration of the therapy, its efficacy, and the criteria used for its evaluation (Bonati 2007). Due to the limited availability of financial and human resources, the reference centers frequently define the multimodal therapy that is then implemented by other clinicians or services; typically, the pediatrician prescribes the medication following the reference center's indications, and local child psychiatrists or, in the majority of cases, private psychologists are responsible for the psycho-behavioral intervention (Maschietto et al. 2012). No specific services are currently available for adults with ADHD, although it is a topic under discussion.

The Social Construction of ADHD in the Italian Context: Discourses of Risk, Blame, and Legitimation

The relative newness of the ADHD diagnosis to the Italian context may have influenced the discourses surrounding ADHD. ADHD is an important area for exploring the current assumptions about childhood and mental illness that characterize a specific socio-ideological context, given that a diagnosis is the social act of attributing meaning to experience and behaviors (Berrios 2006). Regarding the specific Italian context, Frazzetto, Keenan, and Singh (2007) identified four main narratives about ADHD that were circulating in the public debate when methylphenidate was reintroduced into the pharmaceutical market: the right to health, the right to childhood, parents' feelings of guilt, and public stigma. The authors stated that the different positions on ADHD in Italy "are embedded in valued civil and cultural ideas as well and socio-political and governmental practices" (Frazzetto, Keenan, and Singh 2007: 409).

Because there is no organic marker for the disorder, the presence of ADHD is diagnosed by professionals together with parents and teachers, whose interactions determine the diagnosis and management of the condition. The way in which different groups of social actors discursively frame and understand the problems linked to ADHD shapes and provides meaning for this phenomenon and shows how ADHD relates to the larger social, political, and economic contexts of children's lives (Singh 2011).

In this respect, three relevant discursive patterns characterize the narratives of parents, professionals, and teachers regarding ADHD (Frigerio 2013): the rhetoric of risk, related to the positioning of the child diagnosed with ADHD (Frigerio, Montali, and Fine 2013b); the blame embedded in the mutual positioning of these relevant social actors (Frigerio, Montali, and Fine 2013a); and the self-legitimation discourse, as that which emerged in a study on a self-help group of parents linked with the AIFA (Frigerio and Montali 2015).

Discourses of Risk

The discourse and psychological framing of "risk" pervades the structuring of narratives on ADHD among Italian professionals, parents, and teachers. These narratives position the child as at-risk, and risky, in body and mind (Frigerio, Montali, and Fine 2013b). Different stakeholders articulate notions of risk differently. For mental health professionals, children are likely to develop serious psychiatric conditions. For teachers, children mainly pose a potential threat and source of danger for other children and the school's social order; in this sense, teachers' concerns are about the "risk to others" that they feel children with ADHD might represent. For parents, the view of risk is articulated as "risk for the future"; the child is susceptible to marginalization by society and school and is susceptible to being marginalized as an "out-of-society" adult in the future—one who is at risk for becoming a criminal, not having a family, or being unemployed. In this sense, ADHD is characterized according to a variety of risky behaviors and conditions that are not necessarily associated with the specific symptoms of the diagnosis and the spectrum of which ranges from antisocial behavior and marginalization to oppositional conduct, violence, criminality, personality disorder, and low academic performance.

The discursive construction of the child with ADHD as being interwoven with risk resonates with the Western contemporary and pervasive public discourse about childhood that, according to some authors, is focused on risk and fear (Burman 1994; Jackson and Scott 1999; Nybell 2001; Rose 2003; Massumi

2010; Pica-Smith and Veloria 2012). The psychiatric categorization of the child is used to manage the present and stabilize the future in the light of risk, informing future decisions. In particular, the classification of the child as having a structural and innate deficit constructs ADHD as a lifetime and life-defining condition. This construction implies that the child's problems and difficulties will remain forever, and it orients the view of a possible future. The construction of the child as being structurally deficient implies that he is constantly at risk for inadequate development and represents a permanent risk to the contexts he inhabits because of his inability to socialize with others. The three risk discourses are different, but they converge in their construction of the disease as worsening if not treated. Therefore, risk operates as a central regulatory device (Clough 2007) leading from warning and picturing a possible future to action and preventing this future. Indeed, the risky character of the child implies both the necessity and the moral obligation to mobilize to protect her from herself and justifies intervening on the child's behalf. Adhering to these specific ways of protecting and educating the child assigns implied tasks to health service providers, families, and schools; these tasks are implemented based on the idea that they are in the child's "best interest" (Stainton-Rogers and Stainton-Rogers 1992).

The risk associated with genetic susceptibility may result in neglecting psychological and relational factors and, therefore, in the restriction of the options for managing children's behaviors (Hughes 1999). The notion of individual risk may also lead to an underestimation of the role of sociopolitical and economic realities. Underestimation may relieve experts, schools, and families from the responsibility of interrogating themselves about the major sociocultural context in which children express themselves (Finn, Nybell, and Shook 2010) and about their practices regarding education, training, and social inclusion (Lubeck and Garrett 1990). The lack of debate about ADHD that characterized Italy until a few years ago might have influenced parental concerns and fears, as well as childcare professionals' representations and physicians' behavior with respect to ADHD, leading to a tendency to embrace dominant psychiatric conceptualizations and practices as concrete and specific solutions to problems that were previously obscure.

Discourses of Blame

In the Italian context, mutual blame seems to be a constitutive element of relational dynamics among the key adult stakeholders—professionals, teachers, and parents—surrounding ADHD children (Frigerio, Montali, and Fine 2013a).

The conflicting relationships between the social agents who are supposed to work together for the child are not only related to the debate regarding the validity of the ADHD diagnosis. Rather, the mutual blame centers on questions of compliance, recognition of authority, and morality.

The literature on ADHD in Western countries has highlighted that ADHD is discursively placed within a culture of blame (Harborne, Wolpert, and Clare 2004; Singh 2004; Hansen and Hansen 2006). Even though hyperactivity, impulsivity, and inattention are ascribed to biological and genetic causes, this conceptualization does not prevent conflicts among medical, scholarly, and familial institutions.

The circulation of blame is articulated differently across mental health professionals (i.e., psychiatrists, psychologists, and social workers), teachers, and parents. Mental health professionals' construction of their knowledge as objective leads them to devalue teachers' and parents' knowledge and expertise. In particular, experts blame schools and families when they do not conform to their indications. For example, teachers are positioned by mental health professionals as being anchored to an old-fashioned educational outlook and are criticized for their scarce knowledge of the pathology of ADHD. This position is tied to what professionals see as teachers' intentional unwillingness to recognize experts' authority and related negligence toward the child (Frigerio, Montali, and Fine 2013a).

Teachers may not question the medical understanding of ADHD, but a substantial number of them direct blame toward parents and society to account for the child's behavior (Frigerio, Montali, and Fine 2013a). This pattern is consistent with the "toxic childhood" rhetoric that, according to Horton-Salway (2011: 12), characterizes some discourses about ADHD. In particular, the "toxic childhood" rhetoric indicates a psychosocial explanation of ADHD as originating from the social environment and as a symptom of a sick society that is incapable of educating its children. At the same time, the blame pattern discussed above shows that ADHD's biological and psychosocial discursive repertoires (Horton-Salway 2011) are not markedly distinct in the case of Italian teachers, who construct mixed discourses. This process might be indicative of the tension between the tendency to conform to the psychiatric body of knowledge and the effort to maintain a distinct perspective. Therefore, the tendency to integrate the academic and medical agendas, which suggests that medical and psychological knowledge is needed for proper child development (Singh 2006), is supported primarily by professionals and is partially resisted by teachers.

Finally, parents—particularly mothers—counter the blame professionals and teachers place on them by shaping their subjectivity in terms of narratives of sacrifice and by blaming the majority of the "psy-community" (Frigerio, Montali, and Fine 2013a: 594). That is to say, they blame the community of experts and mental health professionals, including psychiatrists and psychologists, for not recognizing ADHD and addressing it in a standardized way. In this sense, parents use their acquired medical knowledge of ADHD as a device to reverse the traditional relationship between passive patients and authoritative specialists, positioning themselves as the real experts and suggesting that many professionals are in need of training. Parents also blame teachers, whom they consider to be culpable for not updating their "obsolete" knowledge on ADHD or adapting their practices to reflect scientific recommendations about ADHD treatment and management.

Therefore, blame not only affects parents but also circulates in the triangle of adults who interact with the child. This blame discourse is the storyline by which all participants inscribe others and themselves, and this blame discourse frames their construction of subjectivity. Through the "blame game," adults negotiate their own and others' subjectivity in ways that simultaneously (re)produce power relationships and resistance efforts. The underlying problem facing key adults frequently shifts from the causes of the child's behavior to questions of true knowledge, compliance with instructions, and recognition of authority. The network of adults does not distribute blame for the child's behavior; rather, social actors distribute blame for the lack of respect toward medical, educational, or parental authority (Frigerio, Montali, and Fine 2013a).

The blame game is a way for adults to negotiate not only what must be done but also by whom—allocating rights, duties, and obligations in ways that (re)produce power relationships and resistance efforts. Indeed, social actors are embedded in a politics of knowledge (Baert and Rubio 2011) that defines medical and psychological statements as legitimate and establishes a priori whose knowledge counts and who has the authority to dictate instructions to others (Fine 2012). These conflicting dynamics outline a constellation of different levels of legitimacy; blame emerges as a way to resist these power inequalities. These topics are linked to the issue of morality. Compliance and recognition of others' authority are framed as assumptions of moral responsibility for the child's best interest. By contrast, the lack of recognition of the roles and authority of the other key stakeholders surrounding children with ADHD is constructed as an immoral act of refusing to behave in the child's interest. In this sense, the ADHD phenomenon constitutes a channel for the expression of opposition between three major social institutions: family, school, and medicine. The relevance of blame in the mutual positioning of those social actors attests to the relevance of moral dimensions related to ADHD (Singh 2011) and shows that morality pervades the relationships between the adults involved.

Discourse of Self-Legitimation

The Italian parental association formed around ADHD—the AIFA—may be viewed as part of a broader social and political movement that aims to penetrate society "in the name of health" (Landzelius 2006: 530). An ethnographic-discursive analysis (Galasiński 2011) of the interpersonal dynamics enacted by parents within this group indicated the association's orientation toward the production of a uniform and safe space for parents, which in turn can allow for the construction of a common narrative around ADHD (Frigerio and Montali 2015). Specifically, the discursive dynamic characterizing the parental association and related self-help groups includes a series of strategies that range from homogenization of the internal space of the group via mirroring (e.g., constructing the experiences of children with ADHD as if they were all "the same" and the pattern of their development as identical and predictable), mutual identification, and differentiation from the outside world, to normalization of ADHD and pharmacological treatment, use of various forms of evidence to support specific accounts of ADHD, and correction of "not allowed" accounts (Frigerio and Montali 2015).

Members of the AIFA interact with ADHD in a way that contributes to the mutual identification of the members and to the related production of a specific and shared narrative. This shared narrative seems to function as a ratified and consensual body of knowledge that constitutes for parents not only a language to narrate what ADHD is and means (within and outside the group) but also a resource for legitimization. In contrast to the stigmatizing social context that leads parents to feel powerless and excluded, the parental association is a setting where parents can find recognition for their experiences and voices.

In this sense, the common narrative used to talk about ADHD provides a resource for supporting parents' subjectivity and a means for parents to reestablish their moral status. Commonality of experience converts troubling experiences into credentialed forms of parenting (Rabeharisoa 2003) and is a resource for self-legitimization. To protect their identities from social blame, parents adopt a medicalized version of hyperactivity and inattention (Conrad and Potter 2000) and perceive any challenge to this account to be a threat to their legitimacy—

despite the fact that biomedical constructions of mental illness "frequently fail to protect individuals from delegitimation and stigma" (Lafrance and McKenzie-Mohr 2013: 124).

The narrative of the association, which acquires its legitimacy from its consensual character, also represents a means by which parents acquire a position that authorizes them to actively enter the social space they inhabit (Allsop, Jones, and Baggott 2004) without feeling less legitimate than other social actors, such as mental health professionals and teachers. Self-disclosure and the sharing of experiences are tools that parents use to produce an empowering story that provides them with access to certain practices—such as the contestation of the authority of medical professionals and teachers, the reclamation of specific rights, and the assertion of their competence as parents (Ryan and Cole 2009). Overall, the parental group provides participants with a language to articulate their experiences and sustain their subjectivity within a stigmatizing social context. However, the tendency to maintain and repair the orderliness of the group's interactions, for example, through the correction of "not allowed" accounts, could have problematic implications. Because the group constructs a narrative that tends to ignore or counteract incongruous information, the group might not value different perspectives, might inhibit the expression of certain opinions, and might emphasize certain aspects of the experience at the expense of others.

The knowledge produced by parents represents a form of "lay expertise" (Novas and Rose 2000: 488). Lay experts are experts by experience because they generate and authorize their own knowledge. Indeed, parents build and claim their own position of authority not through training or membership in a professional group but rather in relation to their experience, which acquires legitimate status because of its shared and consensual character. Parents construct a form of "experiential authority" by associating with one another (Novas and Rose 2000: 503) and act as sort of "proto-professionals" (Hilton and Slotnick 2005) who may position themselves as having more expertise than many mental health professionals.

The self-positioning of parents as lay experts who educate one another also implies a reconfiguration of their relationship with professionals and related power dynamics (Rabeharisoa 2003). Professionals in the mental health field, as well as in education, are not regarded as authorities holding the truth; parents see themselves as active subjects engaged in political action to support the biomedical understanding of ADHD. This phenomenon recalls Darling's (1988) concept of the "parental entrepreneur." Focusing on the development of activism among parents of disabled children, Darling (1988) argued that parental activism can be viewed as a response to the failure of society to provide resources for children and their families; in this sense, these types of advocacy groups represent a challenge to the authority of professional experts.

ADHD: A "Constructed" and "Constructive" Social Object

The connection between the discourses of risk, blame, and legitimation provides the frame for the social construction of ADHD in the Italian context. The construction of children as being potentially at-risk and risky interplays with the mutual attribution of blame among the adults (i.e., mental health professionals, teachers, and parents) who interact with children diagnosed with ADHD. The rhetoric of risk allows adults simultaneously to not consider the problematic behavior of children as being their fault and to blame each other for not being aware of the risk and not behaving properly to manage it. The adult is morally culpable if she does not take responsibility for preventing the risks that the child may encounter in his environment.

The risk discourse creates the conditions for the conflict among three contexts that are deeply engaged with the topic of ADHD: medicine, school, and family. This conflict is primarily based on the transfer of individual responsibility from the self to others. Doctors feel legitimated in blaming teachers and parents who, if not behaving in a compliant way, actually expose children to the risk they embody. Teachers blame parents whom they feel represent a potential connection between a "toxic society" and the children, and they blame doctors whose practices they consider to be potentially dangerous. Parents, worried about the risks they see for their children, blame others for not being able to recognize and manage ADHD. This deep connection between risk and blame problematizes the idea proposed by other authors such as Lakoff (2000), according to which the construction of ADHD as a neurobiological disorder necessarily implies relief from guilt and blame for the social actors involved. In contrast to this hypothesis, within the specific Italian context, risk seems to be a locus of blame, even though the biological model of ADHD ignores questions of personal and social responsibility (Pardeck and Murphy 1993). This is in line with Kildea, Wright, and Davies's (2011: 615) view that "the label ADHD appears to offer an explanation, but this begins to dissolve when the reality of everyday experience starts to attach new (and often negative) meanings and connotations" to the same problem that different stakeholders have to confront.

Mutual blame is also interwoven with issues of authority and different levels of legitimacy, and therefore with the discourse of legitimation. This connection is exemplified by the analysis of the dynamics that take place within the AIFA. The parental association fronts the blame that parents have experienced on a daily basis, producing a common narrative on ADHD that is based on the biomedical model. This common narrative represents a form of knowledge that both reestablishes parents' moral status, reducing their feelings of guilt, and—due to its shared character—gives legitimacy to parents' experiences, claims, and rights. Researchers working in the United Stated (Conrad and Potter 2000; Mayes, Bagwell, and Erkulwater 2008) have also underlined parents' efforts to promote the medical discourse on ADHD and to find a legitimate space for social and political actions to resonate.

Therefore, it is our view that ADHD is socially constructed in relation to specific interests and power dynamics characterizing the contextualized relationships among the social actors that are relevant to the child and her contexts. This conclusion does not imply that genes do not play a role in children's behaviors; rather, it indicates that genetic dispositions express themselves always in interaction with other factors, which are relational, social, and political and which significantly affect the way we understand, represent, and confront specific problems. Subjects cannot be reduced to a mere expression of their genetic complement (Dreyfuss and Nelkin 1992) because illnesses are socially constructed by the bodies of knowledge that aim to explain and describe them (Macey 2000).

In conclusion, ADHD is simultaneously a constructed and a "constructive" object (Frigerio and Montali 2015). The adults surrounding a child are involved not only in the process of constructing the child with ADHD, but they are also constructing themselves and others within a theater of voices struggling for their identity in relation to the "disturbed" child. What is at stake is not only the construction of ADHD and the ADHD child, but also the subjectivity of all the people involved.

Conclusion

In this chapter, we outlined how the Italian scientific community, the public, and political authorities mobilized around ADHD and how different groups tried to exercise social and political influence over the way in which the problem should be conceptualized and treated. The Italian case of ADHD's emergence and development shows that the practices activated around the ADHD diagnosis are not the effect of "medical imperialism"; rather, they result from the "interaction of lay and professionals claims-makers" (Conrad and Potter 2000: 575) and derive from a polyphonic chorus of voices surrounding the child (Frigerio, Montali, and Fine 2013a) whereby diverse social actors actively contribute to shape a common problem. In this sense, the child with ADHD and the adults relevant to him are located in a network of relatedness, commitments, and obligations, where multiple forms of expertise are developed in multiple settings: clinics or hospitals, schools, associations of laypeople, and political institutions.

Therefore, the meanings attributed to the ADHD diagnosis and the practices of diagnosis and treatment are related to power dynamics characterizing the relationships among the social actors that are relevant to the child and her contexts. The ADHD case, and the relatively rapid change of understanding and management regarding ADHD in the Italian context, can be viewed in light of broader social trends regarding the psychiatric field: the established tendency toward a biomedical conceptualization of mental distress; the consumerist trend within the mental field and the demanding orientation of patients and their relatives; and the connection between morality and concepts of health and illness.

NOTE

1. The project was named in English by its founding members; the Italian translation for the project's name is "Genitori per i Genitori." Despite the fact that the parental group was not affiliated with any specific group from an English-speaking country, the choice of naming the project in English might be understood as a way that parents adopt to distance themselves from the Italian context, which parents consider to be not advanced or civilized enough with respect to attention and policies devoted to ADHD.

REFERENCES

Alegret, Joana. 2012. "Un Approccio Sistemico alla Sindrome di ADHD. Revisione della Tipizzazione delle Famiglie di Bambini con ADHD." *Psicobiettivo* 2: 15–39. doi:10.3280/PSOB2012-002002.

Allsop, Judith, Kathryn Jones, and Rob Baggott. 2004. "Health Consumer Groups in the UK: A New Social Movement?" *Sociology of Health & Illness* 26 (6): 737–56. doi:10.1111/j.0141-9889.2004.00416.x.

American Psychiatric Association (APA). 2000. *Diagnostic and Statistical Manual of Mental Disorders (DSM-IV)*. 4th ed. Washington, DC: American Psychiatric Association.

———. 2013. *Diagnostic and Statistical Manual of Mental Disorders (DSM-5)*. 5th ed. Washington, DC: American Psychiatric Association.

Baert, Patrick, and Fernando Domìnguez Rubio. 2011. *Politics of Knowledge*. London: Routledge.

Beck, Ulrich. 1992. *Risk Society: Towards a New Modernity*. London: Sage.

Berrios, German E. 2006. "'Mind in General' by Sir Alexander Crichton." *History of Psychiatry* 17 (4): 469–86. doi:10.1177/0957154X06071679.

Besoli, Giancarlo, and Daniele Venier. 2003. "Il Disturbo di Attenzione con Iperattività: Indagine Conoscitiva tra i Pediatri di Famiglia in Friuli-Venezia Giulia." *Quaderni acp* 10: 8–9.

Bianchini, Rio, Valentina Postorino, Rita Grasso, Bartolo Santoro, Salvatore Migliore, Corrado Burlò, Carmela Tata, and Luigi Mazzone. 2013. "Prevalence of ADHD in a Sample of Italian Students: A Population-based Study." *Research in Developmental Disabilities* 34 (9): 2543–50. doi:10.1016/j.ridd.2013.05.027.

Bonati, Maurizio. 2007. "Disturbi Mentali e Farmaci: il Caso dell'ADHD e degli Psicostimolanti." *Medico e Bambino* 2: 75–76.

Bonati, Maurizio, and Pietro Panei. 2009. "Il Registro dell'ADHD: lo Stato dell'Arte." *Medico e Bambino* 5: 279–81. http://www.medicoebambino.com/?id=0905_277.pdf.

Bonati, Maurizio, and Laura Reale. 2013. "Reducing Overdiagnosis and Disease Mongering in ADHD in Lombardy." *British Medical Journal* 347. doi: 10.1136/bmj.f7474.

Burman, Erica. 1994. *Deconstructing Developmental Psychology*. London: Routledge.

Camerini, Giovanni Battista, Mauro Coccia, and Ernesto Caffo. 1996. "Il Disturbo da Deficit dell'Attenzione-Iperattivita: Analisi della Frequenza in una Popolazione Scolastica attraverso Questionari agli Insegnanti." *Psichiatria dell'Infanzia e dell'Adolescenza* 63: 587–94.

Capuano, Annalisa, Cristina Scavone, Concetta Rafaniello, Romano Arcieri, Francesco Rossi, and Pietro Panei. 2014. "Atomoxetine in the Treatment of Attention Deficit Hyperactivity Disorder and Suicidal Ideation." *Expert Opinion* 13 (1): S69–S78.

Ciotti, Francesco. 2003. "La Sindrome Ipercinetica 'Pura' fra gli Alunni nel Territorio Cesenate." *Quaderni acp* 10: 18–20.

Clough, Patricia Ticineto. 2007. "Introduction." In *The Affective Turn: Theorizing the Social*, edited by Kim Hosu and Jamie Bianco, 1–33. Durham, NC: Duke University Press.

Conners, Keith. 2007. *Conners' Rating Scales—Revised*. Firenze: Giunti-OS.

Conrad, Peter, and Deborah Potter. 2000. "From Hyperactive Children to ADHD Adults: Observations on the Expansion on Medical Categories." *Social Problems* 47 (4): 559–82. doi:10.2307/3097135.

Corbo, Serenella, Federico Marolla, Vittoria Sarno, Maria Giulia Torrioli, and Silvia Vernacotola. 2003. "Prevalenza dell'ADHD in Bambini Seguiti dal Pediatra di Famiglia." *Medico e Bambino* 1: 22–25.

Costabile, Ernesto, Massimiliano Bugarini, Ilaria Itro, Anne-Laure Knellwolf, Massimo Marzi, Chiara Panci, Pietro Panei, and Romano Arcieri. 2007. "Il Disturbo da Deficit Attentivo con Iperattività (ADHD). La Comunicazione del Problema, il Problema della Comunicazione in Sanità Pubblica." *Notiziario dell'Istituto Superiore di Sanità* 20 (7–8): 12–14. http://www.hepatitis.iss.it/binary/publ/cont/lu-ago .1188907080.pdf#page=12.

Darling, Rosalyn Benjamin. 1988. "Parental Entrepreneurship: A Consumerist Response to Professional Dominance." *Journal of Social Issues* 44 (1): 141–58. doi: 10.1111/j.1540-4560.1988.tb02054.x.

D'Errico, Raffaele, and Enzo Aiello. 2003. "Il Progetto ADHD 'Parents for Parents.'" *Medico e Bambino* 22: 25–32. http://www.medicoebambino.com/?id=0301_15.pdf.

Didoni, Anna, Marco Sequi, Pietro Panei, Maurizio Bonati, and the Lombardy ADHD Registry Group. 2011. "Lombardy ADHD Registry Group: One-year Prospective Follow-up of Pharmacological Treatment in Children with Attention-Deficit/Hyperactivity Disorder." *European Journal of Clinical Pharmacology* 67: 1061–67. doi:10.1007/s00228-011-1050-3.

Di Trani, Michela, Stefano Marinucci, and Daniela Tortolani. 2012. "Il Modello Analitico di Fronte alla Diagnosi di Disturbo da Deficit dell'Attenzione ed Iperattività." *Psicobiettivo* 2: 40–56.

Dreyfuss, Rochelle Cooper, and Dorothy Nelkin. 1992. "The Genetics of Jurisprudence." *Vanderbildt Law Review* 45: 313–48.

Fine, Michelle. 2012. "Troubling Calls for Evidence: A Critical Race, Class and Gender Analysis of Whose Evidence Counts." *Feminism & Psychology* 22 (1): 3–19. doi:10.1177/0959353511435475.

Finn, Janet L., Lynn M. Nybell, and Jeffrey J. Shook. 2010. "The Meaning and Making of Childhood in the Era of Globalization: Challenges for Social Work." *Children and Youth Services Review* 32 (2): 246–54. doi:10.1016/j.childyouth.2009.09.003.

Frazzetto, Giovanni, Sinéad Keenan, and Ilina Singh. 2007. "'I Bambini e le Droghe': The Right to Ritalin vs the Right to Childhood in Italy." *BioSocieties* 2 (4): 393–412. doi:10.1017/S1745855207005844.

Frigerio, Alessandra. 2013. "Discourses of Risk, Blame and Legitimation: The Social Construction of Attention Deficit/Hyperactivity Disorder." PhD diss., Università degli Studi di Milano Bicocca.

Frigerio, Alessandra, and Lorenzo Montali. 2015. "An Ethnographic-Discursive Approach to Parental Self-Help Groups: The Case of ADHD." *Qualitative Health Research*. doi:10.1177/1049732315586553.

Frigerio, Alessandra, Lorenzo Montali, and Michelle Fine. 2013a. "Attention Deficit/Hyperactivity Disorder Blame Game: A Study on the Positioning of Professionals, Teachers and Parents." *Health: An Interdisciplinary Journal for the Social Study of Health, Illness and Medicine* 17 (6): 584–604. doi:10.1177/1363459312472083.

———. 2013b. "Risky and At-risk Subjects: The Discursive Positioning of the ADHD Child in the Italian Context." *Biosocieties* 8 (3): 245–64. doi:10.1057/biosoc.2013.19.

Frigerio, Alessandra, Lorenzo Montali, and Gian Marco Marzocchi. 2014. "Italian Teachers' Knowledge and Perception of Attention Deficit/Hyperactivity Disorder (ADHD)." *International Journal of School & Educational Psychology* 2 (2): 126–36. doi:10.1080/21683603.2013.878677.

Frigerio, Alessandra, Paola Rucci, Robert Goodman, Massimo Ammaniti, Ombretta Carlet, et al. 2009. "Prevalence and Correlates of Mental Disorders among Adolescents in Italy: The PrISMA Study." *European Child and Adolescent Psychiatry* 18: 217–26. doi:10.1007/s00787-008-0720-x.

Galasiński, Dariusz. 2011. "The Patient's World: Discourse Analysis and Ethnography." *Critical Discourse Studies* 8 (4): 253–65. doi:10.1080/17405904.2011.601634.

Gallucci, Franco, Hector R. Bird, Carla Berardi, Virgilio Gallai, Pietro Pfanner, and Alain Weinberg. 1993. "Symptoms of Attention Deficit Hyperactivity Disorder in an Italian School Sample: Findings of a Pilot Study." *Journal of the American Academy of Child & Adolescent Psychiatry* 32: 1051–58. doi:10.1097/00004583-199309000-00026.

Germinario, Elena A. P., Romano Arcieri, Maurizio Bonati, Alessandro Zuddas, Gabriele Masi, Stefano Vella, Flavia Chiarotti, Pietro Panei, and the Italian ADHD Regional Reference Centers. 2013. "Attention-Deficit/Hyperactivity Disorder Drugs and Growth: An Italian Prospective Observational Study." *Journal of Child and Adolescent Psychopharmacology* 23 (7): 440–47. doi:10.1089/cap.2012.0086.

Giù le mani dai bambini. 2007. "Allarme Reintroduzione Ritalin: Dichiarazione di Esperti e Parlamentari." http://www.giulemanidaibambini.it/stampa/glm_pressrelease__7.pdf.

———. 2005. "Consensus Internazionale: ADHD ed Abuso nella Prescrizione di Psico-farmaci ai Minori." http://www.giulemanidaibambini.org/consensus/.

Hansen, Dana Lee, and Ebba Holme Hansen. 2006. "Caught in a Balancing Act: Parents' Dilemmas Regarding Their ADHD Child's Treatment with Stimulant Medication." *Qualitative Health Research* 16 (9): 1267–85. doi:10.1177/1049732306292543.

Harborne, Alexandra, Miranda Wolpert, and Linda Clare. 2004. "Making Sense of ADHD: A Battle for Understanding? Parents' Views of Their Children Being Diagnosed with ADHD." *Clinical Child Psychology and Psychiatry* 9 (3): 327–39. doi:10.1177/1359104504043915.

Hilton, Sean, and Henry B. Slotnick. 2005. "Proto-professionalism: How Professionalism Occurs across the Continuum of Medical Education." *Medical Education* 39 (1): 58–65. doi:10.1111/j.1365-2929.2004.02033.x.

Horton-Salway, Mary. 2011. "Repertoires of ADHD in UK Newspaper Media." *Health* 15 (5): 533–49. doi:10.1177/1363459310389626.

Hughes, Leslye. 1999. "How Professionals Perceive AD/HD." In *ADHD: Research, Practice and Opinion*, edited by Paul Cooper and Katherine Bilton, 187–202. London: Whurr.

Istituto Superiore di Sanità (ISS). 2003. "Conferenza Nazionale di Consenso: Indicazioni e strategie terapeutiche per i bambini e gli adolescenti con disturbo da deficit attentivo e iperattività. Cagliari, 6–7 Marzo 2003." http://www.iss.it/binary/wpop/cont/ADHD%20Conf%20Naz%20Consenso%20Cagliari%202003.1174561972.pdf.

———. 2007. "Protocollo diagnostico e terapeutico della sindrome da iperattività e deficit di attenzione per il registro nazionale ADHD." http://www.iss.it/binary/adhd/cont/Protocollo%20diagnostico%20ADHD%20020507.1178184452.pdf.

———. 2012. "Newsletter del Registro Italiano dell'ADHD." http://www.iss.it/binary/adhd/cont/ADHD_Newsletter_Luglio_2012_Curva_arruolamento_2012.pdf.

Jackson, Stevi, and Sue Scott. 1999. "Risk Anxiety and the Social Construction of Childhood." In *Risk and Sociocultural Theory: New Directions and Perspective*, edited by Deborah Lupton, 86–107. Cambridge: Cambridge Press University.

Kaufman, Joan, Borsi Birmaher, Uma Rao, and Neal Ryan. 2004. *K-SADS-PL: Diagnostic Interview for Assessment of Psychopathological Disorders in Children and Adolescents.* Trento: Erickson.

Kildea, Sarah, John Wright, and Julie Davies. 2011. "Making Sense of ADHD in Practice: A Stakeholder Review." *Clinical Child Psychology and Psychiatry* 16 (4): 599–619. doi:10.1177/1359104510390428.

Knellwolf, Anne-Laure, Jean Deligne, Flavia Chiarotti, Guy-Robert Auleley, Serena Palmieri, Claudine Blum Voisgard, Pietro Panei, and Elisabeth Autret-Leca. 2008. "Prevalence and Patterns of Methylphenidate Use in French Children and Adolescents." *European Journal of Clinical Pharmacology* 64: 311–17. doi:10.1007/s00228-007-0401-6.

Knellwolf, Anne-Laure, Pietro Panei, Romano Arcieri, and Stefano Vella. 2006. "Failure to Diagnose ADHD Correctly Puts Children in Danger." *Italian Journal of Pediatrics* 32: 136–37.

Lafrance, Michelle N., and Suzanne McKenzie-Mohr. 2013. "The DSM and Its Lure of Legitimacy." *Feminism & Psychology* 23 (1): 119–40. doi:10.1177/0959353512467974.

Lakoff, Andrew. 2000. "Adaptive Will: The Evolution of Attention Deficit Disorder." *Journal of the History of the Behavioral Sciences* 36 (2): 149–69.

Lambruschi, Furio, and Riccardo Bertaccini. 2012. "Presa in Carico di Casi Clinici nei Servizi ASL: l'ADHD in un'Ottica Cognitivo-Evolutiva." In *Prendersi Cura dei Bambini e dei loro Genitori*, edited by Loredana Cena, Antonio Imbasciati, and Franco Baldoni, 253–72. Milan: Springer.

Landzelius, Kyra. 2006. "Introduction: Patient Organization Movements and New Metamorphoses in Patienthood." *Social Science & Medicine* 62 (3): 529–37. doi:10.1016/j.socscimed.2005.06.023.

Leone, Antonio. 2012. "I Figli Irrequieti di una Società Irrequieta: L'Iperattività." *Minorigiustizia* 3: 287–90. doi:10.3280/MG2012-003036.

Lubeck, Sally, and Patricia Garrett. 1990. "The Social Construction of the 'At Risk' Child." *British Journal of Sociology and Education* 11 (3): 327–40. doi:10.1080/0142569900110305.

Macey, David. 2000. *Dictionary of Critical Theory*. London: Penguin.

Marzocchi, GianMarco, Anna M. Re, and Cesare Cornoldi. 2010. *Batteria Italiana per l'ADHD: BIA*. Trento: Erickson.

Maschietto, Dino, Elisabetta Baioni, Claudio Vio, Federica Novello, Elena A. P. Germinario, Federica M. Regini, and Pietro Panei. 2012. "Prevalenza dell'ADHD in una Popolazione Pediatrica e sua Esposizione al Trattamento Psico-comportamentale e Farmacologico." *Medico e Bambino* 15 (10). http://www.medicoebambino.com/?id=RIC1210_10.html.

Massumi, Brian. 2010. "The Future Birth of the Affective Fact: The Political Ontology of Threat." In *The Affect Theory Reader*, edited by Gregory J. Seigworth and Melissa Gregg, 52–70. Durham, NC: Duke University Press.

Mayes, Rick, Catherine Bagwell, and Jennifer Erkulwater. 2008. "ADHD and the Rise in Stimulant Use among Children." *Harvard Review of Psychiatry* 16 (3): 151–66. doi:10.1080/10673220802167782.

Mazzotta, Silvia, Beatrice Gallai, Riccarda D'Angelo, and Giovanni Mazzotta. 2008. "Impatto Economico del Disturbo da Deficit dell'Attenzione e Iperattività nella Popolazione Umbra." *Giornale di neuropsichiatria dell'età evolutiva* 28: 45–56. http://www.iss.it/binary/uvco/cont/Mazzotta%20Impatto%20economico%20ADHD.1234945781.pdf.

Ministero dell'Instruzione, dell'Università e della Ricerca (MIUR). 2010. "Disturbi da Deficit di Attenzione e Iperattività." http://www.iss.it/binary/wpop/cont/circolare_ADHD_MIUR_2010.pdf.

Mugnaini, Daniela, Gabriele Masi, Paola Brovedani, Chiara Chelazzi, Marzenka Matas, Caterina Romagnoli, and Alessandro Zuddas. 2006. "Teacher Reports of ADHD Symptoms in Italian Children at the End of First Grade." *European Psychiatry* 21 (6): 419–26. doi:10.1016/j.eurpsy.2005.04.011.

Novas, Carlos, and Nikolas Rose. 2000. "Genetic Risk and the Birth of the Somatic Individual." *Economy and Society* 29 (4): 485–513. doi:10.1080/03085140050174750.

Nybell, Lynn. 2001. "Meltdowns and Containments: Constructions of Children at Risk as Complex System." *Childhood: A Global Journal of Child Research* 8 (2): 213–30. doi:10.1177/0907568201008002005.

Paiano, Angela, Elena Boatto, Anna Maria Re, Emilia Ferruzza, and Cesare Cornoldi. 2012. "I Gruppi Cognitivo-Emotivo-Relazionali CERG: Una Sperimentazione con Genitori di Bambini con ADHD." *Disturbi di attenzione e iperattività* 8 (1): 33–54.

Panei, Pietro, Romano Arcieri, Stefano Vella, Maurizio Bonati, Nello Martini, and Alessandro Zuddas. 2004. "Italian Attention-Deficit/Hyperactivity Disorder Registry." *Pediatrics* 114: 514. doi:10.3280/PSOB2012-002003.

Pardeck, John T., and John W. Murphy. 1993. "Postmodernism and Clinical Practice: A Critical Analysis of the Disease Model." *Psychological Reports* 72: 1187–94.

Pezzicca, Sara, Federica Carli, Stefano Berloffa, Roberto Segala, and Giuseppe Capovilla. 2011. "Un Training Autoregolativo di Gruppo per Bambini con ADHD: Un'Osservazione Cognitiva, Comportamentale e Relazionale." *Psicologia clinica dello sviluppo* 15 (2): 479–87. doi:10.1449/35345.

Pica-Smith, Cinzia, and Carmen Veloria. 2012. "'At Risk Means a Minority Kid': Deconstructing Deficit Discourses in the Study of Risk in Education and Human Services." *Pedagogy and the Human Sciences* 1 (2): 33–48. http://www.pedagogyandhumanscience.org/files/Pica-Smith_Veloria_PHSv2.pdf.

Rabeharisoa, Vololona. 2003. "The Struggle against Neuromuscular Diseases in France and the Emergence of the 'Partnership Model' of Patient Organisation." *Social Science & Medicine* 57 (11): 2127–36. doi:10.1016/S0277-9536(03)00084-4.

Reale, Laura, Michele Zanetti, Massimo Cartabia, Filomena Fortinguerra, and Maurizio Bonati. 2014. "Due Anni di Attività del Registro ADHD della Regione Lombardia: Analisi dei Percorsi di Cura Diagnostici e Terapeutici." *Ricerca & Pratica* 30: 198–211.

Rose, Nikolas. 2003. "Neurochemical Selves." *Society* 41 (1): 46–59.

Ruggiero, Simona, Concetta Rafaniello, Carmela Bravaccio, Giampina Grimaldi, Rosario Granato, Antonio Pascotto, Liberata Sportiello, Elisabetta Parretta, Barbara Rinaldi, Pietro Panei, Francesco Rossi, and Annalisa Capuano. 2012. "Safety of Attention-Deficit/Hyperactivity Disorder Medications in Children: An Intensive Pharmacosurveillance Monitoring Study." *Journal of Child and Adolescent Psychopharmacology* 22 (6): 415–22.

Ryan, Sara, and Katherine Runswick Cole. 2009. "From Advocate to Activist? Mapping the Experiences of Mothers of Children on the Autism Spectrum." *Journal of Applied Research in Intellectual Disabilities* 22 (1): 43–53. doi: 10.1111/j.1468-3148.2008.00438.x.

Sarno, Vittoria. 2003. "Il Pediatra alle Prese con i Problemi Psicorelazionali: Uno Studio Pilota." *Medico e Bambino* 1: 9–12.

Singh, Ilina. 2011. "A Disorder of Anger and Aggression: Children's Perspectives on Attention Deficit/Hyperactivity Disorder in the UK." *Social Science & Medicine* 73 (6): 889–96. doi:10.1016/j.socscimed.2011.03.049.

———. 2004. "Doing Their Jobs: Mothering with Ritalin in a Culture of Mother-Blame." *Social Science & Medicine* 59 (6): 1193–1205. doi: 10.1016/j.socscimed.2004.01.011.

———. 2006. "A Framework for Understanding Trends in ADHD Diagnoses and Stimulant Drug Treatment: Schools and Schooling as a Case Study." *BioSocieties* 1 (4): 439–52. doi:http://dx.doi.org/10.1017/S1745855206004054.

Società Italiana di neuropsichiatria dell'infanzia e dell'adolescenza (SINPIA). 2002. "Linee-Guida per la Diagnosi e la Terapia Farmacologica del Disturbo da Deficit Attentivo con Iperattività (ADHD) in Età Evolutiva." http://www.iss.it/binary/wpop/cont/SINPIA_L.g.ADHD.1116940207.pdf.

Stainton-Rogers, Rex, and Wendy Stainton-Rogers. 1992. *Stories of Childhood: Shifting Agendas in Child Concern*. Hemel Hempstead: Harvester Wheatsheaf.

World Health Organization (WHO). 2010. *International Classification of Diseases (ICD-10)*. 10th ed. Geneva: World Health Organization.

12

The French ADHD Landscape

Maintaining and Dealing with Multiple Uncertainties

Madeleine Akrich
Vololona Rabeharisoa

In 2009, a scientific symposium entitled "Confronting European Practices on ADHD" was held in Paris. Organized conjointly by HyperSupers (the main advocacy group for French patients and families affected by ADHD) and ADHD Europe (the main European ADHD advocacy organization), the conference attracted several world-renowned specialists such as Aribert Rothenberger, Eric Taylor, and Tobias Banaschewski. The event served as a platform for some French participants to publicly voice their concerns: Franck Baylé, a psychiatrist, stated that "the [French] situation can be considered dramatic," and Diane Purper Ouakil, another psychiatrist, declared that in France "treatments prescribed to children have not been evaluated nor their efficacy proven" and criticized the French academic community for failing to contribute to research on this topic and provide medical education on ADHD (HyperSupers and CPPS 2010). In a conversation with Christine Gétin, the president of HyperSupers, one of the eminent foreign guests, joked: "I thought that France was years behind. I was wrong. France is only fifteen years behind" (interview).

These observations are not new; in the early 2000s, Carla Sept, a mother of a child with ADHD, posted the following excerpt on her website:

Applied research on neurological problems such as dyslexia, dysphasia, and of course hyperactivity barely exists. Professionals work in their own corners without sharing their knowledge and practices. Speech pathologists don't like neurologists intruding into their domain and think they know best. Psychiatrists think that they can take charge of everything and continue to apply psychoanalytical theories without taking neuroscience into consideration. Teachers distrust speech pathologists . . . and the latter often criticize educational methods and think they are forced to do teachers' jobs.[1]

The fact that France is lagging behind other European countries in the field of ADHD is often pointed to, in both lay and expert discourses. However, this "backwardness" rhetoric overlooks the transformation of the French ADHD landscape over the past 15 years. The purpose of this chapter is to document the emergence of ADHD as a public issue in France in the late 1990s and to examine how this issue has evolved since then. To describe this process, we analyze the content of 13 official reports commissioned by French institutions from 1999 to 2014. This choice was motivated by several factors. First, these reports (almost one each year on average) enable us to precisely follow the evolution of the conceptualization of ADHD and the elaboration of concrete solutions to the difficulties encountered by children with the disorder. Second, these reports are the outcomes of collective work, involving different proportions of representatives of all concerned actors: psychiatrists, neurologists, psychologists, patients and parents, the Ministère de la Santé, the Ministère de l'Education, the Comité Interministériel du Handicap (CIH), and so forth. Third, the drafting and publication of a number of these reports have provoked heated debates, evidenced by the significant number of press articles in which people have commented or taken positions. Finally, these reports provide crucial empirical data on the articulation between scientific knowledge and the politics of care related to ADHD.

Our analysis leads us to three main observations. First, specialists from a variety of disciplines, ranging from neurology to neuropsychiatry, neuropediatrics, child psychiatry, psychology, and the cognitive sciences, participated in expert groups mobilized by French institutions. In contrast to the situation described by the mother on her website, the French field of expertise on ADHD can no longer be reduced to psychoanalytical theories versus the neurosciences. Second, the psychodynamic approach to ADHD that prevailed in the early 2000s in France now coexists with multiple conceptions of the disorder and has even become somewhat marginalized based on the content of the reports we studied. Moreover, as a result of extensive public debate on ADHD, the condition has come to be viewed as a serious disorder, the causes and consequences of which have sparked much discussion. Third, professionals, public authorities, and families today confront difficulties in translating the acknowledged complexity of ADHD into solutions, which requires cooperation between the health system and the school system.

In this chapter, we present these findings in detail. First, we describe the French context, particularly the alleged historical "backwardness" with regard to ADHD, and we provide evidence on the need for a nuanced appreciation of the French situation. Second, we present our empirical material. Drawing on this material, we then explain the formation and consolidation of epistemic communities on ADHD and the problematization of ADHD as a multifaceted, complex condition. Finally, we explore the politics of caring for a person with ADHD and the organizational challenges it presents.

The Unique ADHD Landscape in France
THE BELATED EMERGENCE OF ADHD AS A SCIENTIFIC AND PUBLIC ISSUE IN FRANCE

L'hyperactivité chez l'enfant, edited by Michel Dugas in 1987, was the first book published in France on hyperactivity disorder—what is now known as ADHD. Dugas's professional identity is a bit fuzzy: sometimes he is portrayed as a psychiatrist and a professor of child psychopathology (Tremblay 1987), and at other times he is portrayed as a neuropediatrician (Zarifian 2003). This hybrid identity is symptomatic of the way ADHD emerged in France, at the crossroads of neurology and psychiatry (see below). In any case, Dugas is considered to be the one who pioneered an understanding of ADHD in France: "in the Anglo-Saxon meaning of the term, i.e., as a disease in relation with a neurobiological dysfunction, whereas the French tendency was directed towards an all-psychological approach" (Lecendreux 2013).

Whatever perspective one takes when approaching the issue, one is confronted with convergent facts and figures. It was only during the first half of the 2000s that scientific efforts on ADHD took off in France, at the same time as in Spain and the Netherlands, but 6 to 8 years later than in Germany and England, and 10 years later than in the United States. Although French research efforts had increased significantly, they remained quite modest compared to all of these countries (see fig. 12.1). Public attention to ADHD followed more or less the same pattern, as evidenced by the number of press articles on the subject (see fig. 12.2). HyperSupers, the main advocacy group for French patients and families affected by ADHD, was founded in 2002 by parents who were regular participants in an

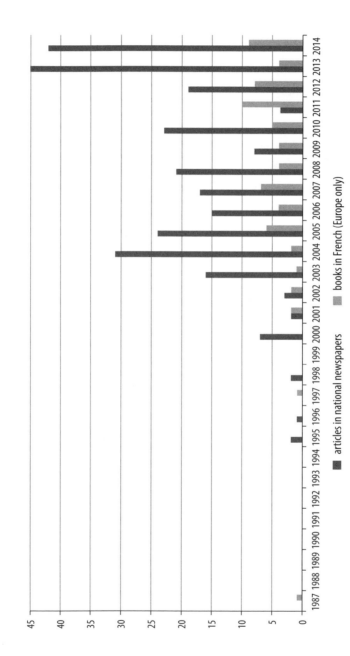

Fig. 12.1. Books and newspaper articles on hyperactivity and attention deficit in the French national press.
Source: Bibliothèque Nationale de France, ©Europresse

articles in national newspapers   books in French (Europe only)

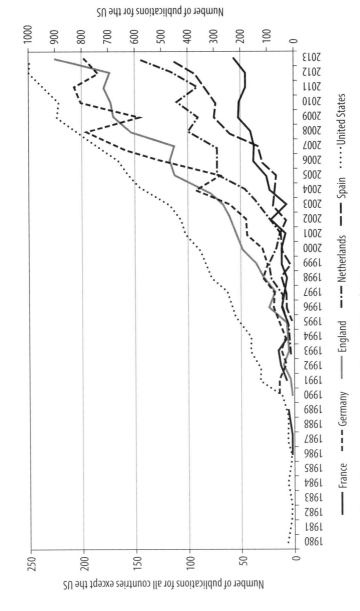

Fig. 12.2. Scientific publications on ADHD. *Source:* Web of Science

Internet discussion group created two years earlier. HyperSupers has contributed significantly to raising public awareness of ADHD (Edwards et al. 2014). As far as medications are concerned, sales of methylphenidate have risen from around 50,000 boxes in 2000 to 280,000 boxes in 2008 and 500,000 in 2013 (ANSM 2013; Proust 2014), an increase that has generated numerous comments in the press. Finally, ADHD has been discussed in a dozen official reports from 1999 to 2014.

Taken together, these facts and figures reveal the belated emergence of ADHD as a scientific and public issue in France. However, the consolidation of ADHD in the public space was not a smooth process since it involved divergent conceptions of the disorder and of the ways it should be treated. Of particular importance were the fierce opposition of some psychiatrists with psychodynamic backgrounds to neurobiological approaches to ADHD and the demonization of medications in public discourses.

THE CHANGING ADHD LANDSCAPE IN FRANCE

For many psychiatrists, the symptoms associated with ADHD were, and still are, either signs of psychological suffering or reactions to social and parenting dynamics. They believe that prescribing methylphenidate is not the answer to the problem because it shifts the focus away from the search for psychological explanations (Vallée 2011). In 2005, Bernard Golse, head of the psychiatry unit at a Parisian children's hospital, declared: "With Ritalin®, the mystery remains unsolved since the meaning of the disorder still has to be worked out in regard to each child's history" (*Le Monde* 2005).

Ritalin has been a "fixation abscess" in public discourses on ADHD. Apparently, it has been prescribed in France for ADHD since the 1980s in the child psychiatry unit (Wodon 2009) headed by Michel Dugas, though its use was limited until the past 10 years. Indeed, obtaining methylphenidate in France is complicated because it is on the list of regulated narcotic drugs; after the first prescription is ordered by a hospital specialist, it is re-prescribed every 28 days by the attending physician and each year by the specialist. As a consequence, many who use methylphenidate have been criticized and even demonized: many parents described the horrified reactions of pharmacists who proceeded to lecture them on their parental duties after being given methylphenidate prescriptions to fill. As the "symbol of all of the drug options in child psychiatry" (*Libération* 2013), methylphenidate is invariably associated with what is viewed as the ideological foundation of American child psychiatry—medicalization, which turns a social or a political issue into a medical one, eventually leading to the individualization and de-politicization of the issue at stake (Conrad 1975).

Despite ongoing tensions between psychodynamic-oriented psychiatrists and other specialists, the ADHD landscape in France has changed considerably over the past 15 years. An examination of press articles on this topic over the period reveals that two-thirds of the papers published between 1998 and 2004 expressed doubts about the reality of ADHD, with one paper even ironically calling the disorder "American democratic disability" (ADD) (Petitnicolas 1998). In contrast, between 2005 and 2012, three-fourths of the papers no longer denied the existence of ADHD and often described the condition from a neurobiological perspective. In short, ADHD has been progressively recognized as a disorder in its own right in the media.

An additional change is the progressive installation of methylphenidate in the French ADHD landscape. A report issued in 2013 by the Agence Nationale de la Sécurité des Médicaments (ANSM) showed significant growth in the consumption of methylphenidate since 2004, rising from a defined daily dose (DDD) of 0.01 per 1,000 inhabitants in 1996 to 0.18 in 2005 and 0.43 in 2012. Despite this increase, however, the use of methylphenidate remains limited as compared with its use in most countries, especially the top-ranking ones: Iceland (13.5 DDD), Canada (11.7 DDD), and the United States (9.12 DDD). Finally, changes also have occurred in medical practices and in public policies, as the reports we studied demonstrate.

How can one make sense of these transformations? Our contention is that the work undertaken by various groups of experts and the public debates they have induced have contributed to reshaping the French landscape of ADHD and facilitated a new scientific and public understanding of the disorder.

Empirical Material

We examined 13 official reports on ADHD that were published between 1999 and 2014. We selected these 13 documents because they explicitly refer to each other, offering insight into the progressive ordering of issues related to ADHD. These reports were commissioned by different institutions and were targeted to a variety of audiences.

The first document, a publication from the Haut Comité de la Santé Publique (HCSP), is not a report per se, but a 40-page dossier on learning impairments, with a special section on ADHD (Vaivre-Douret and Tursz 1999). This document targets actors in the public health sector. In 2000 and 2001, the Ministère de la

Santé and the Ministère de l'Education conjointly commissioned two reports on dysphasia and dyslexia: the first one described the current state of knowledge and practices (Ringard 2000), whereas the second one defined a national plan for children with specific language impairments (Veber and Ringard 2001). Between 2002 and 2009, the Institut National de la Santé et de la Recherche Médicale (INSERM) published four *expertises collectives* (collective expertise reports) on topics including ADHD. They were commissioned by a French social insurance fund with the following aims: (1) to improve the screening and prevention of mental disorders (INSERM 2002) and conduct disorder (INSERM 2005) and to foster the understanding of learning impairments (INSERM 2007); and (2) to provide ideas on how to best help children with these disorders, especially with regard to systematic health assessments and risk factor identification and screening (INSERM 2009). In the years that followed, three reports were published by committees set up by either the Ministère de la Santé, the Ministère de l'Education, or both: (1) a report defining and classifying "cognitive disabilities" (Cecchi Tenerini 2010); (2) e-learning modules on learning impairments and conduct disorder for teachers (EDUSCOL 2012); and (3) a position paper[2] on the organization of screening and provision for children with learning impairments (Commission Nationale de la Naissance et de la Santé de l'Enfant 2013). As mentioned previously, a report on the use of methylphenidate was issued in 2013 by the ANSM at HyperSupers' request. Also at the request of HyperSupers and a sister organization (HAS 2012), a document defining actions to be implemented for children and teenagers with ADHD was published by the Haute Autorité de la Santé (HAS) in 2015. Finally, at the time of the writing of this chapter, the Caisse nationale de solidarité pour l'autonomie (CNSA) was creating a guide[3] to help its professionals manage learning disabilities that was eventually released in 2014.

Collectively, the reports we studied have two main features around which we develop the remaining sections of this chapter. First, with the notable exception of the HAS framework plan for ADHD guidelines, ADHD was not an exclusive focus in any of the other reports. ADHD surfaced in various contexts, sometimes quite marginally, at other times more explicitly, and especially for the last reports, as a result of active lobbying by ADHD advocacy organizations. When scrutinizing the contents of the documents, one is struck by the uncertain positioning of ADHD either within or spanning different categories of disorders—namely, mental disorders, conduct disorders, learning impairments, specific language impairments, and cognitive disabilities. This elusiveness of ADHD was a major preoccupation for members of several expert groups, who continually discussed the nature of the disorder—its causes and effects, its significant manifestations, and the mechanisms underlying its "natural history." This questioning is particularly prominent in the INSERM reports on mental disorders, conduct disorders, and learning impairments, which were based exclusively on the collective expertise of academics, in contrast to the reports published by other expert groups, which included other concerned actors. We devote a section of this chapter to this enduring problematization of ADHD as an unsettled condition, which in turn leads experts to question the very nature of a series of disorders with which it is supposedly associated.

Second, there is a massive difference between the reports that question what ADHD is and the reports that reflect on what to do for the people affected by ADHD (children and families) or for those implicated in the management of the disorder (teachers, health professionals, etc.). As stated previously, in the reports focused on the nature of ADHD, experts seem to be trapped by the complexity of the disorder and fail to provide conclusive answers to the questions posed by the institutions that commissioned the reports. In contrast, in the reports focused on finding solutions for those struggling with ADHD, experts put aside the multiple uncertainties about the definition of the disorder, and rather reflected on how to mutually accommodate ADHD within the existing health and school systems. These reports highlight the deficiencies of the health and school systems when confronting complex and uncertain conditions, as much as scrutinize how ADHD experts and decision makers "act in an uncertain world," to borrow from Callon, Lascoumes, and Barthe (2009). In the final section, we explore the problematization of ADHD as a difficult-to-treat condition that challenges the translation of knowledge into action.

The Problematization of ADHD as an Unsettled Condition

In this section, we concentrate on how reports produced by a multidisciplinary community of experts on ADHD and associated conditions address the question: what is ADHD? Notably, the formation and consolidation of this community of experts was not based on a convergent appraisal of ADHD. Experts did not start with "ADHD" as a category to be explored; rather, drawing on their disciplinary backgrounds and preoccupations, they mobilized categories such as "conduct disorder," "mental disorders," and "learning impairments," and they questioned whether and how an entity named ADHD might fit into the picture. As multiple framings of ADHD were debated, it became clear that the epidemiology of ADHD is as elusive as its natural history and categorization, not only for social scientists, but also for specialists, professionals, and families. Thus, these reports enable us to show that ADHD is not only an unsettled condition in France but is also an "interactive kind" (Hacking 1999) that reopens epistemic and ontological questions about a set of disorders.

The Constitution of a Community of Experts on ADHD and Associated Conditions

The reports we studied do not simply constitute a list of independent, disconnected documents. As shown in figure 12.3, they cite each other. This might be related to the fact that the compositions of the different working groups partially overlapped. Over the years, it seems that these experts progressively formed a community with all of the characteristics that Haas (1992: 3) associated with an epistemic community—that is, "a network of professionals with recognized expertise and competence in a particular domain and an authoritative claim to policy relevant knowledge within that domain or issue-area." This epistemic community did not represent all the scientists, clinicians, and professionals who either worked on or manifested an interest in ADHD and associated conditions; some trenchantly opposed the conclusions of other reports, as will be shown. Rather, this community was a group of people from heterogeneous backgrounds with occasionally conflicting views that was conferred epistemic credentials by institutions and public authorities and struggled to put various conditions, including ADHD, on the political agenda.

To visualize this network of expertise related to ADHD, we listed all individuals who participated in the writing of the reports, and we mapped co-authorship among all these individuals (fig. 12.4). For the sake of clarity, we grouped the reports into four categories: (1) the INSERM report on mental disorders and (2) conduct disorder; (3) various reports on learning impairments; and (4) the HAS guidelines on ADHD. About 60% of all academic experts who took part in producing the various reports are represented on this map, which shows that there indeed exists a community of experts who have multiple bonds with each other. The map also helps distinguish two groups. The first group is mainly composed of psychiatrists who were involved in the reports on mental disorders and conduct disorder. The second group is mainly composed of neurologists who worked on the reports on learning impairments. A few individuals from the two groups helped create the HAS guidelines on ADHD; this provides at least some evidence of the positioning of ADHD at the crossroads of neurology and psychiatry, and as

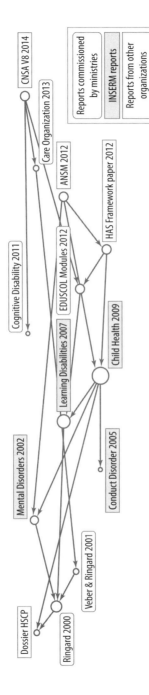

Fig. 12.3. Citation links between the reports.

Legend:
- Reports commissioned by ministries
- INSERM reports
- Reports from other organizations

Node labels:
- CNSA V8 2014
- Care Organization 2013
- ANSM 2012
- HAS Framework paper 2012
- Cognitive Disability 2011
- EDUSCOL Modules 2012
- Learning Disabilities 2007
- Child Health 2009
- Mental Disorders 2002
- Conduct Disorder 2005
- Veber & Ringard 2001
- Dossier HSCP
- Ringard 2000

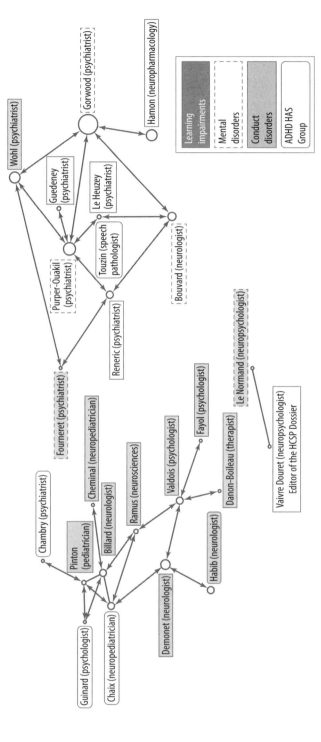

Fig. 12.4. Co-authorships within the expert groups and HyperSupers scientific network.

spanning different conditions—mental disorders, conduct disorder, and learning impairments—at least in this network of expertise. A qualitative analysis of the content of the reports confirms this observation.

ADHD, a Disorder with "Multiple Personalities"

The existence of this epistemic community does not imply that members used a straightforward and consensual definition of ADHD. Actually, until the mid-2000s, most efforts were aimed at identifying the nature of the disorder. Some of these efforts to precisely define ADHD are revealed in descriptions of the disorder that use a variety of competing labels referring to multiple conditions. The question "What is ADHD?" was core to many of the reports we studied.

The variety of labels used in the reports strikingly reveals the uncertainties that prevailed at the time. Although the term "attention deficit/hyperactivity disorder" was specifically used in the dossier published by the HCSP in 1999, a dozen different terms were used to describe the condition in the 2002 INSERM report on mental disorders. In the chapter on epidemiology, experts related these terms to various classifications and epistemic traditions: "hyperkinetic syndrome in the European tradition," "ADDH attention deficit disorder with hyperactivity in the DSM III," "attention deficit/hyperactivity disorders ADHD in the DSM IV," and "hyperkinetic syndrome and attention deficit hyperactivity disorder in the ICD10." In other chapters, new terms appeared, sometimes without references to existing classifications: "attention deficit with hyperactivity/without hyperactivity," "hyperactivity-attention deficit," "hyperactivity disorder with attention deficit," "psychomotor instability," and "minimal brain dysfunction." Thus, through the listing of these terms, the report synthesized the history of ADHD (Conrad 1975; Rafalovich 2001; Singh 2002) without contextualizing it. The report did not make any decisions about the term that should be used; this probably indicates a lack of consensus within the group and even a confrontational atmosphere (Schmit 2007).

At about the same time, a special issue of *Le Carnet Psy* was published on unstable children. In its introduction entitled "Instability of the Instability," the editor (Joly 2003: 78) commented on this multiplicity: "There might be as many instabilities as unstable subjects, and we may use the label ADHD or hyperactive to talk of very diverse children . . . although they display . . . the much talked-about triptych hyperkinesis, inattention and impulsivity." In this issue, maintaining this multiplicity appears to be a way to preserve a plurality of approaches, including psychoanalysis, and to encompass the "pervasive hegemonic trend of the

American DSM IV" (Joly 2003: 78). The issue therefore managed to provide a platform for debate. Some people such as Bernard Golse (2003: 26) remained firmly rooted in their psychodynamic positions. He declared: "Giving up on words, one eventually gives up on ideas . . . Giving up on theories, one eventually gives up on practices." Others, however, called for an integrated approach to ADHD: "Investigating child hyperactivity with a complex psychopathological perspective may result in more than a dispute between schools of thought: a deep reflection on a psychopathology that would neither ignore psychoanalytical intelligence . . . nor the neuro-bio-physiological substrate of any human singularity" (Joly 2003: 78).

The variety of terms decreased in subsequent documents and eventually converged around TDAH (trouble déficit de l'attention/hyperactivité, the French equivalent of ADHD), after a period when THADA (trouble hyperactivité avec déficit de l'attention) prevailed. Thus, the focus moved from hyperactivity—the most disputed concept—to attention deficit. Even psychodynamic-oriented psychiatrists have come to use the term "TDAH," although some limited variability remains in the psychodynamic literature (e.g., "psychomotor instability" [Metz and Thévenot 2010] and "hyperkinetic disorder" [Raffy 2006]). The use of such terms always manifests a contestation of what "ADHD" entails.

Indeed, beyond the "naming" question, the definition of ADHD itself was at the heart of a number of reports, especially those published by INSERM. Two main questions were discussed: (1) To what category of disorders should ADHD be attached? and (2) What are the links between ADHD and other disorders such as learning impairments and conduct disorder? It seems that each of the three INSERM reports constituted a site of problematization within which ADHD was positioned in a specific way. Whereas mental disorders, conduct disorder, and learning impairments supposedly constitute more or less exclusive categories, ADHD was the only disorder considered in each of the three categories/reports.[4] Strikingly, in the 2002 INSERM report on mental disorders, ADHD was considered to be both a learning impairment (in the section entitled "Biological and Cognitive Approach") and a category of its own, deserving a special subsection (in the section entitled "Clinical Approach"). Moreover, the issue of the uniqueness and multiplicity of ADHD was raised in the same report in relation to the various associations of THADA with other disorders:

> THADA is barely isolated. International epidemiological studies have shown a
> very high comorbidity, since more than half of children with THADA have

received at least one additional diagnosis, especially a conduct disorder, an oppositional disorder, a mood disorder and/or an anxiety disorder . . . Clinical studies also point to its co-occurrence with learning impairments (between 10 and 92% depending on the study) . . . It is estimated that 18% of children with THADA have tics . . . Children with a comorbid form of THADA would present special clinical characteristics . . . Comorbidity of THADA with bipolar disorder represents a specific clinical form which is still being discussed. (IN-SERM 2002: 578)

The INSERM reports questioned the very nature of the links between ADHD and other disorders. Is ADHD a precursor of conduct disorder, "suggesting that these two disorders are part of a same clinical entity" (INSERM 2005: 34)? Or is it a different kind of disorder that co-occurs with conduct disorder? More precisely, what is the role of executive dysfunctions in both disorders? Are they common to them or specific to ADHD? The conclusion of the report suggests that "real" antisocial behavior is associated with ADHD, and it deduced that ADHD seems to be constitutive of conduct disorder. But what about the comorbidity between ADHD and learning impairments? Is ADHD a conduct disorder that exacerbates learning impairments, or is it a learning impairment itself?

These reports thus show that experts allowed a variety of interpretations to proliferate without endorsing one or another, except to agree that ADHD has some sort of biological origin, possibly a genetic one. ADHD is chameleon-like, transforming itself when various epistemic lenses are applied. Even more, it seems difficult to discern ADHD from other entities. Does ADHD span the frontiers between different disorders, or do other disorders exacerbate ADHD as a separate entity? Experts left all of these questions unanswered. As they worked on the joint problematization of ADHD and its supposedly associated disorders—namely, mental disorders, conduct disorder, and learning impairments—they instead highlighted the complexity of the involved mechanisms and the multiple uncertainties related to causes and effects.

An Elusive and Disputed Prevalence

Calculating the prevalence of a single disease implies that the disease is recognizable and that there is consensus on the diagnostic criteria. Considering the ADHD landscape in France, it is hardly surprising that until recently, no data were available on this matter. Yet, this did not prevent the topic from being discussed in a variety of arenas. The INSERM reports reflected the multiplicity of

ADHD and presented a set of thresholds, each corresponding to the definition of the disorder according to a single classification:

> Studies drawing upon DSM produce rates ranging from 0.4% to 16.6%, generally between 5% and 10%. Conversely, studies drawing upon the ICD definition of hyperkinetic syndrome result in much lower rates ranging from 0.4% to 4.2%, with an average around 2%. The calculation of this rate does not take gender into consideration. Prevalence seems to be around 3–4% in boys, and 1% in girls. It seems to decrease in teenagers. (INSERM 2002: 17)

The prevalence of comorbidities was discussed in similar terms, with an emphasis on the diversity of methodologies used in the literature.

The press also reflected this uncertainty; newspapers published various rates based on the source of information. Commenting on the 2002 report by INSERM, *Le Monde* and *La Croix* estimated the figure at 1% to 2%. A year later, in an interview with Christine Gétin, the president of HyperSupers, *La Croix* quoted her estimation of 3% to 5% but mentioned that according to some specialists, the prevalence is only about 1%.

Until 2005, ADHD was mainly considered to be a childhood disorder. In 2005, two former students of Michel Dugas published the first book on ADHD in adulthood (Bange and Mouren 2005). In 2009, *Le Monde* published an article on adults with ADHD, stating that "according to various studies, it is estimated that out of the 3 to 8% of children suffering from this disorder, 60% still suffer from the disorder as adults." However, at the end of the article, they quoted Bernard Golse's reaction: "3 to 8%, I consider that to be a big joke and that there are only a few children per thousand. Society cannot stand restless children and thus the problem is eliminated by prescribing amphetamines rather than investigating the symptoms." This argument illustrates the need for finely grained analysis on the social and cultural understanding of ADHD, as proposed by Singh (2006).

In 2010, Michel Lecendreux and Eric Konofal, two French specialists who have developed and sustained a research agenda on ADHD, published the first epidemiological study on ADHD in France together with an American specialist (Lecendreux, Konofal, and Faraone 2011). Data from a phone survey conducted with a sample of about 1,000 families revealed the prevalence of ADHD to be between 3.5% and 5.6% of children. The authors concluded that "the epidemiology of ADHD in French children is similar to the epidemiology of ADHD in other countries"; they therefore reinforced the "reality" of the disorder (Lecendreux, Konofal, and Faraone 2011: 516).

Thus, in less than 15 years, ADHD's status has dramatically changed. Considered to be an American invention in the late 1990s, it is now recognized as a real (albeit controversial) disorder. Concerned people and professionals continue to face a burdensome problem, however: What should be collectively done to help patients, families, and professionals manage the disorder in a context in which multiple uncertainties continue to loom large in expert discourses on ADHD? We explore this question in the following section.

The Problematization of ADHD as a Difficult-to-Treat Condition

In the previous section, we examined reports authored primarily by academic experts whose main focus was defining ADHD. In this section, we analyze reports focused on actions that should be taken in order to help patients and families who are struggling with the disorder. Representatives of patient organizations such as HyperSupers and sister organizations helped author the reports, some of which were produced at their requests. This is why we place a stronger focus on these organizations in this section.

At the beginning of this chapter, we mentioned that HyperSupers asked the ANSM to produce a document on the use of methylphenidate, with the aim of combating ignorance and prejudice among medical and pharmaceutical professionals. In 2013, the ANSM published two documents: (1) a report on the current use of methylphenidate and how to use it safely; and (2) an information leaflet for parents. HyperSupers and sister organizations also contributed to the integration of a new concept—"cognitive disability"—into the 2005 French Disability Act and to its operational translation using the framework provided by the International Classification of Functioning, Disability and Health (ICF). Through this categorization, HyperSupers tried to overcome the fuzziness and ambiguity that had characterized the previous positioning of ADHD within existing disease classifications.

Rather than fighting against the uncertainties into which ADHD is mired, HyperSupers strove to work with these uncertainties in a pragmatic way. Practitioners who encounter ADHD on a daily basis share HyperSupers' pragmatism. However, they are constrained by the organization and functioning of the health system (based on disease classifications and domains of expertise), which hinders the implementation of a global approach to the disorder. Moreover, bridging the health system and the school system is a serious challenge. In practice, the process of creating alternative systems to address conditions such as ADHD and other disorders is so complex that one is left with the impression that actions have yet to be taken.

Distinguishing the Disorder from Learning Difficulties

In 2000 and 2001, two working groups were in charge of producing the reports commissioned by the Ministère de la Santé and the Ministère de l'Education on specific language impairment (SLI). Whereas the aim of the first report was to describe the current state of knowledge and practices, the objective of the second report was to propose a national plan for children with SLI. The president of Coridys—an organization of families and professionals concerned about learning impairments—was a member of these two working groups. Since its creation, HyperSupers had been in contact with Coridys, given the frequency of language impairments associated with ADHD. The president of Coridys approached Christine Gétin, his HyperSupers counterpart, and they agreed that ADHD should be added to the list of conditions addressed by the action plan. In fact, in the document issued to implement the national plan resulting from these reports, ADHD was included in the broader category of learning impairments to which SLI also belongs (Ministère de l'Education 2002).

The plan provided a series of benchmarks in the domain. For example, it stated that "specific learning impairments which comprise dyscalculia, dyspraxia and attention disorders with or without hyperactivity [in addition to SLI, the focus of this document] are considered primary disorders, i.e. their origin is supposed to be developmental, independent from the sociocultural environment on the one hand, and different from a recognized mental impairment or psychic disorder on the other hand" (Ministère de l'Education 2002). It also set up a distinction between difficulties and impairments, given the fact that the identification of a real SLI is not that easy since "symptoms" can be confused with those displayed by children who are having temporary school difficulties. Consequently, the document emphasized the need to develop early screening practices for teachers and school doctors. Another plan recommendation was that in most cases, children with SLI should remain in the standard school system, and that educational plans should be created to define specific learning methods and educational support mechanisms from which children could benefit. Finally, the report recommended the creation of multidisciplinary centers of reference in university hospitals that would be responsible for providing precise diagnoses, defining care, and conducting research.

In support of families and professionals, the plan clearly stated that SLI and ADHD are serious medical problems that should not be regarded as mere temporary difficulties induced by the social or family environment. The plan also recognized that these disorders challenge the capabilities of existing health and education systems. It notably drew attention to the issues of screening and diagnosis, the rationale for which had been endlessly discussed by experts with few conclusive results.

Organizing Screening and Diagnosis

Screening has been, and remains, a contentious and difficult issue. Indeed, the 2000 Ringard report recommended systematically identifying 3- to 4-year-old children who exhibit oral language delays. Although he made several complimentary comments about the report, Jack Lang, the minister of education at the time, declared that he disagreed with this proposition, arguing that "a diagnosis too early can be a catastrophe for a child, and a lot of learning difficulties can be handled by means other than heavy medical management" (Ministère de l'Education 2002).

A massive controversy about screening arose in the aftermath of the publication of the 2005 INSERM report on conduct disorder. In the final chapter, the report outlined a number of recommendations, including health examinations for 3-year-old children:

> At this age, it is possible to identify children with difficult dispositions, hyperactivity and the first symptoms of conduct disorder. This early identification would enable preventive actions to be taken . . . The items [to be added to child health records] may relate to various symptoms of conduct disorder: physical aggression (fighting, biting, hitting, kicking); opposition (refusing to obey, showing no remorse, not changing); hyperactivity (can't stay quiet, is always fidgeting, can't wait for his/her turn). (INSERM 2005: 373)

This measure sparked public outcry, especially from a number of psychiatrists. A group formed to oppose the recommendations, and a petition was created that eventually received nearly 200,000 signatures.[5] The opponents denounced the INSERM report as using care practices to benefit the security policy of Nicolas Sarkozy, the minister of home affairs at the time. The opponents' attack did not stop there, however. In the petition, they stated that the knowledge mobilized by the INSERM report was limited to "theories of behavioral neuropsychology that enable the identification of any deviance from a norm established in accordance with Anglo-Saxon scientific literature" (Lecendreux 2013). Drawing explicitly on social sciences, they also noted that this approach leads to the "medicalization of educational, psychological, and social phenomena, and creates confusion between social unrest and psychic suffering." Finally, they denounced the use of medicines that might "induce a formatting of children behaviors" and "a form of infantile drug addiction."

The controversy lasted several months. The Ministère de la Santé asked INSERM to organize a large conference on conduct disorder in order to foster dialogue among the main protagonists with the goal of producing recommendations. Although various perspectives were voiced during the conference, the end result was a rather spineless consensus on the need for a combined approach to conduct disorder and the recommendation to use extreme caution before labeling children with behaviors that are evocative of conduct disorder. Probably owing to a press release issued in March 2006, the president of HyperSupers was invited to present a paper (Vergnaud Gétin 2007) at the conference. There she criticized some formulations of the report that could be interpreted as validating the idea that ADHD leads to delinquency. However, she also argued for the need to develop prevention, detection, and care policies. In the confrontational atmosphere induced by the INSERM report, however, the association between ADHD and conduct disorder proved to be a dead end. No significant change followed, and the issues of screening and diagnosis were once again postponed until the most recent reports.

Multiple Paralyses: An Ill-Adapted System, Lack of Expertise, and Enduring Suspicion

After years of debate among experts, today there is a shared acknowledgment that the system does not work properly. This statement describes the most recent report we studied from the CNSA initiative, the objective of which was to provide guidelines to the Ministère de la Santé for the organization of care for children with learning impairments. The working group was composed of representatives of all the professions involved in the care of these children (i.e., pediatricians, neurologists, psychologists, speech therapists, teachers, health administrators, and disability administration officers), as well as representatives from patient organizations, including the president of HyperSupers. These representatives were asked to make presentations on what they saw as the main issues at stake.

Drawing on a survey it conducted in 2011 on families' experiences with the health system and the school system (Gétin-Vergnaud and Angenon-Delerue 2011), HyperSupers reported that it took 31 months, on average, for a family to receive a diagnosis and that half of the parents estimated that the first professional they had consulted had no knowledge or poor knowledge related to ADHD. Once they got on the right track, the diagnosis process seemed satisfactory: 79% received a psychometric assessment, 70% received a psychological assessment, 52% received a detailed neuropsychological assessment, 62% received a speech and language assessment, and 53% received a psychomotor assessment. A major issue was the cost of care evaluated at €200 per month since the survey revealed that, among patients, 39% were engaged in psychotherapy, 27% in speech and language therapy, and 19% in psychomotor therapy. Not all of these services were covered by the public health insurance system. Even though 44% of children benefited from a personalized school plan, they encountered a lot of difficulties: 20% had been excluded from school at least once, 30% had repeated at least a grade, and half of the parents had difficult or very difficult relationships with teachers. Remarkably, to date these remain the only available data on how French children and families deal with ADHD and health and educational institutions. Some professionals voiced similar concerns associated with their daily practices:

> We are faced with children with school problems, and more and more often with complex cases that involve a series of different issues, including psychological issues. If we wait for the assessments to be completed it can take up to one year, and in the meantime the children continue to deal with problems, so we want them to start something before the diagnosis is complete. (A pediatrician, working group)

The ideal organization described in the position paper would implement three levels of care. The first level would address difficulties that call for light intervention. These difficulties would be identified and possibly differentiated from more serious disorders. The second level would address diagnosis and care of children with ADHD of medium severity. The third level would handle the most complex or severe cases, which would be referred from other levels for diagnosis and treatment. But as the group admitted throughout the discussion, stable knowledge and expertise that would enable such a division of work are dramatically lacking—training for doctors as well as teachers remains insufficient, and evidence on the efficacy of therapies remains scarce.

Moreover, echoing Georgieff's (2008) analysis of the discrepancies between research and clinical practices in psychiatry, it seems that the categories on which a diagnosis is supposed to be based are not relevant in clinical contexts. Some participants came to question the very notion of diagnosis:

> Why not eliminate the word "diagnosis" and replace it with "review of the situation"? We could then adapt, not to an adult with hemiplegia or to a child with radiotherapy side effects due to leukemia, but to a developing being about whom the only thing we can currently say is: "We observe this; we don't know more for now." But what we know is that if we give this child this therapy for a certain time, it might be life-changing. (A neuropediatrician, working group)

Finally, some participants highlighted that social factors can come into play in a complex way. Children with disadvantaged backgrounds might be ignored because their problems are mistakenly attributed to their situations, whereas children from privileged backgrounds might also be ignored because the environmental support they receive conceals their problems until they simply collapse.

In this context of major epistemic difficulties, implementing the "three-level" ideal organization is clearly not an easy task. On one hand, uncertainties about the disorder and the frequency of comorbidities make it very difficult to delegate screening and diagnosis to first-level practitioners. On the other hand, theoretical conflicts drastically reduce the number of second-level practitioners who recognize ADHD, even though a number of practitioners are confident that various approaches could be reconciled (Barbot 2007; Cohen de Lara et al. 2007; Georgieff 2008).

According to some authors, uncertainties around ADHD engender two major attitudes among practitioners. Some maintain the contested status of the condition, which hinders its recognition as a genuine disorder (Jupille 2014). Others recognize the existence of the disorder and work around its unsettled character; this has the effect of "facilitating" the diagnosis of ADHD and increasing the frequency with which methylphenidate is prescribed (Chamak 2011; Jupille 2011). Our empirical material suggests that both practitioners and families are well aware of this latter risk of misdiagnosis and strive to put together organizational solutions in order to avoid an uncontrolled expansion of the category (Conrad and Potter 2000) that, in the end, may threaten the emerging credibility of the disorder.

Conclusion

We began this chapter by describing the weak and late emergence of ADHD in France. We showed that a unique aspect of the French context was the extreme lack of academic interest in ADHD until the end of the 1990s; this might have delayed its emergence as an issue worthy of debate and inquiry. As a consequence, ADHD emerged as a public issue under peculiar circumstances.

First, the INSERM *expertise collective* on mental disorders, conduct disorder, and learning impairments in which ADHD surfaced as an unsettled condition provided high visibility into international bodies of literature, most notably a significant amount of research in neurology. This resulted in a biologically oriented conception of these disorders and opened up debates on their very nature. This biological approach and the discussions it induced somehow marginalized the French psychodynamic "exception" in a highly confrontational atmosphere.

Second, working groups on disorders associated with ADHD blossomed. Together, these successive groups sustained reflection over the past 15 years and progressively constituted an epistemic community. Their enduring efforts help to ensure the continuing elaboration and re-elaboration of public policies on these conditions.

Third, HyperSupers, the main advocacy group for French patients and families affected by ADHD, formed in 2002 and took the initiative to mobilize scientists and clinicians who showed interest in ADHD. These efforts culminated in an international conference on ADHD that the association jointly organized with ADHD Europe in 2009. HyperSupers also contributed by conducting surveys and producing data on families' experiences with ADHD, which they presented to various groups of experts.

As a result of this problematization work undertaken by certain actors at certain moments in certain settings, the term "TDAH" (the French equivalent of "ADHD") and the epistemic discussions it opened up eventually surfaced in the public space. In France, the term was eventually adopted and is currently used by ADHD specialists, including those who continue to oppose the neurobiological orientation it suggests.

The progressive emergence and installation of ADHD does not imply univocal positioning within the French scientific and medical landscape. Rather, the position of the disorder shifts, and in turn unfolds new relationships among different specialties. Early research on ADHD in France was undertaken by Michel Dugas, who trained most of the psychiatrists who specialize in specific aspects of the disorder (associated sleep disorders, the role of iron deficiency, and medications). In the 2000s, INSERM reports problematized ADHD as an unsettled condition within and between mental disorders, conduct disorder, and learning impairments. When it came to care, HyperSupers partnered with sister organizations concerned with learning impairments; this alliance in turn repositioned the latter within the category of "neurodevelopmental disorders"—similar to the *DSM-5* (APA 2013).

Yet, approaches to care are far from embracing an "all neurological" perspective. As described by Vallée (2011), although psychoanalysis has had a continuing influence in France, many psychiatrists have adopted an "eclectic approach," which has led some of them to develop ADHD care models integrating a variety of interventions. Although the reports we studied are not as conclusive as decision makers would probably have wished, they all reflected on how to organize multidisciplinary diagnosis and care among neurologists, pediatricians, child psychiatrists, paramedics, teachers, education specialists, and, last but not least, families.

This overview of the problematization of ADHD over the past 15 years in France enables us to make two concluding remarks. Our first remark is on the issue of medicalization. One difficulty with this issue is that the notion of medicalization is an analytical category as much as it is a category mobilized in political debate. As an analytical category, this notion depicts the process through which a social or a political issue is turned into a medical one, eventually leading to the individualization and de-politicization of the issue at stake (Conrad 1975). This conceptual framework has been adopted by actors themselves, some of them explicitly quoting social scientists (Gori 2007). In addition, some social scientists have been involved in controversies on the medicalization of certain disorders in the area of mental health (Ehrenberg 2006, 2007; Pignarre 2008; Chamak 2011). Interestingly, by circulating the notion of medicalization from the academic arena to the political arena, social scientists have helped enhance actors' reflexivity on their practices and positioning. Rather than closing debates and restricting the exploration of the disorder, the notion of "medicalization" raised concerns and sensitized different actors to a variety of problems that were previously ambiguous.

Handling such a variety of issues is far from straightforward, however. Our second concluding remark relates to the seemingly "paralyzing" effect of the continuing problematization of ADHD as an unsettled condition. By multiplying their efforts to singularize ADHD and associated disorders, specialists and concerned actors are plunging into the ever-complex bio-psycho-social compositions of these conditions, so much so that finding solutions to the problems they raise often seems impossible. At present, ADHD is difficult to treat, in the sense that diagnosis and care cannot be accurately performed by highly knowledgeable clinicians and professionals. This is an immense problem for public policy makers: what sorts of institutional arrangements and interventions should be designed to accommodate the multiple uncertainties into which certain conditions continue to be mired, due to the endless singularizing processes they are subjected to? Without a doubt, this will soon become a primary concern related to ADHD in France.

NOTES

We warmly thank Kara Gehman and Florence Paterson for their careful reading and editing of our chapter.

1. https://web.archive.org/web/20030619151902/http://carla7.chez.tiscali.fr/.

2. One of us had the opportunity to attend five of the six meetings of the group in charge of preparing this chapter.

3. We were able to access a nearly complete version of the report.

4. Whether this is unique to the French context or not is hard to determine, and such a comparative analysis is beyond the scope of this chapter. Our approach in this chapter is to look at the problematization of ADHD from within the community of experts that has progressively formed around the disorder. This implies that the alleged French context is, in one way or another, embodied in these experts' statements and cannot easily be separated unless these experts explicitly do so.

5. http://www.pasdeodeconduite.org/appel/.

REFERENCES

Agence Nationale de la Sécurité des Médicaments (ANSM). 2013. *Méthylphénidate: données d'utilisation et de sécurité d'emploi en France.* http://ansm.sante.fr/var/ansm_site/storage/original/application/8dd1277a3867155547b4dce58fc0db00.pdf.

American Psychiatric Association (APA). 2013. *Diagnostic and Statistical Manual of Mental Disorders (DSM-5).* 5th ed. Washington, DC: American Psychiatric Association.

Bange, François, and Marie-Christine Mouren. 2005. *Comprendre et soigner l'hyperactivité chez l'adulte.* Paris: Dunod.

Barbot, Françoise de. 2007. "Les diverses approches des troubles de l'attention: sont-elles conciliables?" *La lettre de l'enfance et de l'adolescence* 66 (4): 49–56.

Caisse Nationale de Solidarité pour l'Autonomie (CNSA). 2014. *Troubles Dys: Guide d'appui pour l'élaboration de réponses aux besoins des personnes présentantdes troubles spéci ques du langage, des praxies, de l'attention et des apprentissages.* December.

Callon, Michel, Pierre Lascoumes, and Yannick Barthe. 2009. *Acting in an Uncertain World: An Essay on Technical Democracy.* Cambridge, MA: MIT.

Cecchi Tenerini, Roland. 2010. *Proposition d'écriture: Contribution à la définition, à la description et à la classification des handicaps cognitifs.* http://www.coridys.asso.fr/pages /Coridys/definitioncognitif2010.pdf.

Chamak, Brigitte. 2011. "Troubles des conduites." *L'information Psychiatrique* 87: 383–86.

Cohen de Lara, Aline, Maïa Guinard, Emmanuelle Lacaze, Florence Pinton, Jean Chambry, and Catherine Billard. 2007. "Hyperactivité et psychose de l'enfant: l'intérêt de la méthodologie projective dans l'affinement des diagnostics." *Psychologie clinique et projective* 13 (1): 173–96.

Commission Nationale de la Naissance et de la Santé de l'Enfant. 2013. "Parcours de soins des enfants et des adolescents présentant des troubles du langage et des apprentissages." Ministère de la Santé. http://www.sante.gouv.fr/IMG/pdf/Parcours_de_soins _des_enfants_atteints_de_troubles_des_apprentissages.pdf.

Conrad, Peter. 1975. "The Discovery of Hyperkinesis: Notes on the Medicalization of Deviant Behavior." *Social Problems* 23: 12–21.

Conrad, Peter, and Deborah Potter. 2000. "From Hyperactive Children to ADHD Adults: Observations on the Expansion of Medical Categories." *Social Problems* 47 (4): 559–82.

EDUSCOL. 2012. *Scolariser les enfants présentant des troubles des apprentissages.* Paris: Ministère de l'Education. http://cache.media.eduscol.education.fr/file/Handicap/46 /6/TSA_EDUSCOL_225466.pdf.

Edwards, Claire, Etaoine Howlett, Madeleine Akrich, and Vololona Rabeharisoa. 2014. "Attention Deficit Hyperactivity Disorder in France and Ireland: Parents' Groups' Scientific and Political Framing of an Unsettled Condition." *BioSocieties* 9 (2): 153–72. doi: 10.1057/biosoc.2014.3.

Ehrenberg, Alain. 2006. "Dans trois rapports qui soulèvent la controverse, l'INSERM ignore l'action menée en France et brouille la donne. Santé mentale, trouble de l'évaluation." *Libération*, April 5.

———. 2007. "Épistémologie, sociologie, santé publique: tentative de clarification." *Neuropsychiatrie de l'enfance et de l'adolescence* 55: 450–55.

Georgieff, Nicolas. 2008. "À propos de l'expertise collective de l'INSERM sur le 'trouble des conduits:' quelques problèmes critiques de la pédopsychiatrie contemporaine." *La psychiatrie de l'enfant* 51 (1): 5–42.

Gétin-Vergnaud, Christine, and Katia G. Angenon-Delerue. 2011. "Après 10 ans d'activité, HyperSupersTDAH France dresse un premier bilan de ses actions au travers des résultats d'une enquête menée durant l'été 2011 auprès des familles adhérentes." *ANAE. Approche neuropsychologique des apprentissages chez l'enfant* 114: 358–64.

Golse, Bernard. 2003. "L'hyperactivité de l'enfant: un choix de société." *Le Carnet Psy* 78 (1): 26–28.

Gori, Roland. 2007. "La construction du trouble comme entreprise de normalisation." *La lettre de l'enfance et de l'adolescence* 66 (4): 31–41.

Haas, Peter M. 1992. "Introduction: Epistemic Communities and International Policy Coordination." *International Organization* 46: 1–35.

Hacking, Ian. 1999. *The Social Construction of What?* Cambridge, MA: Harvard University Press.

Haute Authorité de la Santé (HAS). 2012. *Conduite à tenir devant un enfant ou un adolescent ayant un déficit de l'attention et/ou un problème d'agitation.* http://www.tdah-france

.fr/IMG/pdf/trouble-de-lattention-de-lenfant_note_de_cadrage.pdf?683/c366599cf6
57c4f2d0d3c3f1d1af7854716093ee.

HyperSupers TDAH France and Centre Pédiatrique des Pathologies du Sommeil (CPPS) du CHU Robert Debré. 2010. *Confrontation des pratiques européennes au sujet du TDAH— Synthèse des débats.* http://www.tdah-france.fr/confrontation-des-pratiques.html.

Institut National de la Santé et de la Recherche Médicale (INSERM). 2002. *Troubles mentaux. Dépistage et prévention chez l'enfant et l'adolescent.* http://www.ipubli.inserm .fr/handle/10608/46.

———. 2005. *Trouble des conduites chez l'enfant et l'adolescent.* http://www.ipubli.inserm .fr/handle/10608/60.

———. 2007. *Dyslexie, Dysorthographie, Dyscalculie: Bilan des données scientifiques.* http:// www.ipubli.inserm.fr/handle/10608/73.

———. 2009. *Santé de l'enfant : Propositions pour un meilleur suivi.* http://www.ipubli .inserm.fr/handle/10608/82.

Joly, Fabien. 2003. "Instabilité de l'instabilité . . ." *Le Carnet Psy* 78 (1): 12.

Jupille, Julien. 2011. "Hyperactivité et troubles des conduites: des diagnostics controver-sés." *L'information Psychiatrique* 87: 409–16.

———. 2014. "De 'coupables' à 'victimes actives.' Enjeux pour les familles d'un diagnostic de TDA/H." *Socio-logos. Revue de l'association française de sociologie.* http://socio-logos .revues.org/2835.

Lecendreux, Michel. 2013. "Hyperactivité et trouble de l'attention: du diagnostic et des soins." Interview with Michel Lecendreux. *FranceTV Education Online.* March 7. http://education.francetv.fr/psychologie/article/hyperactivite-et-trouble-de-l-attention -du-diagnostic-et-des-soins.

Lecendreux, Michel, Eric Konofal, and Stephen V. Faraone. 2011. "Prevalence of Atten-tion Deficit Hyperactivity Disorder and Associated Features among Children in France." *Journal of Attention Disorders* 15 (6): 516–24.

Le Monde. 2005. "Des enfants sages sur ordonnance." November 23.

Libération. 2013. "Et si la psychanalyse n'avait pas parlé sur les ondes." July 13.

Metz, Claire, and Anne Thévenot. 2010. "Instabilité psychomotrice des enfants: trouble ou symptôme?" *Psychologie clinique* 30 (2): 34–48.

Ministère de l'Education. 2002. *Mise en œuvre d'un plan d'action pour les enfants atteints d'un trouble spécifique du langage oral ou écrit.* February 7. http://www.education.gouv .fr/bo/2002/6/default.htm.

Petitnicolas, Catherine. 1998. "Un comportement qui désoriente les parents. Le difficile diagnostic de l'hyperactivité de l'enfant." *Le Figaro*, February 27.

Pignarre, Philippe. 2008. "Médicaliser/démédicaliser: développer l'expertise des pa-tients." *Cliniques méditerranéennes* 77 (1): 125–36.

Proust, Claudine. 2014. "Hyperactifs: on fait quoi?" *Le Parisien*, May 9. http://www .leparisien.fr/informations/hyperactifs-on-fait-quoi-09-05-2014-3826383.php.

Rafalovich, Adam. 2001. "Psychodynamic and Neurological Perspectives on ADHD: Ex-ploring Strategies for Defining a Phenomenon." *Journal for the Theory of Social Behav-iour* 31: 397–418.

Raffy, Alex. 2006. "L'enfant des limites, l'enfant du DSM." *L'information Psychiatrique* 82 (9): 723–30.

Ringard, Jean-Charles. 2000. *A propos de l'enfant dysphasique et de l'enfant dyslexique.* Paris: Ministère de l'Education. http://media.education.gouv.fr/file/95/7/5957.pdf.

Schmit, Gérard. 2007. "Troubles des conduits: un an de mobilisation constructive." *La lettre de la psychiatrie française* 162: 11–13. http://www.psychiatrie-francaise.com /Data/Documents/files/LLPF%20162%20-%20f%C3%A9v%202007.pdf.

Singh, Ilina. 2002. "Biology in Context: Social and Cultural Perspectives on ADHD." *Children & Society* 16 (5): 360–67.

———. 2006. "A Framework for Understanding Trends in ADHD Diagnoses and Stimulant Drug Treatment: Schools and Schooling as a Case Study." *BioSocieties* 1: 439–52.

Tremblay, Pierre H. 1987. *La dépression chez l'enfant . . . un entretien avec le Professeur Michel Dugas.* Montreal: CECOM HRDP Montréal and Université de Montréal Department of Psychiatry.

Vaivre-Douret, Laurence, and Anne Tursz, eds. 1999. "Les troubles d'apprentissage chez l'enfant. Un problème de santé publique?" *Actualite et dossier en santé publique* 26: 23–66.

Vallée, Manuel. 2011. "Resisting American Psychiatry: French Opposition to DSM-III, Biological Reductionism, and the Pharmaceutical Ethos." *Advances in Medical Sociology* 12: 85–110.

Veber, Florence, and Jean-Charles Ringard. 2001. *Plan d'action pour les enfants atteints d'un trouble spécifique du langage écrit ou oral.* Paris: Ministère de l'Education, Ministère de la Santé, Secrétariat d'Etat aux personnes âgées et aux personnes handicapées. http://www.sante.gouv.fr/IMG/pdf/plandysl.pdf.

Vergnaud Gétin, Christine. 2007. "TDAH, prédictif et/ou facteur de risque?" *Neuropsychiatrie de l'enfance et de l'adolescence* 55 (8): 495–96.

Wodon, Isabelle. 2009. *Déficit de l'attention et hyperactivité chez l'enfant et l'adolescent: comprendre et soigner le TDAH chez les jeunes.* Brussels: Editions Mardaga.

Zarifian, Édouard. 2003. "Les fondements du soin en psychiatrie." In *Droit d'être soigné, droits des soignants*, 27–36. Toulouse: ERES.

13

ADHD in Japan
A Sociological Perspective

Mari J. Armstrong-Hough

Japanese research on ADHD is prolific, and clinical management of this condition in Japan takes place in one of the most accessible and efficient health care delivery systems in the world. It is therefore particularly instructive to examine differences in the identification, management, and social context of ADHD in Japan; these differences can tell us much about the role of "local" cultural, political, and institutional forces in professional and popular perceptions of a global illness. As this subchapter shows, differences in the sociocultural and institutional context of ADHD in Japan lead not only to different experiences of illness among individuals, but also to different choices about its management and treatment for parents and clinicians. Although rates of medication usage for ADHD are on the rise in Japan, they remain low by international standards (Scheffler et al. 2007). The classic formulation of Ritalin, emblematic of the rise of ADHD in the United States, is eschewed completely, and there is evidence that clinicians and regulators alike have a preference for non-stimulant drug therapy. Medicalized understandings of the origins of ADHD symptoms do not seem to have removed the stigma associated with the diagnosis. These differences in the medicalization of ADHD in Japan are particularly notable in the context of the country's notoriously competitive, exam-based educational system and high levels of anxiety surrounding child and adolescent behavioral issues.

This short subchapter responds to three related sociological questions about the rise of ADHD in Japan. First, and most broadly, how has the medicalization of ADHD progressed in Japan? Second, what is the nature of the stigma associated with ADHD in Japan, what are its origins, and how is it changing? And finally, how has the course of its medicalization and its changing association with deviance influenced the identification and treatment of ADHD in Japan?

The Medicalization of ADHD in Japan

Research on inattention has a long history in modern Japan. In the early twentieth century, the founding father of Japanese psychology, Yuzero Motora, theorized inattention and described "ADHD-like symptoms" in his subjects (Takeda, Ando, and Kumagai 2015). Contemporary research on inattention is rooted in a long history of conversation and exchange with international research communities. Nonetheless, the following sections note several features of ADHD in Japan that may be less familiar to researchers outside the country: the relatively narrow rules set by the Ministry of Health, Labor, and Welfare (MHLW) restricting ADHD diagnosis to children, longstanding associations with autism spectrum disorder, the stigma attached to diagnosis, and cultural and institutional constraints on pharmacotherapy.

Current official classifications of ADHD in Japan are narrow: symptoms are expected to emerge by 7 years of age (but cannot be treated until after age 6) and MHLW rules prevent diagnosis and treatment of the disorder after 18 years of age. In line with international prevalence estimates, the MHLW estimates that between 3% and 7% of Japanese children are affected by ADHD and that the disorder disproportionately affects boys (MHLW 2015b). However, adult ADHD is not officially recognized, and no medications from the narrow range of ADHD treatment options are indicated for adult ADHD. This has not necessarily prevented "off-label" prescriptions to help adults manage the disorder, but it does represent a significant institutional hurdle to diagnosis and treatment after age 18.

A further notable feature of ADHD in Japan is its association with autism spectrum disorder through the umbrella term *hattatsu shogai*. *Hattatsu shogai* literally translates as "neurodevelopmental disorder." The anthropologist Junko Teruyama cautions English speakers not to assume that the Japanese term reflects the same classificatory schema that underlies its use in any version of the

Diagnostic and Statistical Manual of Medical Disorders (DSM). In Japan, the professional and popular use of the term *hattatsu shogai* to group together disorders related to autism, inattention, hyperactivity, and learning long predates the *DSM* classification and primarily emerged to distinguish these disorders from intellectual disabilities (Tamekawa et al. 2014; Teruyama 2014). The term groups a wide range of disorders, from mild dyslexia to autism, together into a single category of "developmental disorder." In part because of this classification, there is a longstanding perception among the general public that ADHD and autism spectrum disorder are cousin afflictions. Educational institutions and the professionals who work in them also group these disorders together, so that the same programs and strategies aimed at students with autism spectrum disorder are also aimed at students with ADHD and learning disabilities (Miyahara 2008).

The association of ADHD with autism spectrum disorder in Japan has contributed to its stigmatization. In a society that values harmony and implicit communication, individuals with autism spectrum disorder are easily "othered" in media discourse and associated with antisocial, even violent behavior. Similarly, in Japan's etiquette-fixated social and educational environment, unaddressed behavioral symptoms of ADHD may be particularly debilitating to social wellbeing and academic achievement. As a result, although both disorders have been medicalized, their association with deviance has not necessarily faded. The following section considers the origins and consequences of associations of ADHD with deviance in Japan.

The Stigma Associated with ADHD

The Japanese public had little exposure to media stories about ADHD until the late 1990s. Then, in 1997, a troubled 14-year-old boy kidnapped, murdered, and decapitated an 11-year-old child in Kobe, leaving the victim's head by the gate of his elementary school. The gruesomeness and inexplicability of the crime, the young age of the victim and the murderer, and the relative rarity of violent crime in Japan brought immediate national attention to the case. The murderer's bizarre, taunting interactions with police, later revelations that the boy had eluded capture for a previous murder of a 10-year-old girl, and his controversial trial and subsequent release in 2004 extended media coverage of the crime for years (fig. 13.1). The media soon discovered that the accused murderer had been diagnosed with ADHD; the publication of his diagnosis coincided with and contributed to the first period of sustained popular attention to ADHD in Japan (Teruyama 2014). Thus, some of the earliest mentions of ADD/ADHD in Japanese

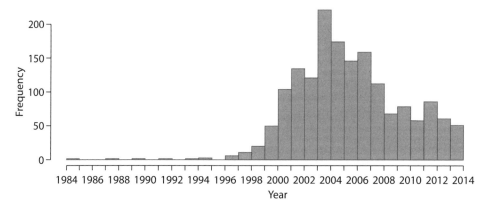

Fig. 13.1. Mentions of ADHD in major Japanese newspapers, 1985–2014.

newspapers occurred in reference to one of the most grotesque crimes of the decade. *Hattatsu shogai*—though not specifically ADHD—continued to be associated with violence and criminal deviance in media discourse into the 2000s.[1]

An analysis of mentions of ADHD in two prominent national newspapers reveals that before 1997 there was almost no popular press attention to ADHD or its predecessor diagnoses.[2] Before 1997, at most 1 article per year mentioned attention deficit or hyperactivity disorders. In 1997 and 1998, a total of 6 and 9 articles, respectively, mentioned these disorders in the wake of the Kobe murders. By 2000, a total of 50 articles mentioned one of the terms, and in 2001, a total of 107 articles mentioned one of the terms. From a sociological perspective, the timing and context of the rise of ADHD in Japan is meaningful because it suggests that the disorder has been associated with deviance from its very introduction to public discourse. Even as public understanding of ADHD and other *hattatsu shogai* has evolved and these conditions have become increasingly medicalized, this group of disorders remains popularly associated with social maladjustment and crime (Tamekawa et al. 2014; Teruyama 2014). As elsewhere, researchers in Japan have noted associations between juvenile crime and ADHD symptom severity (e.g., Matsuura, Hashimoto, and Toichi 2010).

Enduring stigma and misapprehension of ADHD help explain otherwise surprising patterns in treatment-seeking behavior among Japanese parents of children exhibiting symptoms. Given Japan's brutally competitive, evaluation-oriented education system, one might expect that anxious parents would seek diagnosis and psychopharmacological treatment—even overtreatment—for their children. Indeed, Japanese parents demonstrate dramatically greater sensitivity to ADHD symptoms in children than do Japanese teachers. One study found that when Japanese parents were asked to report symptoms in their children, the prevalence of ADHD symptoms reached an astonishing 31.1%; when Japanese teachers were asked to report ADHD symptoms in children, symptom prevalence dropped to 4.3% (Soma et al. 2009). The difference in parent versus teacher evaluations of children's ADHD symptoms may be greater in Japan than in other countries because parents' behavioral expectations are unusually high.

Clearly, Japanese families are sensitive to the emergence of ADHD symptoms and take them seriously. Yet the average lag between parental recognition of symptoms and a first hospital visit to consult with a clinician is 2.6 years (Yamauchi, Fujiwara, and Okuyama 2014); this is relatively long by international comparisons (e.g., Ghanizadeh 2007). More research must be done on how the stigma associated with ADHD; misunderstandings about the nature and severity of its behavioral symptoms; and concerns about future social, educational, or employment discrimination influence parents' treatment-seeking behavior.

Pharmacotherapy and Its Discontents in Japan

Not only has ADHD itself been associated with deviance in Japan, but ADHD medications that are common elsewhere have negative associations specific to the Japanese context. Japanese regulators have long been wary of amphetamines, which have a troubled history in postwar Japan and are strongly associated with substance abuse and organized crime (Tamura 1992). Ritalin prescription is strictly controlled and has never been indicated for ADHD in Japan; current guidelines permit its use only for narcolepsy. In addition, all amphetamine-type stimulants are controlled as narcotics in Japan; this both reflects a prescribing culture that is wary of habit-forming drugs and creates logistic and institutional barriers to obtaining such medications, even when they are considered to be justified. For example, Ritalin (methylphenidate) and Concerta (osmotic controlled-release methylphenidate) are each subject to their own distribution control panels that require that prescribing physicians and dispensing pharmacies register and pledge appropriate use (Takeda 2009). The control panels' measures effectively restrict the number of physicians who are permitted to prescribe these drugs.

Thus, although the MHLW points to pharmacological intervention (along with behavioral modification) as one of the two primary strategies for ADHD, first-line options for medication are limited. Only two psychopharmacotherapies are officially indicated for ADHD in Japan: the non-stimulant Strattera (atomoxetine) and the long-acting stimulant Concerta (MHLM 2015a). Concerta is a methylphenidate formulation designed for slow, sustained release and thus considered less habit-forming than other stimulant formulations. Whereas non-controlled-release methylphenidate formulations are simply not indicated for ADHD, Adderall (amphetamine and dextroamphetamine), a common treatment elsewhere, is completely prohibited—possession of the drug is punishable by a prison sentence. These regulatory constraints necessarily and directly shape clinical options.

Within this narrower range, Japanese clinicians move to medicate children diagnosed with ADHD more slowly than their American counterparts, favoring environmental coordination, parent training, and psychosocial interventions. "Environmental coordination" refers to efforts to redesign children's educational and home environments to better manage ADHD symptoms. In the Japanese algorithm, environmental coordination and psychoeducation are first attempted, then medication is introduced alongside behavior therapy (Takeda 2009). When medication is introduced, dosages are markedly low by international standards and a lower dosage ceiling is indicated than in the United States (Takeda 2009). This is in line with a prescribing culture in Japan that favors lower dosages across a range of medications and diseases (Iizuka 2007; Armstrong-Hough 2011).

Finally, reluctance to medicate in general and aversion to amphetamine-type stimulant treatment in particular extends to parents. Parents in Japan appear to have little expectation of a pharmacological solution; only 23% of respondents to a survey of parents of children with ADHD listed medication as being among their expectations for treatment (Saito 2005). The lack of interest in pharmaceuticals is surprising because, even though average dosages tend to be lower in Japan than elsewhere, Japanese medical culture has long emphasized the dispensing of pharmaceuticals over the dispensing of medical advice (Tomita 2009). Very little research has been conducted on the expectations of parents with respect to ADHD treatment in Japan, but it is possible—even likely—that parental disinterest in pharmacotherapy is linked to the stigma surrounding amphetamine use, general concerns about habit-forming substances, and cultural preference for behavioral and environmental modification.

In short, regulatory choices related to concerns about amphetamine abuse, Japan's prescribing culture, and parent expectations all contribute to lower reliance on pharmacotherapy for ADHD treatment in Japan than elsewhere. Thus, whereas the United States is an outlier because of its high reliance on ADHD medications among children, Japan's ADHD medication usage is lower than would be predicted by its per capita GDP (Scheffler et al. 2007). In this context, strategies for environmental coordination, parent training, and psychoeducation such as those described in the following section have blossomed.

Conclusion

Stigma—both stigma attached to the ADHD diagnosis among the general public and stigma associated with amphetamine-type stimulants—has shaped the course of ADHD in Japan in important ways. First, associations of ADHD with social deviance influence the illness experiences of children and help-seeking behavior of parents. The perception that the illness identity associated with ADHD may be a "spoiled" one (Goffman 1963) may contribute to a delay between symptom recognition and seeking medical help and suggests that AD-HD's route "from badness to sickness" through medicalization has been neither straight nor smooth (Conrad and Schneider 2010 [1992]). As ADHD and other *hattatsu shogai* are increasingly integrated into disability rights discourses in Japan, the association of ADHD with deviance is beginning to fade—but concerns about negative social associations remain relevant.

Second, the role of amphetamine aversion in Japan's regulatory environment and prescribing culture, in part as a result of Japan's particular history of post-war amphetamine abuse and organized crime, should not be ignored. Resulting differences in the availability of and preferences for pharmacotherapies shape patterns in ADHD treatment in important ways. But even more interesting, negative social associations with amphetamine use may shape the hopes and expectations of parents regarding treatment in ways that make it easier for clinicians to direct families toward environmental and psychoeducational interventions. When parents do not expect pharmacotherapy to be a risk-free magic bullet for ADHD, a range of other strategies emerges.

Nonetheless, medication usage for ADHD is increasing. A recent article in the *Journal for the Japanese Society of Psychiatry and Neurology* noted with some concern that the prevalence of ADHD prescriptions for children 12 years of age and younger significantly increased between 2002 and 2010. The odds of a child being prescribed a drug for ADHD in 2008–10 were 84% higher than in 2002–4. For children 13 years or older, the increase was even more dramatic: the odds of an ADHD prescription were nearly 2.5 times higher in 2008–10 than in the earlier period (Okumura, Fujita, and Matsumoto 2014). Perceptions and preferred therapies continue to shift in Japan—and if these trends persist, the social landscape of ADHD may be very different within just a few years.

NOTES

1. These crimes included another bizarre child murder in 2003. For a detailed English-language analysis of media discourse on *hattatsu shogai*, see Teruyama (2014).

2. I searched the digital archives of the *Yomiuri Shimbun* and the *Asahi Shimbun* for all terms popularly and professionally used to refer to ADHD and its predecessors: the roman-letter acronym ADHD, the term 注意欠陥多動障害 (ADHD), the term 注意欠陥多動性障害 (ADHD), the term 注意力欠如障害 (ADD), and the term 多動症候群 (hyperactivity syndrome).

REFERENCES

Armstrong-Hough, Mari. 2011. "Imperial Splenda: Globalization, Culture, and Type 2 Diabetes in the US and Japan." PhD diss., Duke University.

Conrad, Peter, and Joseph Schneider. 2010 (1992). *Deviance and Medicalization: From Badness to Sickness*. Philadelphia: Temple University Press.

Ghanizadeh, Ahmad. 2007. "Educating and Counseling of Parents of Children with Attention-Deficit Hyperactivity Disorder." *Patient Education and Counseling* 68 (1): 23–28. doi:10.1016/j.pec. 2007.03.021.

Goffman, Erving. 1963. *Stigma*. New York: Simon & Schuster.

Iizuka, Toshiaki. 2007. "Experts' Agency Problems: Evidence from the Prescription Drug Market in Japan." *The Rand Journal of Economics* 38 (3): 844–62.

Matsuura, Naomi, Toshiaki Hashimoto, and Motomi Toichi. 2010. "The Characteristics of AD/HD Symptoms, Self-Esteem, and Aggression among Serious Juvenile Offenders in Japan." *Research in Developmental Disabilities* 31 (6): 1197–1203. doi:10.1016/j. ridd.2010.07.026.

Ministry of Health, Labor, and Welfare (MHLW). 2015a. "Hattatsu shogai: ADHD." http://www.mhlw.go.jp/kokoro/know/disease_develop.html Accessed 6/15/2015. (In Japanese)

———. 2015b. "Hattatsu shogai: ADHD to wa?" http://www.mhlw.go.jp/kokoro/know /disease_develop.html. (In Japanese)

Miyahara, Rumiko. 2008. "Educators' Knowledge of and Perception toward Students with ADHD in Japan." Master's thesis, California State University, Northridge.

Noda, Wataru, Ryo Okada, Iori Tani, Masafumi Ohnishi, Mochizuki Naoto, Syunji Naka-jima, and Masatsugu Tsujii. 2013. "Relationship among Inattentive and Hyperactive-Impulsive Behavior, Aggression, and Depression in Japanese Elementary and Junior High School Students." *Shinrigaku Kenkyu: The Japanese Journal of Psychology* 84 (2): 169–75.

Okumura, Yasuyuki, Junichi Fujita, and Toshihiko Matsumoto. 2014. "Trends of Psychotropic Medication Use among Children and Adolescents in Japan: Data from the National Insurance Claims Database between 2002 and 2010." *Seishin Shinkeigaku Zasshi* 116 (11). (In Japanese)

Saito, K. 2005. "Research on a Comprehensive System of Clinical Assessment and Treatment for Attention-Deficit/Hyperactivity Disorder." Research grant (14-A-8) for nervous and mental disorders from the Ministry of Health, Labor, and Welfare. (In Japanese)

Scheffler, Richard M., Stephen P. Hinshaw, Sepideh Modrek, and Peter Levine. 2007. "The Global Market for ADHD Medications." *Health Affairs* 26 (2): 450–57. doi:10.1377/hlthaff.26.2.450.

Soma, Yukio, Kazutoshi Nakamura, Mari Oyama, Yasuo Tsuchiya, and Masaharu Yamamoto. 2009. "Prevalence of Attention-Deficit/Hyperactivity Disorder (ADHD) Symptoms in Preschool Children: Discrepancy between Parent and Teacher Evaluations." *Environmental Health and Preventive Medicine* 14 (2): 150–54.

Takeda, Toshinobu. 2009. "Psychopharmacology for Attention-Deficit/Hyperactivity Disorder in Japan." *Current Attention Disorders Reports* 1 (1): 21–28.

Takeda, Toshinobu, Mizuho Ando, and Keiko Kumagai. 2015. "Attention Deficit and Attention Training in Early Twentieth-Century Japan." *Attention Deficit and Hyperactivity Disorders* 7 (2): 101–11. doi:10.1007/s12402-014-0157-7.

Tamekawa Yuji, Souichi Hashimoto, Akiko Hayashi, and Atsushi Kanno. 2014. *Misunderstandings about Developmental Disabilities in Japan*. Poster.

Tamura, Masayuki. 1992. "The Yakuza and Amphetamine Abuse in Japan." *Drugs, Law and the State*, 99–118.

Teruyama, Junko. 2014. "Japan's New Minority: Persons with Hattatsu Shogai." PhD diss., University of Michigan.

Tomita, Naoko. 2009. "The Political Economy of Incrementally Separating Prescription from Dispensation in Japan." In *Prescribing Cultures and Pharmaceutical Policy in the Asia-Pacific*, edited by Karen Eggleston. Stanford, CA: Walter H. Shorenstein Asia-Pacific Research Center Books.

Yamauchi, Yuko, Takeo Fujiwara, and Makiko Okuyama. 2014. "Factors Influencing Time Lag between Initial Parental Concern and First Visit to Child Psychiatric Services among ADHD Children in Japan." *Community Mental Health Journal*. doi:10.1007/s10597-014-9803-y.

Epidemiology, Treatments, and Cultural Influences

Yasuo Murayama
Hiroyuki Ito
Junko Teruyama
Masatsugu Tsujii

Attention deficit–hyperactivity disorder (ADHD) is a neurodevelopmental disorder that affects approximately 5% of children and adolescents and 2.5% of adults worldwide (Polanczyk et al. 2007). The core characteristics of ADHD—inattention, hyperactivity, and impulsivity—can lead children and adolescents to experience difficulties in many aspects of daily life, such as academic performance and relationships with peers.

ADHD is acknowledged as being a common and chronic neurodevelopmental disorder in many countries. In Japan, numerous children, adolescents, and adults with ADHD, as well as their family members, have some form of distress caused by ADHD symptoms and related problems. In addition, many suffer from social stigma that is in part related to Japanese values regarding child-rearing and discipline. This stigma explains why psychosocial interventions, particularly parent training, are more likely to be used to treat ADHD in Japan. In this section, we describe the epidemiology of this disorder, relevant laws, diagnosis and treatment guidelines, and available types of treatment as well as the specific sociocultural conditions surrounding ADHD in Japan.

The Epidemiology of ADHD in Japan

PREVALENCE

An epidemiological understanding of ADHD may provide insights into its distribution, etiology, and the risk of psychosocial problems, as well as information for intervention planning. In the past two decades, many investigations have been conducted around the world to define the prevalence of the disorder. Although estimated prevalence rates have been highly variable across the literature, meta-regression analyses have shown that the worldwide pooled prevalence was 5.29% among children and adolescents (18 years of age or younger) and 2.5% among adults (Polanczyk et al. 2007; Simon et al. 2009).

In Japan, a few studies have looked at the epidemiology of ADHD (table 13.1). Nomura et al. (2014) examined the prevalence of ADHD among preschool children (5 years of age) and reported that 5.8% of the children were eligible for a diagnosis. The Ministry of Education, Culture, Sports, Science, and Technology (2012) conducted a survey on the prevalence of ADHD among elementary and junior high school students who were enrolled in regular class (6 to 15 years of age). The survey found that 3.1% of students had noticeable ADHD symptoms, although this study was based on behavioral ratings made by class teachers rather than diagnoses made by a specialized physician. Uchiyama, Ohnishi, and Nakamura (2012) looked at ADHD in adults (18 to 49 years of age) and estimated that its prevalence is 1.65%.

The relative dearth of epidemiological studies can be attributed to the fact that widespread public awareness of ADHD grew in Japan only in the past two

Table 13.1. Descriptive Data from Studies on the Prevalence of Attention Deficit–Hyperactivity Disorder in Japan

Study	*n*	Age (years)	Design	Assessment	Estimated Prevalence (%)
Nomura et al. (2014)	583	5	Two-stage sampling Community sample Representative sample	Diagnosis based on *DSM-IV*	5.8
Ministry of Education, Culture, Sports, Science, and Technology (2012)	53,882	6–15	One-stage sampling Regular class[a] students Representative sample	ADHD-RS (Teacher Rating)	3.1
Uchiyama et al. (2012)	3,910	18–49	Two-stage sampling Community sample Non-representative sample	ASRS-Screener (Self-Rating) CAADID Diagnosis based on *DSM-IV*	1.7

Note: ADHD-RS: Attention Deficit Hyperactivity Disorder Rating Scale; ASRS-Screener: Adult ADHD Self-Report Scale-Screener; CAADID: Conners' Adult ADHD Diagnostic Interview for *DSM-IV*.
[a]In Japan, there are two types of classes in a school: regular classes and special needs classes. Students who exhibit academic underachievement or poor adaptation to collective school life are assigned to the special needs classes.

decades (Teruyama 2014). In other words, the diagnosis of ADHD prior to this period was rare and thus there were insufficient data to conduct such studies until recently. As shown in table 13.1, these studies adopt different designs from each other. In addition, the assessment tools and the procedure for the identification of cases varied from study to study. Likewise, studies in other countries have used a variety of design and assessment procedures. Therefore, direct comparison of the results about prevalence estimates is limited, and it is difficult to discuss the impact of geographical and demographic factors. However, despite these methodological variations, the results of the studies conducted in Japan are similar to the worldwide pooled prevalence estimated in the meta-analytic studies (Polanczyk et al. 2007; Simon et al. 2009).

CORRELATES OF ADHD

Although several studies have investigated the prevalence of ADHD (as mentioned above), few studies have systematically examined the relationship between ADHD symptoms and demographic or psychosocial variables in Japan. This is mainly because standardized assessment tools for ADHD symptoms, which are used internationally and have sufficient reliability and validity, have not existed until recently in Japan. However, in the past decade, several international scales have been imported into Japan. These include the Attention Deficit Hyperactivity Disorder Rating Scale (ADHD-RS) (DuPaul et al. 1998; Ichikawa and Tanaka 2008), Conners' 3rd Edition (Conners 2008; Tanaka 2011), Conners' Adult ADHD Rating Scales (CAARS) (Conners, Erhardt, and Sparrow 1999; Nakamura 2011), and Conners' Adult ADHD Diagnostic Interview for DSM-IV (CAADID) (Epstein, Johnson, and Conners 2001; Nakamura 2011). Therefore, it is now possible to conduct systematic epidemiological studies of ADHD, and the results of these studies can be compared internationally.

The use of these internationally standardized scales has been instrumental in benchmarking foreign epidemiological data, comparing them with domestic surveys, and contextualizing the Japanese situation from a global perspective. Such comparability has, on the one hand, fostered communication and exchange regarding diagnosis and treatment among clinicians, epidemiologists, and other professionals across national boundaries. On the other hand, it has substantiated ADHD as an internationally recognized (and thus credible/legitimate) diagnostic category within Japan, where the rapid rise of the prevalence rate could have otherwise been received with suspicion and skepticism.

The Hamamatsu School Cohort

As in many other cultures and societies, ADHD in Japan is manifested as psychosocial maladaptation, particularly in school-age children. The difficulty that they face in fulfilling academic expectations, establishing and maintaining appropriate social relationships, and building healthy self-esteem is a concern that teachers, parents, and professionals share. In this section, we introduce a study that we conducted on this issue to better understand the correlation of ADHD to the experience of maladaptation among children.

Our research group (Research Center for Child Mental Development in the Hamamatsu University School of Medicine, located in Shizuoka Prefecture) has implemented a school cohort study, Hamamatsu School Cohort, from 2007 to the present. The Hamamatsu School Cohort aims to reveal both the risk and protective factors of mental health problems among children and adolescents. In this study, we focus on the symptoms of developmental disorders (including ADHD, autism spectrum disorder [ASD], and developmental coordination disorder [DCD]) as risk factors of psychosocial maladaptation. We then introduce the findings about ADHD symptoms obtained by the Hamamatsu School Cohort.

We collected data from all nursery, elementary, and junior-high schools in a suburban city located in the central area of Japan. Although the study has been conducted in August and September each year since 2007, ADHD-related data have been collected since 2009. The response rate was more than 90% every year. Since 2009, a total of 12,663 students have participated in at least one investigation. The ADHD symptoms were measured with the use of the Japanese version of the ADHD-RS (DuPaul et al. 1998). The parents of the students completed the questionnaire. The presence of ADHD and its subtypes was determined with the use of the cut-off points of the ADHD-RS subscales (Inattention and Hyperactivity/Impulsivity). To examine comorbid conditions, the ASD and DCD symptoms were measured with the use of the Autism Spectrum Screening Questionnaire (ASSQ) (Ehlers, Gillberg, and Wing 1999) and the Developmental Coordination Disorder Questionnaire (DCDQ) (Wilson et al. 2009), which were completed by the parents.

Psychosocial maladaptation was also assessed with the use of standardized achievement tests including the Social Maladaptation Scale for Children and Adolescents (SMS) (Ito et al. 2014), the Birleson Depression Self-Rating Scale for Children (DSRS-C) (Birleson 1981), and the Buss-Perry Aggression Questionnaire (BAQ) (Buss and Perry 1992). These questionnaires were completed by the students.

Gender and Age

Table 13.2 shows the prevalence of ADHD according to gender and grade in the Hamamatsu School Cohort. Boys showed higher rates in the three subtypes: predominantly inattentive, predominantly hyperactive/impulsive, and combined. The prevalence rates of the subtypes decreased with grade, although this decline was more prominent for the predominantly hyperactive/impulsive and combined subtypes than the predominantly inattentive subtype. This suggests that hyperactivity symptoms attenuate with age, but inattention symptoms continue into adulthood to some extent. This pattern is consistent with previous findings confirmed around the world (APA 2013). The decrease in the total prevalence rate with grade is also in accordance with the previous findings in

Table 13.2.   Prevalence of Attention Deficit–Hyperactivity Disorder in the Hamamatsu School Cohort, according to Gender and Grade (%)

Grade	Boys				Girls				Total
	PI	PHI	Com-bined	Total	PI	PHI	Com-bined	Total	
Nursery school									
Grade 1 (3–4 y)	2.05	2.66	3.07	7.79	2.81	1.30	0.86	4.97	6.41
Grade 2 (4–5 y)	1.88	2.82	2.82	7.52	0.99	1.42	0.99	3.41	5.52
Grade 3 (5–6 y)	2.06	3.44	3.03	8.53	0.67	0.94	0.54	2.15	5.31
Elementary school									
Grade 1 (6–7 y)	2.94	2.37	2.57	7.88	0.80	0.38	0.48	1.66	4.83
Grade 2 (7–8 y)	3.65	2.10	2.97	8.72	1.69	0.33	0.66	2.68	5.64
Grade 3 (8–9 y)	3.04	1.16	2.31	6.51	1.20	0.24	0.84	2.27	4.37
Grade 4 (9–10 y)	2.63	1.38	1.32	5.33	0.92	0.43	0.25	1.60	3.49
Grade 5 (10–11 y)	2.50	0.65	1.72	4.87	0.94	0.24	0.12	1.30	3.08
Grade 6 (11–12 y)	2.19	0.63	1.15	3.97	0.75	0.06	0.44	1.25	2.66
Junior high school									
Grade 7 (12–13 y)	3.86	0.74	0.80	5.40	1.11	0.13	0.52	1.76	3.63
Grade 8 (13–14 y)	2.54	0.07	0.41	3.02	1.02	0.00	0.41	1.42	2.22
Grade 9 (14–15 y)	2.20	0.28	0.43	2.92	0.94	0.14	0.14	1.22	2.08

Note: PHI: predominantly hyperactive/impulsive; PI: predominantly inattentive.

Japan (Ministry of Education, Culture, Sports, Science, and Technology 2012; Nomura et al. 2014).

OTHER DEVELOPMENTAL DISORDERS

ADHD often coexists with other developmental disorders. Table 13.3 shows the association of ADHD with other developmental disorders. It shows that about 30% to 40% of students with any of the subtypes of ADHD have coexisting ASD and, conversely, about half of students with ASD have a subtype of ADHD. Also, it shows that about 20% to 30% of students with any subtype of ADHD have coexisting DCD and about 40% of students with DCD have a subtype of ADHD. These results indicate that there is a considerable rate of comorbidity with other disorders among students with any developmental disorder. Students with the predominantly inattentive subtype of ADHD had a higher rate of comorbidity with both ASD and DCD, as compared with those with the predominantly hyperactive/impulsive subtype. This suggests that the inattention symptom tends to coexist with symptoms of other disorders more than the hyperactivity/impulsivity symptom.

Table 13.3.   Association of Attention Deficit–Hyperactivity Disorder
with Other Developmental Disorders

	ASD			
	Students with ASD Who Had ADHD		Students with ADHD Who Had ASD	
ADHD Status	%	95% CI	%	95% CI
Not eligible	2.88	2.52–3.24	54.34	49.67–59.00
PI	40.37	34.52–46.22	24.89	20.84–28.93
PHI	31.68	24.49–38.86	11.64	8.64–14.65
Combined	43.96	33.76–54.15	9.13	6.43–11.83

	DCD			
	Students with DCD Who Had ADHD		Students with ADHD Who Had DCD	
ADHD Status	%	95% CI	%	95% CI
Not eligible	3.22	2.84–3.60	60.05	55.31–64.78
PI	30.22	24.82–35.61	19.18	15.37–22.98
PHI	23.27	16.70–29.84	8.45	5.76–11.14
Combined	29.35	20.04–38.65	6.16	3.84–8.49

Note: ASD: autism spectrum disorder; DCD: developmental coordination disorder; PHI: predominantly hyperactive/impulsive; PI: predominantly inattentive.

PSYCHOSOCIAL MALADAPTATION

ADHD symptoms affect psychosocial adaptation in various contexts. Because ADHD symptoms are associated with the symptoms of other developmental disorders, it is necessary to account for the symptoms of the other disorders when evaluating the effect of ADHD symptoms on psychosocial maladaptation. Therefore, we conducted a multiple-regression analysis in which the symptom scores of ASD and DCD were entered together with the ADHD symptom scores.

First of all, we conducted the multiple-regression analysis for academic achievement for each three-grade segment. Based on the analysis, in grades 1–3, inattention did not show a significant effect ($\beta = -0.031$, $p > 0.05$) and hyperactivity/impulsivity showed a significant but weak effect ($\beta = -0.077$, $p < 0.05$). Also, significant main effects were found for the ASD and DSD symptom scores (ASD symptom $\beta = 0.055$, $p < 0.05$; DCD symptom $\beta = -0.136$, $p < 0.001$). In grades 4–6, the effect of hyperactivity/impulsivity disappeared ($\beta = 0.047$, $p > 0.05$) and inattention showed a weak effect ($\beta = -0.137$, $p < 0.001$). The main effects of ASD and DCD symptoms were not significant (ASD symptom $\beta = -0.039$, $p > 0.05$; DCD symptom $\beta = -0.041$, $p > 0.05$). In grades 7–9, the effect of inattention increased to a moderate level and was greater than that for the ASD and DCD symptoms (inattention $\beta = -0.303$, $p < 0.001$; ASD symptom $\beta = -0.033$, $p > 0.05$; DCD symptom $\beta = -0.071$, $p < 0.001$). The main effect of hyperactivity/impulsivity was significant ($\beta = -0.049$, $p < 0.05$). These results suggest that inattention symptoms become a central risk factor of academic failure with increasing grade.

Table 13.4 shows the results of the multiple-regression analysis of social relationships and emotional/behavioral problems. For peer relationships, although the ASD and DCD symptoms showed moderate and weak effects, respectively, the ADHD symptoms showed no significant effect. However, the ADHD symptoms showed effects for relationships toward teachers and family. These results suggest that the ADHD symptoms themselves have an adverse effect on the relationship to surrounding adults but not to coeval peers.

Table 13.4 also shows the results of the multiple-regression analysis of emotional and behavioral problems. With respect to depression, the ADHD symptoms did not show a consistent effect. That is, although inattention showed a very weak positive effect, hyperactivity/impulsivity showed a negative effect. However, the two ADHD symptoms consistently showed a positive effect on aggression. These results suggest that the ADHD symptoms lead to externalizing problems rather than internalizing problems.

Although the Hamamatsu School Cohort study is limited in its scope, its findings speak to the experience of a large population of school-age children with ADHD in Japan. Their symptoms and the entailing problems that they face in terms of interpersonal relationships, academic performance, and behavioral tendencies have triggered concerns over the range of support and resources that are made available to them. In the following section, we discuss some of the legal measures taken to this end.

Laws Relating to ADHD and Other Neurodevelopmental Disorders

The enactment of two laws has offered the people of Japan more opportunities to obtain information about ADHD as well as other neurodevelopmental disorders. One of the acts—the Act on Support for Persons with Developmental Disabilities—was established in 2005. The other act that concerns ADHD is the revised School Educational Act, which sets out specific provisions for special needs education in elementary and middle schools in Japan. This law describes

Table 13.4. Results of the Multiple-Regression Analysis of Social Relationships and Emotional/Behavioral Problems

| | Social Relationships | | | | | | Emotional/Behavioral Problems | | | |
| | Peer | | Teacher | | Family | | Depression | | Aggression | |
Symptom	β	p	β	p	β	p	β	p	β	p
ADHD symptoms										
Inattention	0.013	0.473	0.128	<0.001	0.126	<0.001	0.039	0.022	0.082	<0.001
Hyperactivity/impulsivity	0.002	0.900	0.093	<0.001	0.061	<0.001	-0.093	<0.001	0.068	<0.001
ASD symptoms	0.297	<0.001	0.009	0.557	0.045	0.002	0.168	<0.001	0.074	<0.001
DCD symptoms	0.099	<0.001	-0.023	0.087	0.041	0.003	0.092	<0.001	-0.037	0.005
R^2	0.126		0.040		0.049		0.046		0.031	

Note: ASD: autism spectrum disorder; DCD: developmental coordination disorder.

the importance of early identification of symptoms and potential neurodevelopmental disabilities and the initiation of supports to the affected individuals, soon after identification. In addition, the Act on Support for Persons with Developmental Disabilities requires schools and local governments to provide sufficient and appropriate support for individuals with developmental disabilities.

Developmental disabilities, as described in this act, include ADHD, pervasive developmental disorders, and learning disabilities. In Japan, this inclusive term, *hattatsu shogai* (developmental disabilities), has gained more currency than the individual diagnostic categories that it contains. By using this generic term in the legal framework, it has been possible to extend support to individuals based on their specific needs rather than insisting on the strict categorization based on the biomedical diagnosis. When the Act on Support for Persons with Developmental Disabilities was established, ADHD was not included as a neurodevelopmental disorder in the *Diagnostic and Statistical Manual of Mental Disorders*, fourth edition, text revision (*DSM-IV-TR*). As we know, the *DSM-5* has revised its conceptualization of neurodevelopmental disorders, and ADHD has been classified as one of them. This change indicates that the Act on Support for Persons with Developmental Disabilities in Japan could pioneer advancements in this area of health care.

The enactment of the Act on Support for Persons with Developmental Disabilities has led to the partial amendment of the School Education Law (Ministry of Education, Culture, Sports, Science, and Technology 2004). Formerly, schools were differentiated according to types of developmental disability and their severity (e.g., schools for the blind, schools for the deaf, and schools for the intellectually disabled, the physically disabled, and the health impaired [students with chronic illnesses that require intermittent and often long-term hospitalization]). Under the new system, these designations according to disability type were loosened. In addition, the new system made a major shift from segregated education to inclusive education, opening up regular schools to students with certain disabilities including ADHD and other developmental disabilities. In order to meet their academic requirements, students with special needs who are enrolled in regular schools are assigned to special needs classes, which have small numbers of students (usually five) (Special Needs Education Division and Elementary and Secondary Education Bureau, Ministry of Education, Culture, Sports, Science, and Technology 2006).

Another program uses resource rooms in regular elementary and secondary schools; children with disabilities who are enrolled in regular classes may visit these rooms a few times a week to receive special instruction. The disabilities addressed in this program include autism, emotional disturbance, learning disabilities, ADHD, and other disorders. Students with ADHD, who are likely to have low academic achievement, utilize this program to "catch up" with schoolwork and to meet the required academic levels of performance. These programs are instrumental in preventing the development of secondary symptoms, such as low self-esteem.

Guidelines for the Treatment of ADHD

In Japan, the Working Group for Guidelines on the Diagnosis and Treatment of ADHD (2008)—a study group entrusted by the government to conduct research on ADHD—has published clinical guidelines for the assessment, diagnosis, and treatment of ADHD. The document is composed of two parts. The first part provides information and advice on the best practices for the assessment and diagnosis of ADHD, and the second part provides guidelines with a focus on the types of treatment for ADHD. This section provides a brief overview of their contents.

The guidelines on assessment/diagnosis comprise (or list) 15 items. For example:

- ADHD is defined as a disorder that is composed of three symptoms: inattention, hyperactivity, and impulsivity. ADHD is caused mainly by inborn brain dysfunctions. Since ADHD is one of the developmental disorders included in the Act on Support for Persons with Developmental Disabilities in Japan, we consider ADHD as one of the developmental disorders in this guideline.
- The following tools provide useful information for the diagnosis and assessment of ADHD: the Attention Deficit Hyperactivity Disorder Rating Scale (ADHD-RS), the Child Behavior Check List (CBCL), and the Oppositional Defiant Behavior Inventory (ODBI).
- Although the comorbidity of ADHD and pervasive developmental disorders has not been acknowledged in the *DSM-IV-TR*, children and adolescents with ADHD also have symptoms of pervasive developmental disorders. Thus, this guideline recommends that physicians and psychiatrists keep in mind the comorbidity of ADHD and pervasive developmental disorders.
- When diagnosing children and adolescents who manifest ADHD symptoms, physicians and psychiatrists must discriminate symptoms of

ADHD from symptoms of emotional conditions associated with maltreatment by caregivers. Physicians and psychiatrists should evaluate intellectual disabilities (which are sometimes associated with neglect by caregivers), attachment problems (which are symptoms of reactive attachment disorders), symptoms of trauma, and conduct problems.

- In Japan, there are few epidemiological research studies on ADHD in adults. Therefore, we currently state that only "some adults show symptoms of ADHD." Since ADHD is an inborn rather than an acquired disorder, it is unlikely that ADHD develops in adulthood. Thus, it is rational to think of adults diagnosed with ADHD as two groups: the continuing group and the newfound group. The continuing group consists of adults who have been diagnosed with ADHD in childhood or adolescence and exhibit symptoms of ADHD in adulthood. The newfound group is composed of adults whose symptoms were not prominent in childhood and adolescence but have surfaced in adulthood because of stressors, deteriorating mental conditions, and other factors.

The Working Group for Guidelines on the Diagnosis and Treatment of ADHD also has published guidelines specifically for the treatment of children and adolescents with ADHD. These guidelines are described in table 13.5.

Psychosocial Treatment for Children and Adolescents with ADHD

In Western countries, there is empirical evidence of the efficacy of pharmacotherapy and behavioral interventions or a combination of these therapies for children and adolescents with ADHD (see Smith et al. 2000). Therefore, both therapies are likely to be administered in Japan to treat children, adolescents, and adults with ADHD. As part of the pharmacotherapy regimen, psychiatrists can prescribe methylphenidate and atomoxetine for patients with ADHD. Usually, adults with ADHD are treated with the same stimulant medications. However, many parents in Japan whose children have ADHD have negative attitudes about pharmacotherapy (Tanaka et al. 2010).

This may be partly due to Japanese cultural beliefs regarding the biomedical control of features or tendencies that one is born with. Ohnuki-Tierney (1984) argues that terms such as *jibyo* (chronic/constantly present illness) and *taishitsu* (inborn weaknesses of constitution) speak to the cultural understanding that certain chronic conditions are considered to be deeply embedded in one's character and must be embodied and dealt with throughout one's life. Efforts to

Table 13.5.   Summary of Guidelines for the Treatment of ADHD

Item	Content
1	All treatments for ADHD should be administered based on a definitive diagnosis of ADHD. When administering pharmacotherapy, physicians and psychiatrists must comply with this guideline.
	When treating and supporting children and adolescents with ADHD, it is common for physicians and psychiatrists in Japan to combine clinical guidance for parents, cooperation with schools, individual therapy, and pharmacotherapy based on the clinical presentation of children and adolescents with ADHD. This is the standard treatment for ADHD in clinical practice.
2	Accumulated evidence has shown that the following strategies have been effective tools for children with ADHD: social skills training to modify inappropriate and problematic behaviors; parent training that provides parents with behavior modification skills; close cooperation with child consultation centers; and hospitalization. Medical institutions, educational facilities, social service agencies, and governments in each area ensure that these treatments are provided to children and adolescents with ADHD and to their parents in an appropriate manner.
3	To treat children and adolescents with ADHD who exhibit increased conflicts and deterioration in their self-esteem, individual psychotherapy, such as play therapy, is effective.
4	◆ Physicians and psychiatrists should not select pharmacotherapy until they reach the conclusion that this treatment modality will improve the symptoms and psychological condition of the patient. Physicians and psychiatrists should pay close attention to the risks entailed in pharmacotherapy, such as side effects.
	◆ If a rating on the Global Assessment of Functioning (GAF) scale is below 50, pharmacotherapy should be administered with psychosocial treatment and support.
	* The range of GAF is from 0 to 100; higher scores indicate higher psychological, social, and occupational functioning that an individual exhibits.
	◆ If a rating on the GAF is between 51 and 60, medical guidance for parents should be provided at the first psychological treatment visit. Physicians and psychiatrists should initiate pharmacotherapy if the patient's symptoms and environment remain invariant after a few months or if she worsens.
	◆ If a rating on the GAF is above 61, children and adolescents with ADHD should be treated with psychosocial methods only. Pharmacotherapy is administered only in exceptional cases.
	◆ In pharmacotherapy, methylphenidate is regarded as a first-line therapy. Among the prescriptions of methylphenidate, only Concerta is approved for the treatment of ADHD. Thus, Concerta is the first-line drug.
5	◆ In pharmacotherapy, Concerta is the first-line drug.
	◆ Children younger than 6 years of age should not take Concerta.
	◆ Physicians and psychiatrists must be careful when prescribing Concerta for adolescents older than 13 years of age.
	◆ Physicians and psychiatrists should attempt to discontinue prescriptions of Concerta before children with ADHD enter junior-high school.

(continued)

Table 13.5. (*continued*)

Item	Content
	♦ They must discontinue the prescription before their patients are 18 years of age.
	♦ Concerta should be taken once a day, before or after breakfast. Concerta should not be taken in the afternoon.
	♦ At first, Concerta should be administered at a dose of 18 milligrams per day. On the basis of the examination of symptoms patients exhibit, physicians and psychiatrists may increase or decrease daily doses by 9 or 18 milligrams.
	♦ A daily dose of Concerta must be less than 54 milligrams.
	♦ Physicians and psychiatrists must discontinue prescribing doses of Concerta if patients show side effects, such as reduced appetite.
	♦ Concerta should not be prescribed to children and adolescents with Tourette's syndrome. The prescription may be administered to children with epilepsy but with extreme caution.
	♦ Before prescribing Concerta, physicians and psychiatrists should screen patients for physical problems with the use of electrocardiography and blood tests. These check-ups should be performed periodically.
6	The following goals for the treatment of ADHD are recommended:
	♦ The treatment of ADHD should not focus on the complete elimination of the three ADHD symptoms, but on breaking the vicious cycle of symptoms and deterioration in the patient's current environments, such as school and family settings.
	♦ Physicians and psychiatrists should support children and adolescents with ADHD; they also should support the parents' view of their children's ADHD symptoms as personality characteristics, such as "active," which have positive rather than negative meanings.
	♦ Physicians and psychiatrists must provide a sufficient number of maintenance treatment periods as needed with consideration of the level of mental development and maturity of the children and adolescents being treated for ADHD.
	♦ After patients have received maintenance treatment, physicians and psychiatrists should examine them for the worsening of ADHD symptoms and psychosocial adaptation that may have occurred when they were without medication. When few or no signs of deterioration are confirmed, physicians and psychiatrists can determine that patients are fully recovered.
7	♦ When administering pharmacotherapy, physicians and psychiatrists should consider the risks of methylphenidate abuse.
	♦ Physicians and psychiatrists should understand that the probability of abuse increases after late adolescence, which means that adolescents and adults have a higher risk of addiction to methylphenidate than children do.
	♦ Physicians and psychiatrists who prescribe methylphenidate must always be aware of the possibility that individuals with drug addiction see doctors in order to obtain prescriptions of methylphenidate.
	♦ Physicians and psychiatrists should bear in mind the possibility that even though methylphenidate is prescribed for patients with ADHD, the patient's family members and friends can also become addicted to it.
	♦ When signs of drug abuse are found, the prescription of methylphenidate should be discontinued immediately.

"fix" these conditions through forceful measures such as biomedical intervention, therefore, are often met with resistance as going against the natural order of the body. In the case of pharmacotherapy for ADHD, such sentiments are voiced as concerns over the long-term side effects and the possibility of irreversible influences, particularly on a child's body. Thus, some of them refuse pharmacological treatments for the ADHD symptoms of their adolescents and children. For this reason, many clinical facilities proactively administer psychosocial interventions in order to treat ADHD in children and adolescents.

In 2007, Tanaka (2010) investigated the types of treatment that 433 psychiatrists, physicians, and pediatricians who were members of the Child Psychiatry and Child Neurology Associations in Japan selected for children and adolescents with ADHD. Pharmacotherapy, childcare advice, advice and liaison services in nursing and educational facilities, and psychological counseling accounted for 70% of the therapeutic interventions. Of the treatments currently used in Japan, pharmacotherapy and parent training were considered to be effective by more than 70% of the respondents. Furthermore, among the procedures that psychiatrists, physicians, and pediatricians reported that they had not administered, 40% of them reported that parent training was the treatment they wished to adopt in the future, followed by group therapy and social skills training. These results suggest that parent training is becoming a major treatment modality for children and adolescents with ADHD in Japan.

One reason for this is that familial support and care are highly valued in Japan, and parents and particularly mothers are seen as the primary caretakers of children with ADHD. Not only is their cooperation toward intervention practices essential in providing consistent feedback to children beyond the clinical setting, but also mothers are often held responsible for the successful implementation of such practices. The other reason is that mothers have been a highly visible and vocal group of activists and advocates for children with ADHD, forming parents' organizations and lobbying groups. Particularly during the early years when ADHD only began to gain currency in Japan, they suffered from unfounded criticism that their children's behavior was caused by lack of discipline or inappropriate child-rearing practices. Although ADHD is not caused by particular child-rearing practices, many parents took this criticism to heart and considered ways in which they could change how they relate to their children. It is against this backdrop that parents became actively involved in intervention practices, not simply as family members but also as victims and co-sufferers of social stigma. In the following section, we explain parent training as it is practiced in Japan.

Parent Training in Japan

Parent training is one of the main behavioral interventions in Japan. Two forms of parent training are most frequently practiced in Japan. One form of parent training was developed by the National Institute of Mental Health and the National Center of Neurology and Psychiatry (NCNP Form). The other approach to parent training was developed by the Hizen Psychiatric Center (Hizen Form). Since both programs are based on theories of behavior modification and cognitive-behavioral therapy, the parents participating in these programs can learn professionally developed techniques. These forms of parent training target parents whose children are in middle childhood because problem behaviors that children exhibit in an earlier developmental stage can be modified more readily than those that appear in a later one, such as adolescence.

The forms of parent training that are practiced in Japan differ from those in the United States. As compared with parent training in the United States, the NCNP and Hizen Forms place more emphasis on the development of parental skills and practices such as praising and encouraging children for their positive behavior. This practice of "complimenting" does not come naturally for many Japanese parents. Parents and teachers in Japan are less likely to directly praise their children or students for their individual achievement because there is a strong emphasis on conforming to the collective group of peers, which should also be the primary source of mutual monitoring, respect, criticism, and other forms of feedback (Lewis 1995). As a result, Japanese culture can contribute to a parenting style that has less positive reinforcement (such as praising) than other cultures. Both the NCNP and Hizen Forms provide parents with many chances to learn how and when they should praise and encourage their children in everyday life.

Although both of the parent training programs utilize techniques of behavioral therapy as noted above, there are differences between them. On the one hand, since the Hizen Form was originally designed to train parents who have children with intellectual disabilities or ASD, it focuses on the improvement of academic skills and the modification of inappropriate learning styles (Ohsumi and Ito 2005). Parents who participate in the program have opportunities to attend many individual lectures with trainers to identify and set up target behaviors and to discuss issues related to homework assignments. The Hizen Form provides individual rather than group training sessions. Because of its background, the Hizen Form usually is practiced in small groups, with fewer than five participants. On the other hand, the NCNP Form is based on the parent-training program developed in the UCLA Neuropsychiatric Institute and the program that Barkley (1987) has developed.

Therefore, the NCNP Form focuses on modifying inappropriate parenting behaviors and learning skills to modify children's problem behaviors (Kanbayashi et al. 2009). The NCNP Form consists of approximately 10 sessions and is conducted with a group of about 10 parents (the themes and content of each session in the NCNP Form are available in the article by Nakata [2010]). Even though the NCNP Form of parent training can efficiently provide a group of parents with parenting skills in one session, many parents who have children with ADHD are on a waiting list to participate in parent training because the number of qualified instructors is insufficient in Japan (Nakata 2010). The NCNP Form is more likely to be held in educational facilities, welfare institutions, and medical institutions.

Conclusion

This section aimed to provide an overview of the epidemiology, relevant laws, and clinical guidelines for the diagnosis and treatment of ADHD in Japan. Epidemiological studies conducted in Japan have shown prevalence rates similar to those in other countries in Europe, North America, and Asia. However, the amount of research on the epidemiology of ADHD in Japan is insufficient, and more research will be needed to determine its prevalence rate. We also presented the Hamamatsu School Cohort project that was initiated by our research team in 2007. The study has indicated that some children and adolescents with ADHD also have other neurodevelopmental disorders, and that ADHD symptoms in children and adolescents are associated with academic performance and social relationships.

In the second part of this section, we described the findings of a study that investigated the types of treatments that psychiatrists and physicians selected for children and adolescents with ADHD. More than half of the respondents considered parent training to be an effective treatment. This suggests that parent training is the primary psychological (or cognitive-behavioral) intervention used to treat children and adolescents with ADHD in Japan. However, in Japan, there are a limited number of practitioners who are qualified to provide parent training in medical, educational, or welfare institutions. Thus, there is a need to develop programs that will train practitioners or psychologists to provide parent training to parents who are distressed by their children's symptoms. We mentioned the spread of the social stigma of ADHD in Japan. Therefore, in the future, we also need to provide appropriate information about ADHD to people in Japan in order to prevent discrimination against children and adolescents with ADHD and their parents in the community.

REFERENCES

American Psychiatric Association (APA). 2013. *Diagnostic and Statistical Manual of Mental Disorders (DSM-5)*. 5th ed. Washington, DC: American Psychiatric Association.
Barkley, Russell A. 1987. *Defiant Children: A Clinician's Manual for Assessment and Parental Training*. New York: Guilford.
Birleson, Peter. 1981. "The Validity of Depressive Disorder in Childhood and the Development of a Self-Rating Scale: A Research Report." *Journal of Child Psychology and Psychiatry* 22: 73–88.
Buss, Arnold H., and Mark Perry. 1992. "The Aggression Questionnaire." *Journal of Personality and Social Psychology* 63: 452–59.
Conners, Keith C. 2008. *Third Edition Manual*. Toronto, ONT: Multi-Health Systems.
Conners, Keith C., Drew Erhardt, and Elizabeth Sparrow. 1999. *Conners' Adult ADHD Rating Scales*. Toronto, ONT: Multi-Health Systems.
Du Paul, George J., Tomas J. Power, Arthur D. Anastopoulos, and Robert Reid. 1998. *ADHD Rating Scale-IV: Checklist, Norms, and Clinical Interpretation*. New York: Guilford.
Ehlers, Stephan, Christopher Gillberg, and Lorna Wing. 1999. "A Screening Questionnaire for Asperger Syndrome and Other High-Functioning Autism Spectrum Disorders in School Age Children." *Journal of Autism and Developmental Disorders* 29: 129–41.
Epstein, Jeff, Diane E. Johnson, and Keith C. Conners. 2001. *Conners' Adult ADHD Diagnostic Interview for DSM-IV*. Toronto, ONT: Multi-Health Systems.
Ichikawa, Hironobu, and Yasuo Tanaka. 2008. *Shindan taiou no tameno ADHD hyouka suke-ru: ADHD-RS (DSM junkyo)—Check list, hyoujunchi to sono rinsyo-teki kaisyaku*. Akashi Syoten.
Ito, Hiroyuki, Yoshihiro Tanaka, Yasuo Murayama, Shunshi Nakajima, Nobuya Takayanagi, Wataru Noda, Naoto Mochizuki, Kaori Matsumoto, and Masatsugu Tsujii. 2014. "Development and Validation of a Scale of Social Maladjustment for Elementary and Junior High School Students." *Clinical Psychiatry* 56: 699–708.
Kanbayashi, Yasuko, Michiko Kita, Miho Kawachi, and Kazuko Fujii. 2009. *Kousureba Umakuiku Hattatsu Shyogai no Parent Training Zissenn Manual*. Tokyo: Chuohoki.
Lewis, Catherine C. 1995. *Educating Hearts and Minds: Reflections on Japanese Preschool and Elementary Education*. Cambridge: Cambridge University Press.
Ministry of Education, Culture, Sports, Science, and Technology. 2004. "Tokubetsu sienn kyouiku ni tsuite." http://www.mext.go.jp/a_menu/shotou/tokubetu/material/001.htm.
———. 2012. "Tsuujou no gakkyu ni zaiseki suru hattatsu syogai no kanousei no aru tokubetsu na kyouikuteki sien wo hitsuyou to suru jidou seito ni kansuru chousa kekka ni tsuite." http://www.mext.go.jp/a_menu/shotou/tokubetu/material/1328729.htm.
Nakamura, Kazuhiko. 2011. *CAARS nihongo ban*. Kaneko Syobo.

Nakata, Yoji. 2010. "Usefulness of the Shortened Program for Parent Training of Developmental Disorder." *Rissho University Shinrigaku Kenkyuuzyo Kiyo* 8: 1–63.

Nomura, Kenji, Kaori Okada, Yoriko Noujima, Satomi Kojima, Yuko Mori, Misuzu Amano, Masayoshi Ogura, Chie Hatagaki, Yuki Shibata, and Rie Fukumoto. 2014. "A Clinical Study of Attention-Deficit/Hyperactivity Disorder in Preschool Children—Prevalence and Differential Diagnoses." *Brain and Development* 36: 778–85.

Ohnuki-Tierney, Emiko. 1984. *Illness and Culture in Contemporary Japan: An Anthropological View*. Cambridge: Cambridge University Press.

Ohsumi, Hiroko, and Keisuke Ito, eds. 2005. *Hizen-shiki Oya Kunnrenn Program AD/HD wo Motsu Kodomo no Okaasann no Gakusyuushitsu*. Tokyo: Niheisha.

Polanczyk, Guiherme, Mauricio S. de Lima, Bernardo L. Horta, Joseph Biederman, and Luis A. Rohde. 2007. "The Worldwide Prevalence of ADHD: A Systematic Review and Metaregression Analysis." *American Journal of Psychiatry* 164: 942–48.

Simon, Viktoria, Pal Czobor, Sara Balint, Agnes Meszaros, and Istvan Bitter. 2009. "Prevalence and Correlates of Adult Attention-Deficit Hyperactivity Disorder: Meta-Analysis." *British Journal of Psychiatry* 194: 204–11.

Smith, Bradley H., Daniel A. Waschbusch, Michael T. Willoughby, and Steven Evans. 2000. "The Efficacy, Safety, and Practicality of Treatments for Adolescents with Attention-Deficit/Hyperactivity Disorder (ADHD)." *Clinical Child and Family Psychology Review* 3: 243–67.

Special Needs Education, Elementary and Secondary Education Bureau, Ministry of Education, Culture, Sports, Science, and Technology. 2006. http://www.mext.go.jp/english/elsec/1303763.htm.

Tanaka, Yasuo. 2010. "Steppingstones to the Psychosocial Treatment of ADHD." *Japanese Journal of Child and Adolescent Psychiatry* 51: 54–66.

———. 2011. *Conners 3 nihongo ban manual*. Kaneko Syobo.

Tanaka, Yasuo, Takayuki Hisakura, Tomomichi Kawamata, Masashi Uchida, Maki Fukuma, Mari Ito, and Yumiko Kanai. 2010. *ADHD no Sogouteki Chiryou—Oya to Honnninn to Sennmonnka no tameni*. Sapporo: Hokkaido Printing Planning.

Teruyama, Junko. 2014. "Japan's New Minority: Persons with Hattatsu Shōgai (Developmental Disability)." PhD diss., University of Michigan.

Uchiyama, Satoshi, Masafumi Ohnishi, and Kazuhiko Nakamura. 2012. "Nihon ni okeru seijinki ADHD no ekigaku chousa: seijinki ADHD no yuubyouritsu ni tsuite." *Kodomo No Kokoro to Nou no Hattatsu* 3: 34–42.

Wilson, Brenda N., Susan G. Crawford, Dido Green, Gwen Roberts, Alice Aylott, and Bonnie J. Kaplan. 2009. "Psychometric Properties of the Revised Developmental Coordination Disorder Questionnaire." *Physical and Occupational Therapy in Pediatrics* 29: 182–202.

Working Group for Guidelines on the Diagnosis and Treatment of ADHD. 2008. "Kodomo no chuui ketuzyo tadou sei syogai (ADHD) no sinndann chiryou guideline." In *Chuui ketuzyo tadousei syougai—ADHD—no sinndann chiryou guideline*, edited by K. Saito and K. Watabe, 1–27. 3rd ed. Tokyo: JIHO.

14

Pharmaceuticalization through Government Funding Activities

ADHD in New Zealand

Manuel Vallée

Worldwide medication consumption has expanded significantly in recent decades, particularly in Western societies, such as France, the United Kingdom, and the United States, and in rapidly developing middle-income countries, including China, Brazil, and India (Busfield 2010). For example, worldwide prescription drug sales nearly tripled between the early 1980s and 2002, reaching a figure of US$400 billion (Angell 2005). Moreover, worldwide sales grew from US$350 billion in 2000 to US$700 billion by 2007, a doubling in the span of seven years (Busfield 2010).

As this pertains to medications for attention deficit–hyperactivity disorder (ADHD), while American consumption skyrocketed during the 1980 and 1990s (Drug Enforcement Agency 1981–2006), in recent decades significant increases have also occurred in other countries. According to the International Narcotics Control Board (INCB), a UN agency charged with tracking the consumption of controlled substances, between 2000 and 2012, Switzerland's methylphenidate (the generic form of Ritalin) consumption grew 422% (from 2.79 to 14.7 standard doses per 1,000 inhabitants), Iceland's grew 529% (from 2.29 to 14.8 standard doses), and Israel's grew 1,077% (from 0.58 to 8.48 standard doses) (for more details, see table 14.1). Sociologists (Abraham 2010; Busfield 2015) view such increases as evidence of the pharmaceuticalization of society, "the process

Table 14.1. Methylphenidate Use by Country (standard daily dose per 1,000 inhabitants/day)

Rank 2012		2000	2001	2002	2003	2004	2005	2006	2007	2008	2009	2010	2011	2012
1	Iceland	2.29	2.35	3.56	5.27	7.53	7.91	4.53	10.6	11.15	11.25	4.72	14.07	14.8
2	Switzerland	2.79	2.82	2.72	2.23	1.97	1.36	3.66	2.36	3.44	3.58	n/a	n/a	14.72
3	Israel	0.58	0.72	0.97	1.31	1.62	2.69	2.26	3.13	4.45	6.05	7.38	7.4	8.48
4	United States	3.69	5.11	5.88	5.21	7.14	7.61	9.18	5.21	12.03	9.3	15.5	19.93	7.94
5	Sweden	0.1	0.16	0.21	0.35	0.58	0.89	1.59	1.72	2.51	3.53	4.92	6.22	7.19
6	Norway	0.74	0.78	0.95	2.13	2.23	2.61	3.66	4.38	4.4	5.9	n/a	n/a	6.94
7	Denmark	n/a	0.22	0.27	1.77	0.63	0.88	1.3	1.77	3.55	2.79	5.09	5.88	6.37
8	Canada	4.74	0.29	1.59	4.24	4.22	2.55	4	5.42	6.12	2.07	n/a	n/a	5.51
9	Spain	0.24	0.66	0.55	0.78	0.49	1.11	1.26	0.02	1.18	1.49	n/a	n/a	2.82
10	New Zealand	1.72	1.29	1.54	1.23	1.93	1.35	1.35	1.75	1.79	n/a	n/a	n/a	2.70
11	Belgium	0.47	0.51	0.79	1.12	0.99	1.24	1.45	1.93	2.06	1.97	n/a	n/a	2.54
12	Australia	0.99	0.89	0.79	1.34	1	1.44	1.36	1.39	1.53	1.78	n/a	n/a	2.33
13	Germany	0.56	0.67	0.78	0.99	1.11	1.47	1.39	1.92	2.19	2.07	1.98	1.97	2.08
14	Chile	0.15	0.24	0.22	0.35	0.33	0.44	0.53	0.75	n/a	1.13	1.1	1.54	1.70
15	Finland	0.04	0.07	0.07	0.29	0.33	0.57	0	0.54	n/a	1.56	n/a	n/a	1.47
16	South Africa	n/a	0.16	0.23	0.27	0.11	0.51	0.3	0	n/a	n/a	n/a	n/a	1.02
17	United Kingdom	1.31	1.04	1.35	0.95	1.38	1.32	0	0.01	3.67	0.39	0.15	0.5	0.68
18	Netherlands	0.99	1.11	1.21	1.38	1.82	1.81	2.75	2.71	4.02	n/a	n/a	6.63	n/a
19	Ireland	0.26	n/a	0.35	0.36	0.66	0.35	0.65	0.59	n/a	n/a	n/a	n/a	n/a

Sources: United Nations 2005, 2006, 2007, 2008, 2009, 2010, 2011, 2013.
Note: n/a: not available.

by which social, behavioural or bodily functions are treated, or deemed to be in need of treatment, with medical drugs" (Abraham 2010: 604).

Although medications can be beneficial to those who need them, it is widely acknowledged that some are used too liberally (WHO 2011), and this might well be the case for ADHD medications. Stuart Kirk (2004) argues that the ADHD diagnostic criteria in the fourth edition of the *Diagnostic and Statistical Manual* (*DSM-IV*) (AOA 1994) are overly inclusive and that for every child who is accurately diagnosed as having ADHD, eight are falsely diagnosed. In the United States, the problem is compounded by the fact that approximately 70% of children diagnosed with ADHD are treated with medications (Robison et al. 2004; Visser et al. 2014). As Busfield (2015) outlines, medication overuse incurs numerous social costs, including health side effects as well as higher health care service costs. ADHD medication side effects include suppressed appetite, growth impairment, restlessness, tremors, headaches, insomnia, symptoms of anxiety and depression, increased blood pressure and heart rate, and cardiac arrest (Rappley 1997; Hamed, Kauer, and Stevens, 2015), each of which can lead to the prescription of additional medications for side effect suppression. Given these problems, it behooves sociologists to better understand the forces that contribute to ADHD's pharmaceuticalization.

To shed light on these issues, I examine New Zealand's growing consumption of medications to treat ADHD. While geographic and linguistic accessibility are two motivations behind this case selection, the case also has strategic value because New Zealand was one of the first countries outside the United States and Canada to experience a dramatic increase in ADHD medication consumption (Berbatis, Sunderland, and Bulsara 2002). Indeed, the nation's methylphenidate consumption grew 1,800% in eight years, from fewer than 3,500 prescriptions in 1993 to nearly 65,000 by 2001 (PHARMAC 1998, 2003), establishing the country as one of the top three consumers in the world (Berbatis, Sunderland, and Bulsara 2002).

To shed greater light on the New Zealand case, I draw from Joan Busfield's (2010) work on pharmaceutical consumption. Although she finds pharmaceutical manufacturers to be the major driving force in the pharmaceuticalization process, she argues that government can be a significant countervailing force through its regulatory and funding activities (Busfield 2010). Following her lead, I analyze the role played by New Zealand funding agencies and maintain that they have shaped the process in two major ways. First, far from being a countervailing force, their decision to subsidize ADHD medications set the stage for a rapid increase in consumption. Second, funding decisions have steered consumption toward lower-cost generic medications and away from the more expensive patent medications. Beyond elucidating the specific case, this analysis provides insights that help us better understand how governments can shape the pharmaceuticalization of ADHD in other countries, as well as the pharmaceuticalization of other medical conditions.

Conceptual Framework

Conceptually, my analysis of the New Zealand case is mainly guided by the work of Cohen and colleagues (2001), which provides a useful overarching framework for studying medication use, and that of Busfield (2010), which provides a more tangible assessment of the forces shaping medication use.

Cohen and colleagues (2001) posit medication use as a "socially embedded phenomenon" (442) and pursue a critical analysis of the "rational use of drugs" view (which portrays medications as technological products to be consumed to satisfy precisely identified health needs). Cohen et al. (2001) consider the "rational use" perspective to be a simplistic technological determinism, which ignores the way medication usage is driven by varied and legitimate rationalities, which change over time and place. Instead, they offer a "systemic" conception, which views medication use as being shaped by a complex interplay of social forces, including socio-historical tendencies, "diverse actors, social systems, and institutions," which determine "who uses what medications, how, when and why" (441). Moreover, they espouse a biographical approach to studying medications in which one traces the medication's lifecycle, and identifies how that lifecycle has been influenced by actors, institutions, and social systems. Although Cohen et al. (2001) provide a useful overarching conception of medication consumption, I used Busfield's (2010) work for a more fine-grained discussion of the social forces shaping medication use.

Busfield (2010) examines five sets of agents who mediate medication use: pharmaceutical manufacturers, doctors, the public, governments, and insurance companies. She argues that while pharmaceutical manufacturers are the primary drivers of medication consumption, the success of their efforts is mediated by the activities of the other four agents, which can act as countervailing forces. Moreover, she highlights the instrumental role played by the state, which influences consumption through both its regulatory and funding activities. As regulators, governments play a determining role in deciding which medicines are available to consumers. They evaluate medications for safety and efficacy, determine whether they should be sold, monitor them after licensing, and pull them off the market when necessary. Regarding funding, the state determines "how easy it is to see a doctor, any charge for a consultation, which medicines require a prescription, whether prescribed medicines are available without cost to some or all groups, and whether costs are to be shared" (Busfield 2010: 939). In other words, their decisions mediate the public's financial accessibility to the medications, which can considerably influence consumption.

Even though regulatory and funding activities are both important to the pharmaceuticalization process, the main focus in this chapter is on the latter since it has received relatively less attention in the pharmaceuticalization literature. Although I do discuss regulatory activities, it is in the context of how they mediate government funding activities.

The Globalization of ADHD and Its Medications

Hyperactive behavior first became a commonly diagnosed problem in the 1960s in the United States, after financial pressures prompted American pediatricians there to add children's behavioral problems to their professional jurisdiction (Pawluch 2009). Although it remained a mostly American phenomenon for decades, the situation has changed in recent decades. First, International Narcotics Control Board (INCB) data (see table 14.1) show that by 2000, methylphenidate was being consumed in numerous countries, which suggests ADHD was being increasingly diagnosed. Similarly, Berbatis, Sunderland, and Bulsara (2002) demonstrated increased consumption in Anglo-Saxon countries, including Australia, New Zealand, and Canada. Additionally, sociologists have demonstrated the spread outside the Anglo-Saxon world. For example, Vallée's work (2010) demonstrated modest consumption growth in France, while Conrad and Bergey (2014) have traced the migration of the ADHD concept in numerous countries, including Germany, Italy, Brazil, and the United Kingdom.

Prevalence in New Zealand

In New Zealand, ADHD prevalence has varied profoundly over time. In the 1970s, Werry and Hawthorne (1976) estimated the prevalence (based on the Conners questionnaire [Conners 1969]) to be 1.07% among boys and 0.58% among girls. A decade later, Anderson and colleagues (1987) investigated the prevalence among 11-year-old children in a rural population and, using the *DSM-III* criteria (APA 1980), reported a prevalence of 6.7%. Using the *DSM-III-R* criteria (APA 1987), McGee and colleagues (1990) then estimated a 2.1% prevalence among 15-year-olds. Their work was followed by that of Fergusson, Horwood, and Lynskey (1993), who estimated a prevalence of 2.8% to 4.8% for the same age group. In 2000, based on his decades-long familiarity with the New Zealand case, John Werry suggested a 5% prevalence among those younger than 18 years (Ministry of Health 2001), which would put the prevalence in line with the United States' range of 6 to 11% (Winterstein et al. 2008; Visser et al. 2014). However, this comparison should be used cautiously. Whereas the American figure is based on epidemiological data, Werry's figure was a heuristic estimate made for the New Zealand ADHD Clinical Practice Guidelines. As the guideline authors (2001) emphasized, studies similar to those in the United States had yet to be produced for New Zealand. The Ministry of Health (2001) also emphasizes that establishing reliable and comparable ADHD prevalence estimates is difficult for a number of reasons, including differing sampling methods; differing diagnostic methods; a high level of subjectivity in the diagnostic process; and varying degrees of agreement between evaluators on what constitutes ADHD.

The 6.7% estimate of Anderson et al. (1987) is anomalous in the context of New Zealand's other studies. Moreover, if that estimate is bracketed, the rest of the data suggests that ADHD prevalence has gradually grown over time. However, this interpretation should also be used cautiously because diagnostic criteria have not remained constant over time. Although the initial research was based on the Conners questionnaire, subsequent research was based on the *DSM* criteria, which has expanded considerably over time. Specifically, whereas the American Psychiatric Association (APA) estimated the *DSM-III* criteria would produce a 3% prevalence, it estimated the *DSM-III-R* and *DSM-IV* criteria would produce estimates of 4.2% and 7%, respectively (August and Garfinkel 1989; Kirk 2004). Thus, all other things being equal, one should expect the ADHD prevalence to have increased over time.

The Globalization of the Pharmaceutical Approach

The extensive use of psychostimulants to address children's behavioral problems can be traced to the United States, where pediatricians seized control of and continue to dominate the ADHD treatment field (Robison et al. 2004; Pawluch 2009). Given their disciplinary background, pediatricians are inclined to see behavioral problems through a biomedical lens and, following the US Food and Drug Administration's (FDA) 1955 approval of methylphenidate (the generic name for Ritalin) for the US market, began prescribing Ritalin for hyperactive behavior (Safer and Zito 1999). By 1970, it is estimated that 150,000 American children were consuming the medications (Gadow 1981). In subsequent decades, growing numbers of American children were medicated with Ritalin, Dexedrine, and other psychostimulants, and it is now estimated that 3.5 million US children (6.1%) are consuming psychostimulants or other ADHD medications (Visser et al. 2014).

For decades, treating children with psychostimulants remained an American phenomenon. In fact, as of the mid-1990s, the use of Ritalin was banned in several European countries (including France, Sweden, and Italy), and as late as 2003, the United States still accounted for at least 80% of worldwide methylphenidate (the generic name for Ritalin) consumption (Shrag and Divosky 1975; Bonati, Impicciatore, and Pandolfini 2001; Larrson 2005; Scheffler et al. 2007). However, during the 1990s psychostimulant consumption grew considerably in English-speaking countries (see table 14.1). For instance, between 1994 and 2000, Canada's psychostimulant consumption grew 375%, Australia's grew 846%, and New Zealand's grew 1500% (from 3,500 to 54,600 prescriptions) (PHARMAC 2001; Berbatis, Sunderland, and Bulsara 2002). Moreover, recent INCB data suggest that the practice has spread beyond these English-speaking countries, with significant growth occurring in Iceland, Switzerland, and Israel, which are now among the world leaders in methylphenidate consumption (see table 14.1).

As mentioned earlier, the growing use of psychostimulants is problematic. Beyond the high rate of false diagnoses provided by an overly inclusive ADHD category, the medications are associated with numerous side effects, they contribute to medical inflation, and they are a controlled substance in many countries, such as France (Vallée 2010).

New Zealand's Growing Consumption of ADHD Medications

Eight ADHD medications have been significantly prescribed in New Zealand: Ritalin, Dexedrine, Rubifen (generic version of Ritalin), Ritalin-SR, Rubifen-SR; Concerta (a sustained-release formulation of Ritalin); Atomoxetine; and Strattera (a nonstimulant medication). Even though other medications can be prescribed, the aforementioned are the only ones whose costs have been subsidized by the country's national health plan.

In New Zealand's health care system, general practitioners are the first to assess children for ADHD. If a general practitioner suspects ADHD is present, she then refers the patient to a specialist, such as a pediatrician or psychiatrist, who is required to pursue a comprehensive assessment of the patient (Ministry of Health 2001). Since March 1999, prescriptions for ADHD medications can only be obtained if the specialist confirms the initial diagnosis (Ministry of Health

2001). This practice departs significantly from that in the United States, where ADHD medications can be prescribed by general practitioners and, in four states, nurse practitioners (Safer 2000).

Although New Zealand is more restrictive regarding who can prescribe ADHD medications, its treatment approach seems to align almost seamlessly with the pharma-centric approach favored in the United States, as suggested by the New Zealand 2001 Clinical Practice Guidelines, which state that "as a general rule, monotherapy with a stimulant drug (methylphenidate or dexamphetamine) is the first line of treatment" (Ministry of Health 2001: viii). The authors of the guidelines do acknowledge the studies (in particular, the Multimodal Treatment Study of Children with ADHD [MTA Cooperative Group 1999]) that found better results when behavioral therapy was combined with a stimulant drug. However, they systematically deemphasize this option, arguing it is "more labour intensive and costly" and that "the resources involved in the MTA study would not normally be available in New Zealand" (ix).

It is difficult to trace the origins of New Zealand's psychostimulant use because there are little reliable data predating the 1993 period. However, New Zealand psychiatrists have been studying methylphenidate's effects on New Zealand children since at least 1974 (Werry and Sprague 1974), which suggests that the country's medication use dates back to at least that period. In contrast to the US case, however, New Zealand consumption took longer to grow. Whereas US consumption rates increased dramatically within 15 years after methylphenidate's first use (Gadow 1981), in New Zealand, consumption rates were still low in 1993 (see table 14.3), two decades after it was first used. However, as table 14.2 demonstrates, between 1993 and 2001, New Zealand's psychostimulant prescriptions grew 1,853%.

This growth slowed considerably over the following decade, inching up to a peak of 69,000 prescriptions in 2004, when prescriptions plateaued until 2009 (see table 14.2). However, between 2008 and 2012, New Zealand experienced a sharp increase in the per capita consumption of methylphenidate, which grew from 1.79 to 2.7 standard daily doses per 1,000 inhabitants (United Nations 2009, 2013). This consumption increase seems to mimic that of other industrialized countries, such as Australia, Israel, Spain, Sweden, and Switzerland, whose consumption increased 52%, 91%, 139%, 187%, and 328%, respectively, during the period (see table 14.1).

Another international trend occurring in New Zealand is the growing number of adults who are being treated for ADHD. This trend emerged in the United

Table 14.2.   Psychostimulant Use in New Zealand, 1993–2009

Year	Prescriptions	Growth Year over Year (%)	Growth since 1993 (%)
2009	69,820	7	2,002
2008	65,153	−3	1,861
2007	67,058	−2	1,919
2006	68,746	−1	1,969
2005	69,678	1	1,997
2004	69,084	3	1,980
2003	67,260	5	1,925
2002	64,317	−1	1,836
2001	64,874	19	1,853
2000	54,681	2	1,546
1999	53,496	18	1,510
1998	45,306	36	1,264
1997	33,213	33	900
1996	24,922	94	650
1995	12,817	112	286
1994	6,038	82	82
1993	3,322		

Sources: PHARMAC 1998, 2000, 2001, 2003, 2007, 2008a, 2009.

Table 14.3.   New Zealand Psychostimulant Use by Region, 1993–2001

	North Region	Change since 1993 (%)	Mid-land Region	Change since 1993 (%)	Central Region	Change since 1993 (%)	Southern Region	Change since 1993 (%)
2001	15,559	1,746	13,282	2,756	17,953	2,066	18,079	1,426
2000	12,357	1,366	11,317	2,334	15,467	1,766	15,476	1,206
1999	12,020	1,326	11,517	2,377	14,496	1,649	15,463	1,205
1998	9,642	1,044	10,614	2,183	11,826	1,327	13,294	1,022
1997	5,156	512	8,803	1,793	8,689	948	10,756	808
1996	4,778	467	6,204	1,234	5,481	561	8,459	614
1995	2,554	203	2,239	382	2,913	251	5,111	331
1994	1,356	61	942	103	1,636	97	2,104	78
1993	843		465		829		1,185	

Source: PHARMAC 2001.
   Note: Totals reflect methylphenidate and dexamphetamine prescriptions.

Table 14.4.   Percentage of Scripts Dispensed to Patients between the Ages of 0 and 14 Years

2006	2007	2008	2009	2010	2011	2012	2013
65.60	63.10	60.90	58.20	56.30	54.00	52.70	51.00

Source: Ministry of Health 2014.

States in the late 1990s, when changes to the *DSM* diagnostic criteria allowed adults to be diagnosed with ADHD, thereby resulting in a stream of adults seeking treatment for the condition (Conrad 2007). This seems to also be a trend in New Zealand, as DuPaul et al. (2009) report that 8.1% of male and 1.7% of female college students self-report clinically significant ADHD symptoms. Moreover, the percentage of prescriptions for persons younger than 15 years of age has dropped from 65.6% in 2006 to 51% in 2013, which suggests a higher percentage of the medications are now being consumed by those older than 14 (see table 14.4).

Government Funding Activities and the Pharmaceuticalization Process

According to Busfield (2010: 940), government funding policy helps determine "how easy it is to see a doctor, any charge for consultation, which medicines require prescription, and whether prescribed medicines are available without cost to some or all groups." Access to health care is reasonably good in New Zealand, thanks to its universal health care system. This is particularly true for children younger than 6 years, for whom doctor consultations are free. For older populations, cost is more of an issue. Prior to July 2015, those in the 6- to 17-year-old age range paid NZD$11 to NZD$50 per visit, and those older than 17 years paid NZD$45 to NZD$60 per visit (Johnston 2013). Given that most children treated for ADHD are in the 6- to 17-year-old age range, New Zealand's funding scheme could have impeded access to care in the past, particularly for children from lower economic classes. In turn, this could have impeded medication consumption. However, in July 2015 this became less of an issue for children between 6 and 12 years, who became eligible for free consultations with general practitioners (Ministry of Health 2016).

Beyond consultation charges, Busfield (2010) argues that medication consumption is also mediated by medication costs. She maintains that these costs are not a major deterrent in England, where medications are free to large groups of people, including those younger than 16 or older than 60 years, pregnant women, women who have given birth in the previous 12 months, war pensioners, and low-income populations (NHS Information Centre 2009). In contrast, medications were slightly less accessible in New Zealand: prior to July 2015 they were only free to children younger than 6 years (Ministry of Health 2015). However, although the rest of the population has to pay a co-pay for each subsidized prescription item, the amount is a relatively low NZD$5 (Ministry of Health 2015).

Regarding ADHD medications, the government increased accessibility to Ritalin and Dexedrine in the early 1990s, when they began subsidizing both. The subsidies meant that parents only had to pay a small co-pay for the prescription, which enabled the rapid consumption growth that occurred during the 1990s. While the pre-2015 co-pay scheme meant the majority of children diagnosed with ADHD had to pay for medications, the amount was relatively small. Moreover, in July 2015 the cost ceased being an issue for children between 6 and 12 years because the government made subsidized medications free of charge to all children younger than 13 (Ministry of Health 2016).

PHARMAC—Steering Consumers to Less Expensive Options

Even though government funding facilitates access to medications, Busfield (2010) emphasizes that governments also have a strong interest in controlling medication prices, in order to limit skyrocketing medical expenditures. In 1993, 10% to 20% annual increases in pharmaceutical expenditures led the New Zealand government to try reining in expenses by establishing PHARMAC (PHARMAC 1995; Davis 2004). PHARMAC is the government agency that decides which medications are to be subsidized for use in public and community hospitals (PHARMAC 2014). As part of its decision-making process, PHARMAC tries to "balance the needs of patients for equitable access to health care with the needs of tax payers for responsible management of costs" (PHARMAC 1995: ii).

One cost-limiting government strategy is steering consumption toward lower-cost generic medications, and away from the more expensive patent medications (Busfield 2010). This phenomenon is well illustrated by the New Zealand case, where PHARMAC funding policies have tended to favor generic medications over their more expensive brand-name predecessors (Davis 2004). Regarding ADHD medications, in November 2006, PHARMAC started subsidizing Rubifen-SR (a less-expensive, generic form of Ritalin), with the intention of stopping subsidizing Ritalin-SR by April 2007; this decision was intended to save more than NZD$1 million per year (Johnston 2007).

Beyond funding generics, the New Zealand case demonstrates other cost-limiting government strategies. For example, PHARMAC has avoided subsidizing "me-too" drugs: new brand-name drugs that are the same formulation as preexisting brand-name medications but with a minor cosmetic change, such as changes in pill color or shape. Although these medications have brand-name prices, they offer no additional therapeutic value, and PHARMAC has steadfastly avoided funding them. It has also delayed or avoided funding new patent medications, which would have been more costly and could have replaced the consumption of generic medications. For example, while Adderall became one of the top-prescribed ADHD medications in the United Kingdom and the United States, severely eroding Ritalin's market share in the process (Dorfman 2006), PHARMAC never subsidized it for the New Zealand market. In addition, PHARMAC did not subsidize Strattera (a non-stimulant medication) until 2009, a full three years after the FDA approved it for the American market. Moreover, even though PHARMAC eventually subsidized Strattera, it limited access to the medication by stipulating it would only be subsidized in cases where (1) stimulant medications posed an unacceptable medical risk, (2) a subsidized stimulant resulted in worsening substance abuse or if there existed a significant diversion risk with the subsidized stimulant, or (3) stimulant treatments were tried but found to be ineffective or associated with serious adverse reactions (PHARMAC 2008b).

Mediated by Economic Context

While Busfield (2010) is correct in saying that government funding decisions can strongly affect pharmaceutical consumption, it bears noting that the degree of influence will be mediated by the country's underlying economic context. Specifically, a government's influence is likely to be stronger in areas where citizens have less disposable income and are more dependent on government subsidies. This is particularly true in countries like New Zealand, where the cost of living is very high. In particular, the country has a high wage-to-housing ratio (in 2012, the average income was NZD$48,600 and the average home cost NZD$410,000; Tait 2013; Ninness 2014), which has led the country's housing market to be rated "among the most overvalued in the developed world" (Nichols 2014). This means citizens have less disposable income and would be hard-pressed to afford out-of-pocket medication costs for unsubsidized ADHD medications, which in 2007 dollars ranged from NZD$50 to NZD$100 per month (depending on the dosing) (Ford 2007; Johnston 2007). This point was underscored in 2006, when PHAR-

MAC stopped subsidizing Ritalin-SR in favor of Rubifen-SR. Although many parents would have preferred to keep their children on Ritalin-SR (due to the side effects of Rubifen-SR), many could not afford the unsubsidized out-of-pocket cost (Ford 2007; Johnston 2007).

The Mediating Effect of Regulatory Agencies

Funding agency decisions can amplify and channel the use of medications, but their influence can be strongly mediated by the activities of regulatory agencies. First, the regulatory agency power supersedes that of funding agencies because a decision to subsidize a medication is contingent on the regulatory agency's safety assessment of the medication. For example, even though PHAR-MAC approved the subsidization of Strattera in 2008, its availability on the New Zealand market was contingent on the safety assessment by the Medicines and Medical Devices Safety Authority (MEDSAFE) (PHARMAC 2008b).

Additionally, if a newly subsidized generic medication becomes associated with adverse drug reactions, MEDSAFE can take it upon itself to reinvestigate and, if necessary, order PHARMAC to continue subsidizing the brand-name medication. This is precisely what took place with Rubifen-SR in 2006–7, when the New Zealand Centre for Adverse Reaction Monitoring received more than 200 reports of either reduced therapeutic effect or adverse psychiatric reactions, which prompted MEDSAFE to reexamine Rubifen-SR and to order PHARMAC to continue subsidizing Ritalin for patients who were suffering reactions to Rubifen-SR (Kiong 2007; Fraser and Tilyard 2009).

Comparative research shows that beyond determining a medication's legal access to the market, regulatory agencies can mediate the restrictiveness of prescribing conditions. For example, while New Zealand regulations stipulate ADHD medications can only be obtained when specialists (child psychiatrists, neurologists, and pediatricians) sign off on the ADHD diagnosis (Ministry of Health 2001), regulations are more restrictive in France, where methylphenidate can only be prescribed by specialists practicing in hospital settings (Debroise 2004; Vallée 2010). In contrast, the situation is far less restrictive in the United States, where the medications can be prescribed by general practitioners and, in four states, nurse practitioners working in any setting (Safer 2000). In turn, such variation can powerfully influence medication prescribing.

Apart from setting regulations for a drug's first approval, regulatory agencies can also introduce new prescribing restrictions for a previously approved medication, which happened in 2010 when MEDSAFE restricted the prescribing of all methylphenidate-containing products. Specifically, after reviewing European product information for methylphenidate, MEDSAFE changed the approved uses of methylphenidate products and barred them from being prescribed to people with preexisting cardiovascular or cerebrovascular disorders or a "history of severe depression, anorexic disorders, suicidal tendencies, psychotic symptoms, severe mood disorders, mania, schizophrenia, or psychopathic personality disorder" (MEDSAFE 2010). MEDSAFE also stipulated that patients prescribed methylphenidate products should be closely monitored, which was to include: (1) recording blood pressure at least every six months and at every dose adjustment; (2) recording the height, weight, and appetite at least every six months; (3) treatment holidays for patients who did not meet weight and height standards for their age; and (4) a cardiac evaluation for all patients with symptoms suggesting heart disease (MEDSAFE 2010).

Social Consequences of Government Funding Activities

Subsidizing ADHD medications is a double-edged sword for patients and their families. On the one hand, subsidies provide access to symptom-suppressing treatments, which can be a significant short-term aid for both children and their parents. However, to the degree that medications become the main treatment option, encouraging the use of pharmaceuticals can be problematic. First, the medications can have side effects. In the case of methylphenidate, these include suppressed appetite, growth impairment, restlessness, tremors, headaches, insomnia, symptoms of anxiety and depression, increased blood pressure and heart rate, and cardiac arrest (Rappley 1997; Hamed, Kauer, and Stevens, 2015). In turn, the use of medications can lead to the prescription of other medications to suppress those side effects. Then there is the question of the medication's long-term safety. According to the European Medicines Agency (2009), methylphenidate's long-term safety has never been systematically evaluated in controlled trials.

Another problem with encouraging pharmaceutical use is that the medications do not cure the patient. The best they can do is suppress symptoms, and there are serious questions about their ability to do so over the long term. For instance, the European Medicines Agency (2009) reports that methylphenidate's long-term efficacy has never been assessed in controlled trials. Additionally, while the much-hyped Multimodal Treatment Study of ADHD initially suggested that psychostimulants were significantly more effective than behavior therapy, follow-up studies showed that any perceived superiority had vanished by the 14-month mark (Molina et al. 2009). Moreover, some patients develop a tolerance to the medications, which diminishes their efficacy and necessitates stronger doses to stave off symptoms (Breggin 2001). In turn, the stronger doses increase the child's risk of suffering side effects (Breggin 2001).

More insidiously, however, by encouraging the use of pharmaceuticals, the subsidies encourage a reductionist and individualizing approach to the condition, where the source of the symptoms is located in the body and contextual sources are obscured. Contextual contributors to ADHD symptoms can include exposure to toxicants (such as lead, mercury, cadmium, polychlorinated biphenyls [PCBs], dioxins, or organophosphate pesticides) (Schettler et al. 2000; Boucher et al. 2012) or dietary factors (Jacobson and Schardt 1999; McCann et al. 2007). In turn, failing to address underlying causes condemns patients to being re-exposed to environmental factors that may be contributing to the symptoms, thereby creating a continual need for medical care. In a sense, strongly encouraging pharmaceuticals has the effect of steering people away from the care they need and deserve.

Beyond the individual families, channeling patients to pharmaceuticals also incurs societal costs, such as contributing to medical inflation due to the medication's cost and the costs of treating the medication's side effects. This is a particularly salient point considering the ADHD criteria's high rate of false positives (Kirk 2004). Additionally, the INCB (United Nations 2011) considers methylphenidate and other psychostimulants to have significant abuse potential, and that widespread consumption opens the door to trafficking, drug abuse, and other social problems.

This is an important point for New Zealand, where financial considerations seem to be key to the country's high consumption of ADHD medications. For instance, the New Zealand clinical practice guidelines (Ministry of Health 2001) suggest that financial considerations make it unlikely that New Zealand patients can access the behavioral therapy that has been shown to enhance treatment effectiveness (MTA Cooperative Group 1999). However, the reason pharmaceuticals typically prevail in cost considerations is that analysts use a narrow lens, which only considers costs at the point of treatment and externalizes all other costs associated with pharmaceutical use. The calculus changes significantly if one starts to internalize the costs of medication side effects, the social costs associated with psychostimulant abuse, and the environmental costs of producing and disposing of the medications.

While subsidizing ADHD medication usage has important societal costs, it benefits industry in important ways. First, encouraging a reductionist treatment approach benefits industries that poison the environment through their use of toxicants, such as lead, mercury, cadmium, manganese, dioxins, PCBs, and organophosphate pesticides (Schettler et al. 2000; Boucher et al. 2012). John McKinlay (2005) refers to such industries as "manufacturers of disease," and he argues that continuing to emphasize a treatment paradigm, instead of a preventive one, obscures the disease-causing activities of such industries, which allows them to continue harming humans and their environments. In turn, a society's failure to prevent such activities undermines efforts to stem the growing tide of chronic disease and reduce burgeoning health care budgets.

Second, subsidies favor the pharmaceutical industry, which benefits when patients are encouraged to consume medications rather than pursue other treatment approaches. Admittedly, the subsidies don't benefit all players equally. For example, the manufacturer of Rubifen-SR, AFT Pharmaceuticals, benefited when its product was subsidized, whereas Ritalin-SR's manufacturer, Novartis, was placed at a disadvantage when its product ceased to be subsidized. As well, the refusal to subsidize Adderall had important implications for its manufacturer (Shire Labs) and benefited the manufacturers whose products were being subsidized by the government. The same is true for the delayed subsidization of Strattera. What this highlights is that each funding decision has significant market implications and should be seen as a site of struggle between those with a stake in the outcomes.

Conclusion

This chapter's overarching aim has been to elucidate how government-funding activities can shape ADHD's pharmaceuticalization. New Zealand's medication subsidies have increased patient access to ADHD medications, thereby enabling the 1990s rapid consumption expansion. Additionally, funding agencies have steered consumption toward low-cost generics and away from the more expensive patent medications.

This analysis underscores that governments can significantly influence the pharmaceuticalization process. Moreover, it suggests that, far from being a countervailing force, governments are central pillars to the pharmaceutical hegemony, which encourages symptom suppression instead of addressing either underlying causes or preventive approaches. This should encourage social scientists to continue analyzing government influences on pharmaceuticalization processes. In particular, it would be useful to know how funding policies have shaped the pharmaceuticalization of ADHD in other countries.

Additionally, we need analyses that reveal the process by which funding decisions are made, which includes identifying the decision makers, the rationales that guide them, and the ways in which pharmaceutical manufacturers try to influence that process. Given the importance of funding policy to pharmaceuticalization processes, it is safe to assume that manufacturers try to influence such policy and social scientists need to explain how they do so. Such explanations should elucidate their tactics, the activities' impact, and the contextual factors that mediate that impact.

Even though financial accessibility is necessary for pharmaceutical consumption to increase, it is an insufficient condition because there has to also be a demand for that product. Thus, analyses of the state should be coupled with those elucidating how the ADHD diagnosis migrated to New Zealand, the process through which the medical profession came to rely primarily on pharmaceuticals, and the role government agencies played in both of those processes. Shedding light on these many issues, both for ADHD and other medicalized conditions, will help us better understand the processes that enable the pharmaceutical industry to reinforce and reproduce its hegemony. In turn, such knowledge can provide the insight with which to decrease our reliance on pharmaceutical options, to increase our reliance on effective non-pharmaceutical treatment options, and, most important, to prioritize preventive approaches that tackle diseases at their source, rather than downstream (McKinlay 2005).

REFERENCES

Abraham, John. 2010. "Pharmaceuticalization of Society in Context: Theoretical, Empirical and Health Dimensions." *Sociology* 44 (3): 603–22.
American Psychiatric Association (APA). 1980. *Diagnostic and Statistical Manual of Mental Disorders (DSM-III)*. 3rd ed. Washington, DC: American Psychiatric Association.
———. 1987. *Diagnostic and Statistical Manual (DMR-III-R)*. 3rd ed., revised. Washington, DC: American Psychiatric Association.
———. 1994. *Diagnostic and Statistical Manual of Mental Disorders (DSM-IV)*. 4th ed. Washington, DC: American Psychiatric Association.
Anderson, Jessie, Sheila Williams, Rob McGee, and Phil Silva. 1987. "DSM-III Disorders in Preadolescent Children: Prevalence in a Large Sample from the General Population." *Archives of General Psychiatry* 44: 69–76.
Angell, Marcia. 2005. *The Truth about Drug Companies: How They Deceive Us and What to Do about It*. New York: Random House.
August, Gerald J., and Barry D. Garfinkel. 1989. "Behavioral and Cognitive Subtypes of ADHD." *Journal of the American Academy of Child and Adolescent Psychiatry* 28 (5): 739–48.

Berbatis, Constantine, Bruce Sunderland, and Max Bulsara. 2002. "Licit Psychostimulant Consumption in Australia, 1984–2000: International and Jurisdictional Comparison." *Medical Journal of Australia* 177 (10): 539–43.

Bonati, Maurizio, Piero Impicciatore, and Chiara Pandolfini. 2001. "Reintroduction of
Methylphenidate in Italy Needs Careful Monitoring." *British Medical Journal* 322
(7285): 556.

Boucher, Olivier, Sandra Jacobson, Pierrich Plusquellec, Eric Dewailly, Pierre Ayotte,
Nadine Forget-Dubois, Joseph Jacobson, and Gina Muckle. 2012. "Prenatal Methyl-
mercury, Postnatal Lead Exposure, and Evidence for Attention Deficit/Hyperactivity
Disorder among Inuit Children in Arctic Québec." *Environmental Health Perspectives*
120 (10): 1456–61.

Breggin, Peter. 2001. *Talking Back to Ritalin: What Doctors Aren't Telling You about Stimulants and ADHD*. Cambridge, MA: Da Capo.

Busfield, Joan. 2010. "'A Pill for Every Ill': Explaining the Expansion in Medicine Use."
Social Science & Medicine 70: 934–41.

———. 2015. "Assessing the Overuse of Medicines." *Social Science & Medicine* 131:
199–206.

Cohen, David, Michael McCubbin, Johanne Collin, and Guilhème Pérodeau. 2001.
"Medications as Social Phenomenon." *Health* 5 (4): 441–69.

Conners, Keith. 1969. "A Teacher Rating Scale for Use in Doing Studies with Children."
American Journal of Psychiatry 126: 152–56.

Conrad, Peter. 2007. *The Medicalization of Society: On the Transformation of Human Conditions into Treatable Disorders*. Baltimore: Johns Hopkins University Press.

Conrad, Peter, and Meredith Bergey. 2014. "The Impending Globalization of ADHD:
Notes on the Expansion and Growth of a Medicalized Disorder." *Social Science &
Medicine* 122: 31–43.

Davis, Peter. 2004. "'Tough but Fair?': The Active Management of the New Zealand
Drug Benefits Scheme by an Independent Crown Agency." *Australian Health Review*
28: 171–81.

Debroise, Anne. 2004. "Ritaline: Un Feuilleton à la Française (Ritalin: A French Series)." *La Recherche* 16: 34–36.

Dorfman, Natalia. 2006. "Attention Grabbers." *Medical Marketing & Media* 41 (6):
62–66.

Drug Enforcement Agency. 1981–2006. Automation of Reports and Consolidated Orders
System (ARCOS) Database, "Cumulative Distribution by State in Grams per 100,000
Population." US Department of Justice. http://www.deadiversion.usdoj.gov/arcos
/retail_drug_summary/index.html.

DuPaul, George, Lisa Weyandt, Sean O'Dell, and Michael Varejao. 2009. "College
Students with ADHD: Current Status and Future Directions." *Journal of Attention
Disorders* 13: 234–50.

European Medicines Agency. 2009. "EMEA 2010 Priorities for Drug Safety Research:
Long-Term Effects in Children and in Young Adults of Methylphenidate in the
Treatment of Attention Deficit Hyperactivity Disorder (ADHD)." London: European Medicines Agency. http://www.emea.europa.eu/htms/human/phv/commu
nications.htm.

Fergusson, David, John Horwood, and Michael Lynskey. 1993. "Prevalence and Comorbidity of DSM-III-R Diagnoses in a Birth Cohort of 15 Year Olds." *Journal of the American Academy of Child and Adolescent Psychiatry* 32 (6): 1127–34.

Ford, Joel. 2007. "ADHD Medicine Made Son Angry, Says Woman." *Bay of Plenty Times,* July 2. http://www.nzherald.co.nz/bay-of-plenty times/news/article.cfm?c_id=1503343 &objectid=10957896.

Fraser, Tony, and Murray Tilyard. 2009. *Best Practice Special Edition: Generics.* Dunedin, New Zealand: Bpac^nz Ltd. http://www.pharmac.govt.nz/2009/08/25/bpjse_generics _2009.pdf.

Gadow, Kenneth. 1981. "Prevalence of Drug Treatment for Hyperactivity and Other Childhood Behavior Disorders." In *Psychosocial Aspects of Drug Treatment for Hyperactivity,* edited by Kenneth Gadow, 13–76. Boulder, CO: Westview.

Hamed, Alaa, Aaron Kauer, and Hanna Stevens. 2015. "Why the Diagnosis of Attention Deficit Hyperactivity Disorder Matters." *Frontiers in Psychiatry* 6: 168. doi:10.3389/ fpsyt.2015.00168.

Jacobson, Michael, and David Schardt. 1999. *Diet, ADHD, & Behavior: A Quarter-Century Review.* Washington, DC: Center for Science in the Public Interest. http://www .nzherald.co.nz/nz/news/article.cfm?c_id=1&objectid=10904685.

Johnston, Martin. 2007. "Drug Switch Plunges Boy into Hell." *New Zealand Herald,* July 30. http://www.nzherald.co.nz/nz/news/article.cfm?c_id=1&objectid=10454549.

———. 2013. "Doctor's Fees for School-age Children Too High, Say Critics." *New Zealand Herald,* July 29.

Kiong, Errol. 2007. "Parents Victors in Ritalin Fight." *New Zealand Herald,* September 28. http://www.nzherald.co.nz/nz/news/article.cfm?c_id=1&objectid=10466334.

Kirk, Stuart. 2004. "Are Children's DSM Diagnoses Accurate?" *Brief Treatment and Crisis Intervention* 4 (3): 255–70.

Larrson, Janne. 2005. "Ritalin—the Cover-Up of Suicides." *24-7 Press Release,* October 29. http://www.24-7pressrelease.com/view_press_release.php?rID=9094.

McCann, Donna, Angelina Barrett, Alison Coope, Debbie Crumpler, Lindy Dalen, Kate Grimshaw, Elizabeth Kitchin, Kris Lok, Lucy Porteous, Emily Prince, Edmund Sonuga-Barke, John Warner, and Jim Stevenson. 2007. "Food Additives and Hyperactive Behaviour in 3-Year-Old and 8/9-Year-Old Children in the Community: A Randomised, Double-Blinded, Placebo-Controlled Trial." *The Lancet* 370: 1560–67.

McGee, Rob, Michael Feehan, Sheila Williams, Fiona Partridge, Phil Silva, and Jane Kelly. 1990. "DSM-III Disorders in a Large Sample of Adolescents." *Journal of the American Academy of Child and Adolescent Psychiatry* 29: 611–19.

McKinlay, John. 2005. "A Case for Refocusing Upstream: The Political Economy of Illness." In *The Sociology of Health & Illness: Critical Perspectives,* edited by Peter Conrad, 551–64. Duffield, UK: Worth, 2005.

MEDSAFE. 2010. "Methylphenidate—Updated Guidance When Treating Children." New Zealand Medicines and Medical Devices Safety Authority. http://www.medsafe .govt.nz/profs/PUArticles/Methylphenidate.htm.

Ministry of Health. 2001. *New Zealand Guidelines for the Assessment and Treatment of Attention-Deficit/Hyperactivity Disorder.* Wellington, NZ: Ministry of Health. http:// www.moh.govt.nz.

———. 2014. Email message to the author from an information analyst at the Ministry of Health.

———. 2015. "Prescription Charges." Wellington, NZ: Ministry of Health. http://www .health.govt.nz/your-health/conditions-and-treatments/treatments-and-surgery /medications/prescription-charges.

———. 2016. "Zero Fees for Under-13s." Wellington, NZ: Ministry of Health. http://www .health.govt.nz/our-work/primary-health-care/primary-health-care-subsidies-and -services/zero-fees-under-13s.

Molina, Brooke, Stephen Hinshaw, James Swanson, Eugene Arnold, Benedetto Vitiello, Peter Jensen, Jeffrey Epstein, Betsy Hoza, Lily Hechtman, Howard Abikoff, Glen Elliott, Laurence Greenhill, Jeffrey Newcorn, Karen Wells, Timothy Wigal, Robert Gibbons, Kwan Hur, Patricia Houck, and the MTA Cooperative Group. 2009. "The MTA at 8 Years: Prospective Follow-Up of Children Treated for Combined-Type ADHD in a Multisite Study." *Journal of the American Academy of Child and Adolescent Psychiatry* 48 (5): 484–500.

MTA Cooperative Group. 1999. "A 14-Month Randomized Clinical Trial of Treatment Strategies for Attention-Deficit/Hyperactivity Disorder." *Archives of General Psychiatry* 56: 1073–86.

NHS Information Centre. 2009. "Prescriptions Dispensed to the Community: Statistics for 1998 to 2008: England." UK Government Statistical Service. http://www.hscic .gov.uk/catalogue/PUB01396/pres-disp-com-stat-1998-2008-rep.pdf.

Nichols, Lane. 2014. "NZ Housing among the Most Overvalued in World." *New Zealand Herald*, September 2. http://www.nzherald.co.nz/nz/news/article.cfm?c_id =1&objectid=11317934.

Ninness, Lane. 2014. "Average Property Price up 10pc in 2013." *Stuff.co.nz*, January 14. http:// www.stuff.co.nz/business/money/9608412/Average-property-price-up-10pc-in-2013.

Pawluch, Dorothy. 2009. *The New Pediatrics: A Profession in Transition.* New Brunswick, NJ: AldineTransaction.

PHARMAC. n.d. "About PHARMAC." New Zealand: Pharmaceuticals Management Agency. http://www.pharmac.health.nz/about.

———. 1995. *Annual Review for the Year Ended 30 June 1995.* Wellington, NZ: Pharmaceuticals Management Agency.

———. 1998. *Annual Review for the Year Ended 30 June 1998.* Wellington, NZ: Pharmaceuticals Management Agency.

———. 2000. *Annual Review for the Year Ended 30 June 2000.* Wellington, NZ: Pharmaceuticals Management Agency.

———. 2001. *Annual Review for the Year Ended 30 June 2001.* Wellington, NZ: Pharmaceuticals Management Agency.

———. 2003. *Annual Review for the Year Ended 30 June 2003.* Wellington, NZ: Pharmaceuticals Management Agency.

———. 2007. *Annual Review for the Year Ended 30 June 2007.* Wellington, NZ: Pharmaceuticals Management Agency.

———. 2008a. *Annual Review for the Year Ended 30 June 2008.* Wellington, NZ: Pharmaceuticals Management Agency.

———. 2008b. "Consultation—Proposal for Strattera (atomoxetine), Humalog Mix 25 and Humalog Mix 50 (insulin lispro with insulin lispro protamine suspension),

Zyprexa and Zyprexa Zydis (olanzapine), and Actos (pioglitazone)." Pharmaceuticals Management Agency. http://www.pharmac.govt.nz/2008/08/27/Proposal%20for%20 Strattera,%20Humalog%20Mix,%20Zyprexa%20and%20Actos.pdf.

———. 2009. *Annual Review for the Year Ended 30 June 2009*. Wellington, NZ: Pharmaceuticals Management Agency.

Rappley, Marsha. 1997. "Safety Issues in the Use of Methylphenidate: An American Perspective." *Drug Safety* 17 (3): 143–48.

Robison, Linda, David Sclar, Tracy Skaer, and Richard Galin. 2004. "Treatment Modalities among US Children Diagnosed with Attention-Deficit Hyperactivity Disorder: 1995–99." *International Clinical Psychopharmacology* 19: 17–22.

Safer, Daniel. 2000. "Are Stimulants Overprescribed for Youths with ADHD?" *Annals of Clinical Psychiatry* 12 (1): 55–62.

Safer, Daniel, and Julie Zito. 1999. "Psychotropic Medication for ADHD." *Mental Retardation and Developmental Disabilities Research Reviews* 5: 237–42.

Scheffler, Richard, Stephen Hinshaw, Sepideh Modrek, and Peter Levine. 2007. "The Global Market for ADHD Medications." *Health Affairs (Millwood)* 26 (2): 450–57.

Schettler, Ted, Jill Stein, Fay Reich, Maria Valenti, and David Wallinga. 2000. *In Harm's Way: Toxic Threats to Child Development*. Cambridge, MA: Greater Boston Physicians for Social Responsibility. http://www.igc.org/psr/.

Shrag, Peter, and Diane Divosky. 1975. *The Myth of the Hyperactive Child: And Other Means of Child Control*. New York: Pantheon.

Tait, Morgan. 2013. "Income Gap Growing across the Ditch." *New Zealand Herald,* March 27. http://www.nzherald.co.nz/nz/news/article.cfm?c_id=1&objectid=10873868.

United Nations. 2005. International Narcotics Control Board. *Psychotropic Substances 2005—Statistics for 2004: Assessments of Annual Medical and Scientific Requirements*. Austria: United Nations.

———. 2006. International Narcotics Control Board. *Psychotropic Substances 2006—Statistics for 2005: Assessments of Annual Medical and Scientific Requirements*. Austria: United Nations.

———. 2007. International Narcotics Control Board. *Psychotropic Substances 2007—Statistics for 2006: Assessments of Annual Medical and Scientific Requirements*. Austria: United Nations.

———. 2008. International Narcotics Control Board. *Psychotropic Substances 2008—Statistics for 2007: Assessments of Annual Medical and Scientific Requirements*. Austria: United Nations.

———. 2009. International Narcotics Control Board. *Psychotropic Substances 2009—Statistics for 2008: Assessments of Annual Medical and Scientific Requirements*. Austria: United Nations.

———. 2010. International Narcotics Control Board. *Psychotropic Substances 2010—Statistics for 2009: Assessments of Annual Medical and Scientific Requirements*. Austria: United Nations.

———. 2011. International Narcotics Control Board. *Psychotropic Substances 2011—Statistics for 2010: Assessments of Annual Medical and Scientific Requirements*. Austria: United Nations.

———. 2012. International Narcotics Control Board. *Psychotropic Substances 2012—Statistics for 2011: Assessments of Annual Medical and Scientific Requirements*. Austria: United Nations.

———. 2013. International Narcotics Control Board. *Psychotropic Substances 2013—Statistics for 2012: Assessments of Annual Medical and Scientific Requirements*. Austria: United Nations.

Vallée, Manuel. 2010. "Deconstructing America's Ritalin Epidemic: Contrasting US-France Ritalin Usage." PhD diss., University of California, Berkeley.

Visser, Susanna, Melissa Danielson, Rebecca Bitsko, Joseph Holbrook, Michael Kogan, Reem Ghandour, Ruth Perou, and Stephen Blumberg. 2014. "Trends in the Parent-Report of Health Care Provider-Diagnosed and Medicated Attention-Deficit/Hyperactivity Disorder: United States, 2003–2011." *Journal of the American Academy of Child and Adolescent Psychiatry* 53 (1): 34–45.

Werry, John, and Daniel Hawthorne. 1976. "Conners' Teacher Questionnaire—Norms and Validity." *Australia and New Zealand Journal of Psychiatry* 10 (3): 257–62.

Werry, John, and Robert Sprague. 1974. "Methylphenidate in Children—Effect of Dosage." *Australian and New Zealand Journal of Psychiatry* 8 (1): 9–19.

Winterstein, Almut, Tobias Gerhard, Jonathan Shuster, Julie Zito, Michael Johnson, and Huazhi Liu. 2008. "Utilization of Pharmacologic Treatment in Youth with Attention Deficit/Hyperactivity Disorder in Medicaid Database." *Annals of Pharmacotherapy* 42 (1): 24–31.

World Health Organization (WHO). 2011. *The World Medicines Situation: Rational Use of Medicines*. Geneva: World Health Organization.

15

From Problematic Children to Problematic Diagnosis

The Paradoxical Trajectories of Child and Adolescent ADHD in Chile

Sebastián Rojas Navarro
Patricio Rojas
Mónica Peña Ochoa

What are the specific trajectories of ADHD in Chile? What is the current situation? How does the past express itself in the present, and what does this point toward in the future? These are some of the questions that we explore throughout this chapter as we discuss some of the social and historical processes that have shaped the way ADHD is currently diagnosed, treated, and contextualized in Chile.

In a broad sense, the Chilean history of ADHD in children and adolescents can be portrayed as one of contrasts. ADHD and the use of stimulant medication have been matters of concern for experts in the medical and educational fields, social scientists, and the general public. The main concern regarding the diagnosis is rooted in the fact that ADHD has become one of the leading reasons for mental health consultation for both children and young adults (Vicente et al. 2012a), and stimulant medication is one of the key ways to treat the disorder. Regardless of the concern, these high rates of ADHD and requisite stimulant consumption have been mostly omitted from official records. Governmental institutions such as the Ministerio de Salud and the Ministerio de Educación have produced little significant and coherent data on the subject. Although guidelines for treatment and management of the disorder have been produced for medical and educational purposes (Ministerio de Salud 2008; Ministerio de Educación

2009), these documents are mainly technical and provide procedural protocols. There is no attempt to explain how ADHD became a widespread phenomenon or to provide the catalyst to produce research related to the topic.

Some scholars who are independent from the government have tried to engage with the topic of ADHD in universities across the country. These studies vary in their aims and methods. Some are interested in the epidemiological aspects of the disorder (Vicente et al. 2012a; De la Barra et al. 2013), whereas others focus on the lived experiences of children diagnosed with ADHD (Peña, Rojas Navarro, and Rojas Navarro 2014; Rojas Navarro and Rojas 2015) or on the neurobiology of the disorder (Aboitiz and Schröter 2005). However, there has been little integration of these efforts. This lack of integration, in combination with the scarce production of official data about the subject by governmental institutions or by institutions working in relation to the Chilean government, produces considerable gaps in the understanding of this phenomenon. The existing data are at most partial, and occasionally contradictory.

Throughout this chapter, we work under the assumption that the abovementioned difficulties—the lack of systematic studies, data production, and research agendas—are not reasons to dismiss the study of ADHD in Chile as being impossible, partial, or irrelevant, but rather constitute a phenomenon in and of itself. Our work here contributes to organizing the dispersed elements of the past and present history of ADHD in Chile, in the form of a "bricolage." The anthropologist Claude Lévi-Strauss (1966) defined the "bricoleur"—the maker of a bricolage—as someone using a heteronomous repertoire in order to elaborate a patchwork. Likewise, we found ourselves in need of bringing together different materials, observations, and experiences across policy, lay, and scientific resources in order to convey meaning (Lincoln and Denzin 2003). We are not aiming for a coherent whole; indeed, one of our core arguments is that ADHD in Chile is, for now and perhaps for the foreseeable future, a heterogeneous object that defies coherence (Whitehead 1968). For these reasons, this chapter follows some of the trajectories ADHD has traveled in the Chilean context and explores the key factors and actors involved in its shaping.

In order to tackle how ADHD has been understood in medical and educational contexts, we systematically reviewed the Chilean *Boletín de la Sociedad de Psiquiatría y Neurología de la Infancia y Adolescencia* (*Bulletin of the Society of Psychiatry and Neurology of Childhood and Adolescence*), searching for articles that addressed the topic of ADHD from 1993 to 1999. We decided to start in 1993 because it is then that, according to the editorial of the 1993 June issue, the journal "became of age," turning more "mature and responsible" (Devilat 1993). In the educational context, we explored how ADHD has been integrated into different policies and how these policies have shaped the ways in which schools have managed children diagnosed with ADHD since the introduction of a new educational finance law called Decreto 170, or "differentiated grant for special educational needs," in 2010.

As a way to understand how ADHD has circulated in the social imagination of Chilean people, we focused our analysis on exploring how ADHD emerged and became a topic of concern for mothers and families according to reports and articles brought together by *Revista YA* since 1981. In order to do so, we systematically reviewed every issue of *Revista YA* published during the 1980s, searching to determine how behavioral issues in children became slowly framed in a biomedical manner. We aimed to explore how biomedical categories such as "ADHD" became widespread according to experts interviewed by the magazine and in accordance with opinion columns published in the magazine by medical and educational experts. This magazine is published on a weekly basis along with the newspaper *El Mercurio. El Mercurio* has systematically been a key political actor in Chilean history. This newspaper has represented the voice of the Chilean elite since 1900, articulating dominant and conservative discourses (Cabalin 2014). Its pages were used to support the implementation of the current neoliberal system of governance in Chile by framing topics in a particular manner. As Cabalin (2014) suggests, such framing and characterization of news stories in specific sources may influence the ways in which news is assimilated by audiences. Therefore, reporting on ADHD in a magazine distributed by *El Mercurio* is highly relevant to understanding the social translations ADHD has undergone in the Chilean context.

In addition to the written sources we consulted about the social, educational, and medical circulation of ADHD, interviews were held with key actors involved in the evolution of ADHD in Chile since the 1950s.

Global Problems, Local Trajectories, and Particular Stories

To our knowledge, there has been no attempt to write a history of ADHD in Chile. When referencing what ADHD is or how this disorder came into being, Chilean articles and experts usually reference what we call the "global history of ADHD." This is the history narrated by American authors such as Barkley (2005) and Mayes and colleagues (Mayes, Bagwell, and Erkulwater 2009), who emphasize a trajectory that begins with the lectures given by the British pediatrician

George Still in 1902 and published in *The Lancet* (Still 1902), through to the official designation of the classification "attention deficit/hyperactivity disorder" in 1987 in the third revised edition of the *Diagnostic and Statistical Manual of Mental Disorders (DSM-III-R)* (Lange et al. 2010). Typically, no references are made as to how, when, and by what means ADHD emerged in Chile, and what its trajectories and implications were at the time.

In 1955, methylphenidate began to be commercialized under the name Ritalin by the pharmaceutical company Ciba in the United States (Mayes, Bagwell, and Erkulwater 2009), but it was only in the 1960s that Ritalin found its way into the Chilean environment. According to reports gathered by the Chilean historian Jorge Rojas (2010) after interviewing pediatricians, child psychiatrists, and other medical experts, the entry point for the medication was the Servicio de Psiquiatría Infanto-Juvenil of the Luis Calvo Mackenna Hospital.[1] This psychiatric ward had contacts in Argentina who helped to bring the medication into Chile as a way of treating hyperactive children. However, Ritalin was not immediately accepted. Rojas (2010) argues that the prescription and use of stimulant medication only became common practice in the 1980s, whereas media articles point out that it was in the 1990s that the use of Ritalin became widespread (Jaque and Rodríguez 2011).

Since the 1980s, Ritalin has become one of the most common ways to treat not only children whose behavior matches the criteria for diagnosing ADHD, but also to treat children with generalized problematic behaviors that eventually did not match the diagnostic criteria. After interviewing health practitioners and social workers in public health at the time, Rojas (2010) found that children labeled as "weird" or "problematic" were also being treated with Ritalin. The wider use of stimulant medication was driven by the misconception that it could be used to target any kind of unpleasant or deviant behavior. Media articles from the 1980s reflected on these concerns. Articles began to suggest that children were being medicated because their behavior was considered problematic, not because that behavior necessarily overlapped with a medical category. According to some of these news items—which we will examine next—the more salient basis for medicating children appeared to be social: they did not meet adult behavioral standards. Although it is unknown to us to what extent these reports were accurate, the mere fact that they were being published is telling of a certain sensitivity toward the topic of behavioral problems in the 1980s.

Revista YA illustrates the points made above. This magazine—the target audience of which is middle-class and upper-class women—has counseled and given suggestions, based on expert opinion, about motherhood, parenting styles, fashion and cooking advice, and related topics for more than three decades. During the 1980s, *Revista YA*'s articles about behavioral problems focused on the problems of children. In 1983, Hernán Montenegro, a child psychiatrist and a columnist and consultant for the magazine, suggested that it could be harder for parents to accept behavioral or learning disorders in their children than to accept other conditions such as mental retardation or cerebral palsy (Montenegro 1983). The opinions of Montenegro reflect a certain problematic found throughout the 1980s in Chile toward children with ADHD: how could children who seemed physically and mentally normal behave in such troublesome ways?

According to articles published in *Revista YA*, schools were key actors in identifying the disorder, and they became concerned with the need to identify and treat the disorder as fast as possible (Araya 1987b). This urgency was driven by the fact that potential outcomes of untreated ADHD at the time clashed with what was expected from school-age children in terms of academic performance and socialization. Mass media described multiple possible outcomes for children diagnosed with ADHD in the 1980s; these outcomes ranged from poor educational achievement and work stability to an increased rate of divorce. As a consequence of these negative projections, the argument for treatment was "the sooner the better" (Araya 1987a: 9).

Most Chilean experts interested in the topic of ADHD agree that the increase in the number of children diagnosed with ADHD has led to an excessive use of medication as the primary treatment in Chile (EducarChile n.d.; Rojas 2010; Jaque and Rodríguez 2011). Juan Sepúlveda, lecturer in child psychiatry at the medical school of the Universidad de Chile, remembers that until the late 1980s the trend among medical practitioners was to prescribe amphetamines to treat behavioral issues in children. He also recalls how medication—amphetamines, and later on methylphenidate—was considered by most of the population, including medical practitioners, as the first line of treatment:

> For the general public, the use of medication was a solution that served everyone. Medication allowed avoiding questioning about parenting styles, or any other etiological possibility not treatable with medication that could be the foundation of the behavioral issues. There was no opposition to this way of procedure; in fact, it was well appreciated by everyone. (Interview with Juan Sepúlveda, July 2014)

What was being treated was not a unified medical entity. Descriptions of who should visit a medical practitioner and the reasons behind the visit varied over time. Most medical experts and psychologists interviewed by the media during the 1980s agreed on core symptoms that could indicate the possibility of a child having ADHD, such as the inability to remain focused for long periods, being too impulsive, or being restless. However, the descriptions of symptoms varied greatly when they encompassed other signs beyond the core symptoms. A child neurologist claimed that a telltale symptom of ADHD is how children with this disorder may present "mechanisms of evasion when they are forced to pay attention: They can get irritable, distracted, and drowsy. They can even turn pale and look haggard" (Araya 1987b: 7). Other experts, such as the psychologist Alfredo Ruiz (1985), indicated that symptoms beyond the core symptoms ranged from arrogance and having low tolerance to frustration to presenting low self-esteem to a lack of response to discipline. Despite these variations in symptoms, experts commonly referred to these children with words such as "public danger," "unbearable" (Araya 1986: 13), "restless," "obstinate," and "naughty" (Ruiz 1985: 5). We believe that the wide variation in the expected potential manifestations of symptoms of ADHD is telling of how loosely the diagnosis was understood at the time. ADHD was still not a cohesive medical entity in practice. By this we mean that, when it came to making the diagnosis, ADHD was understood differently according to different medical experts. Beyond the core symptoms, it appears— as it is possible to observe in the above-mentioned descriptions—that different medical practitioners and mental health experts differed widely in their expectations of how ADHD presented itself, how it was revealed in children's everyday lives, and how it could be detected by their families.

Although there was no consensus regarding the manifestations of symptoms of ADHD, its causes, and the potential effects of stimulant medication—or maybe because of the lack of consensus—diagnoses in Chile kept increasing. In 2011, Jaque and Rodríguez, two journalists working for *La Tercera*, wrote a front-page story about the "Ritalin generation." Looking back at the 1990s, when ADHD became a major diagnostic trend in child psychiatry, psychology, and the educational environment, they interviewed former patients treated with the medication, their family members, and medical practitioners and experts. Their article, which focused on the issue of overmedication and its perils, quickly gained notice from laypeople and medical experts. According to their research, by the beginning of the 1990s it was customary for schools to ask parents to take their children to a neurologist because of their behavior (Jaque and Rodríguez 2011). By this time, Ritalin was the most accepted way to treat children who were "difficult" and had a hard time focusing during class or remaining still in the classroom.

The expectations for children with ADHD who did not use Ritalin were catastrophic at the time. "It was said that almost 80% of children with ADHD would not get better with time without medication, that 30% of children with ADHD would probably fail at school, and 24% might become alcoholics when growing up" (Jaque and Rodríguez 2011: 11). However, the use of Ritalin was starting to be questioned as result of a series of rumors and suspicion about other effects the medication could produce. The testimony of the mother of a child diagnosed with ADHD, interviewed by Jaque and Rodríguez, portrays this complex scenario: "There was a controversy. It was said that [Ritalin] turned children dumb, that it was being overused and that scared me" (Jaque and Rodríguez 2011: 4).

The fear of the potential side effects linked to the use of psychostimulants did not discourage schools from referring children to clinical experts when children were considered to be "annoying, relentless and intolerable" (Jaque and Rodríguez 2011: 4). Most children were referred to child neurologists since child psychiatry was still new in Chile and was experiencing difficulties positioning itself in the local arena.[2] Child psychiatrists at the time only had a few tools with which to tackle ADHD:

> [The] observation of relentless behavior was the key criterion, along [with] the "Conners Test," which is today widely used by schools, almost as a diagnostic proof. Thus, considering the immaturity of child psychiatry, behavioral and hyperactivity disorders were referred to neurologists, who acted as the reference authority for other health practitioners such as psychologists. (Interview with Juan Sepúlveda, July 2014)

In the 1990s, ADHD gained further visibility in the Chilean medical community, particularly in the domain of neurology and psychiatry. Various seminars and workshops were held in relation to the topic of ADHD. In addition, the *Boletín de la Sociedad de Psiquiatría y Neurología de la Infancia y Adolescencia* published original research and articles about the subject on a regular basis (see Marzouka and López 1994; Rojas and Imperatore 1994). In addition, the 12th Chilean Congress of Psychiatry and Neurology of Childhood and Adolescence was dedicated to ADHD, under the telling title of "ADHD: Myth or Reality" (Schlager and Keith 1993). However, almost none of this scholarship discusses key issues in relation to the disorder. ADHD was mostly taken as a given, despite the doubts about its etiology, the consequences of medication, and the heterogeneous protocols and tests used to perform the diagnosis.

It has been argued that the multiple—and not always rigorous—methods used in diagnosis, a lack of reflection on these methods, and the indiscriminate prescribing of Ritalin ended up shaping what the media called the "Ritalin generation" during the 1990s (Jaque and Rodríguez 2011). The term refers to children who grew up being considered as problematic and were stigmatized during their school years by being identified as impossible to deal with by educators and peers. During the early 1990s, schools were still unprepared to deal with children diagnosed with ADHD since teachers and educators lacked the required training to understand what this meant in practice and how to engage with children diagnosed with the disorder. What they observed were forms of restlessness and motor activity that had to be tamed and controlled by any possible means—from particular pedagogies to disciplinary actions. This led to the use of certain practices inside the classroom that ranged from humiliating the child in order to make her stop disturbing others, strapping her to a desk, to even locking her inside a closet (Jaque and Rodríguez 2011).

In addition to these school-related disciplinary actions, Ritalin continued to gain popularity as a way to deal with children's behavioral issues. As Jaque and Rodríguez (2011) argue, the use of Ritalin helped expand the belief that biological causes were at the root of the problematic behaviors and children's mischievous actions. Their argument was that if a pharmaceutical drug produced an effect on the children's behavior, the cause of the behavior had to be a biological disorder. It is due to this that by the mid-1990s mass media began to widely use the label of "ADHD" (a biomedical label), instead of using terms such as "hyperkinesia" (commonly used in the Chilean media in a more descriptive way), in an attempt to explain and refer to children's behavior. By 1995, it is estimated that 5% to 10% of Chilean children were diagnosed with ADHD (Galvez 1995a), and an even larger percentage of children were being taken by their families to consult medical experts, looking for advice and medication.

By the mid-1990s, despite a socially accepted biomedical explanation of ADHD and awareness within educational establishments, children diagnosed with ADHD still faced discrimination at school. Children could be punished if they forgot to bring their medication. Interviews held by Karim Galvez, a journalist working for *Revista YA*, with parents of children diagnosed with ADHD reflected that at times they felt that they were being forced to medicate their children (Galvez 1995a). A mother interviewed by Galvez says:

> I think that it sucks that he [her child] has to take Ritalin, but at the same time I realized that it had helped him. Moreover, if I consider that he should

take more in order to prepare for his school assessments, I should give him more, but I refuse. Maybe it is foolish, but I am not convinced about giving him so much stuff . . . now they [schools] send them [children] to the doctor for any reason. I don't have any family members whose sons have not been sent to visit the *psicopedagogo*.[3] If he [the child] is active, they immediately say that he is hyperactive and it turns out that children are normally supposed to be like that [active]. Maybe it is that some schools are now taking distance from the problem. (Galvez 1995b: 7)

It is this same feeling of having their children unfairly treated by schools and of facing stigmatization and discrimination that led to the constitution of the Asociación Nacional de Padres y Amigos de Niños con Déficit Atencional, or ANPANDA, in 1998. ANPANDA had played a crucial role in pushing the government for modifications aimed at changing and introducing a series of educational policies to tackle how children diagnosed with ADHD—along with children with other learning difficulties—were to be dealt with in schools. Of these modifications, Decreto 170 was probably the most emblematic. We will review some of these educational and policy changes in order to understand the effects they had on the current trajectories of ADHD.

Educational and Policy Changes around ADHD

Chile is recognized as the first neoliberal experiment in the world (Harvey 2007). The dictatorship of Augusto Pinochet (1973–90) implemented educational reform that fostered the incorporation of free-market logic into education. This dramatically changed the Chilean educational system, which was provided by the state.

The cornerstone of the reform was the implementation of a voucher system in 1981. In general terms, the Chilean educational system divides schools into three different types: public schools, state-subsidized schools, and private schools. The resources allocated to the first two are dependent on how many students are attending those schools. Each student "owns" a voucher that, as Sapelli and Aedo (2001) explain, is implicitly transferred to the school in which she is enrolled. If the student moves to a different school, the voucher moves along with her. The idea behind the voucher system was to foster competition between schools that are dependent on state funding in order to "attract and retain students, by making the income of the school dependent on the choice made by students and their families" (Sapelli and Aedo 2001: 37). Private schools are funded almost exclusively by the tuition fees that are charged to students. So far, the use of vouchers has had a clear outcome: private education is growing while public education is decreasing (Cabalin 2014). Today, 92% of Chilean students use vouchers (Elacqua 2012), which means that most of the Chilean educational system is financed by a demand subsidy.

Because of segregation and its effects on families with low income, a change was implemented in 2008, when the Chilean Congress passed an adjusted voucher bill called Ley de Subvención Escolar Preferencial, or Ley SEP. This act increased the amount of money included in the voucher for students who are considered "vulnerable" because of their socioeconomic background. In other words, the Ley SEP considered that educating children from low socioeconomic status is more difficult and expensive than educating children from other socioeconomic backgrounds. However, the increase of resources allocated to "vulnerable" children via the Ley SEP did not change the essence of the voucher system. The Ley SEP was an attempt to modify the idea of "flat vouchers" under the consideration that different children have different needs. However, Ley SEP outcomes were not as beneficial as expected: socioeconomic segregation only declined slightly across all school sectors (Elacqua 2012).

In 2010, during President Michelle Bachelet's first term as head of state, a new educational finance law, Decreto 170, was implemented. This law attempts to increase subsidies for children requiring special financial support because they present problems or face conditions that prevent them from continuing their education in a "normal" way. This additional economic support is aimed at encouraging the acquisition of special education teachers and psychologists by schools. The specialists hired are placed in charge of supporting the education of so-called problematic children. Crucially, in order for a school to attain this benefit, a child must first undergo a diagnostic process. Once a diagnosis is completed, the school receives a grant for the diagnosed child; the amount of this funding can be triple that for a student without a diagnosis.

Within the remit of this law, a student who has special educational needs is recognized by the law as entitled to additional help and resources. Resources, which can be material, human, or pedagogical, are given in order to enhance the child's development and learning process. The law considers two different kinds of educational needs: "permanent needs" such as autism, visual impairment, and severe intellectual disability, and "temporary needs." By "temporary needs," the law refers to nonpermanent needs that students face at some point in their educational career as a result of a disorder or disability. Temporary needs must be "diagnosed by a competent professional" in order for children to obtain "additional help and support to access in order to progress in the curriculum for a certain period of their schooling" (Ministerio de Educación 2009: 3). ADHD is an accepted diagnosis that is considered for the special voucher. One of the key problems in relation to this system, implemented by the Decreto 170, is that it incentivizes the labeling of students for schools because of the potential for access to additional resources.

The effects of this policy have not been officially evaluated. One of the few attempts to evaluate and assess the implementation of the law was made by an employee of the Secretaría Regional Ministerial de Educación de Valparaíso, who attempted to give an account of the diagnostic processes completed under the Decreto 170 during the 2011–12 period in first-grade students (Torres 2013). The study shows that the prevalence of ADHD ranges between 8% and 9% of the total of diagnoses of students in primary school. In 2009, the same Ministerio de Educación department that created the Decreto 170 bill focused on the needs of the classroom itself and published a guide for understanding and developing strategies to support children with ADHD in the basic educational level (6- to 13-year-old students) from an inclusive approach (Ministerio de Educación 2009). As of this writing, this document has acted as the only ADHD-related official guideline in relation to education and how teachers and educators should handle children diagnosed with the disorder.

Although the guideline makes no explicit reference to the *DSM-IV*, which it uses as its primary source, the etiology and symptoms of ADHD listed in the guideline exactly match those listed in the *DSM*. This guideline, which is designed for teachers and educators, recommends certain ways to approach children diagnosed with ADHD. Typically it suggests individual work focused on the students' self-esteem, their potential, or the special skills that teachers should have—or develop—in order to work with children who have special educational needs. This includes interventions within the classroom climate, "internal" organizational school relationships, and particularly relationships between the child with ADHD and her peers and teachers. Thus, the guideline operates more as a broad description of the problems and possibilities of ADHD children than as an actual set of recommendations for the promotion of child mental health or intervention through educational practices. However, it insists on the importance of integrating children and addressing their educational potential and special education needs.

The systemic diagnosis of ADHD is not only the result of Decreto 170. Previously, in 1998, another program in which diagnosis also played a crucial role was implemented in schools: Habilidades para la Vida (Skills for Life), which is usually described as a model of psychosocial intervention, incorporating remedial actions and risk prevention. The program targets children who are 4 to 9 years old and depends on the Ministerio de Educación through the Junta Nacional de Ayuda Escolar y Becas, or JUNAEB. Habilidades para la Vida has been working in low-income schools, and one of its goals is to seek and refer students with ADHD. Its rationale in doing this stems from the belief that the condition increases school dropout rates; has detrimental effects in terms of children's relational, emotional, and social skills; and in the long term affects the psychosocial wellbeing of children. In addition to this, ADHD has a negative effect on the future adults' mental health since it is considered to be associated with illnesses and conditions such as depression, suicide, alcohol and drug abuse, and violent behavior (JUNAEB 2015). Therefore, Habilidades para la Vida considers children with ADHD to be part of a vulnerable group of children "presenting psychosocial risk factors and maladaptive behaviors in school and home" (JUNAEB 2015).

ADHD as a Landscape of Contrasts

The proclamation of the Decreto 170 and the introduction of a series of policies have been mentioned as key factors in shaping the current state of ADHD in Chile. Currently, ADHD still retains characteristics attributed to it from previous decades. Despite growing awareness of the disorder among the general public, media, and educational and medical experts, research and data on ADHD are still scarce and fragmented. This appears to be slowly changing, with several different studies on child mental health emerging in the past five years. These studies touch on the topic of ADHD from an epidemiological approach (Vicente et al. 2012, 2012b; De La Barra et al. 2013).

In 2008, the Chilean Ministerio de Salud stated that the official prevalence of ADHD in Chile was 6.2%. However, it also stated that this rate was prone to change since different studies conducted, using different methodologies, have arrived at other figures (Ministerio de Salud 2008). Chile has yet to overcome this inconsistency in relation to information about ADHD.

One source of confusion over national prevalence estimates is that the public health system and the private health sector in Chile follow different record-keeping practices. There is no publicly available account of the prevalence of ADHD in the private health care system, which provides coverage to more than 20% of the population (Aravena and Inostroza 2015). For its part, the public health system does not make prevalence data available publicly, although this information can be requested via the Ley de transparencia de la función pública y de acceso a la información de la Administración del Estado, or Ley N°20.285. Data obtained this way reveal that, between 2009 and 2013, the number of persons aged 19 years or younger who were treated nationwide for ADHD in the public health system almost doubled, increasing from 27,659 in 2009 to 52,895 in 2013. The most affected age group, ranging from 10 to 14 years, has seen an increase from 9,700 in 2009 to 20,018 in 2013. More than 50% of the people receiving treatment in the public health system were diagnosed and treated in the Metropolitan Region, which contains almost 35% of the country's total population.[4]

Data that were undoubtedly linked to the increase in the rates of diagnosis and that were provided by the Central de Abastecimiento del Sistema Nacional de Servicios de Salud reveal that the amount of money spent by the Chilean government on methylphenidate doubled from 2011 to 2012. The money spent on procurement of the drug doubled during that time, and yet there is no record on how many doses of methylphenidate were purchased in 2011 (i.e., there is no information on how that money was spent). Nevertheless, the International Narcotic Control Board (INCB) placed Chile among the top 10 countries in the world for consumption of methylphenidate, with a stated demand of 400,000 grams in 2013 (INCB 2013). This makes methylphenidate the second highest psychotropic substance procured by the Chilean government.

Newspaper and radio reports have expressed concern about the high rates of psychostimulant consumption among children diagnosed with ADHD, and they have denounced the very existence of the disorder. In its March 16, 2014, edition, *La Tercera*—one of the most traditional Chilean newspapers—published an article entitled "El doctor que dice que el Déficit Atencional no existe" ("The Doctor Who Says ADHD Does Not Exist") . . . Just one day before, *El Mercurio* published an article about the same subject: "Médico se lanza contra el Déficit Atencional con Hiperactividad y asegura que es un mito" ("Medical Doctor Charges against Attentional Deficit Hyperactivity Disorder and Claims It Is a Myth"). Both articles are centered on the opinions of the American doctor Richard Saul, who claims the nonexistence of the disorder and attributes the symptoms usually related to ADHD to other biological determinants such as a poor diet. In addition, both articles disputed the efficacy of medication such as psychostimulants in tackling the symptoms.

Other media articles have also addressed the topic. In its June 16, 2013, edition, *La Tercera* published the results of research conducted in Québec under the revealing headline "Estudio muestra que el Ritalín no mejora el rendimiento academic" ("Study Reveals that Ritalin Use Does Not Improve Academic Performance"). According to the article, Ritalin not only failed to improve school performance, but it also fostered a feeling of unhappiness in children using the medication. Similarly, another article by the same newspaper, this time in its February 13, 2013, edition, was entitled "Estudio dice que fármacos no ayudan a niños con deficit atencional" ("Study Reveals Medication Does Not Help Children with Attentional Deficit Disorder"). That article reported the results of another study, this time conducted in the United States at Johns Hopkins Hospital, which questions the efficacy of the medication.

The attempts to resist the use of stimulant medication, which run alongside the contestation of the diagnosis itself, are normally driven by the same fears described by Rojas (2010) in past decades about the uncertainties surrounding the potential side effects of psychostimulant medication; these feared potential effects include long-term substance abuse and neurological damage. In response to these fears, some parents are starting to treat their children with "traditional medicines," self-healing techniques, and naturalistic approaches (Rojas 2010).

Despite the existence of these groups and their resistance, the use of pharmaceutical stimulants is becoming increasingly common in Chilean schools. As suggested by Amanda Céspedes, a renowned Chilean child psychiatrist, nearly 9% of Chilean children are consuming Ritalin at school (EducarChile n.d.). This rate is similar to that of the United States, according to an article entitled "More Diagnosis of A.D.H.D Causing Concern" published by *The New York Times* in its March 31, 2013, edition. In contrast to countries where research has been conducted to explore the causes and possible outcomes of these figures, there has been little debate on the implications of the widespread use of psychostimulants in Chile.

The widespread practice of treating ADHD with stimulant medication is something to be reflected on, particularly when the guidelines provided by the Chilean government clearly promote the idea that the treatment should also include other measures in an attempt to create an "ecologically grounded" approach to the disorder (Ministerio de Salud 2008). As stated in the guidelines, stimulant medication such as methylphenidate should not be used indiscriminately. Rather, it should be one component of a more complex approach to the disorder, which should also include psychological, educational, and social interventions. Likewise, psychostimulant medication should be discontinued and reevaluated every year. The risks regarding the use of methylphenidate are such that the Instituto

Chileno de Salud Pública launched an "alert campaign" in 2009, warning of potential risks linked to the abuse and misuse of the medication. The fact that such a campaign was necessary is surprising considering that there were no official rates of consumption of the medication at the time.

To the best of our knowledge, only two studies have addressed the topic of the use of stimulant medication by Chilean children. In 2004–5, the World Health Organization (WHO) conducted the Global School Student Health Survey, which included one question regarding the use of Ritalin during the previous 12 months. When answered by children who were 15 years old or younger, 8.3% claimed to be receiving Ritalin (Ministerio de Salud 2005).

In 2012, Soledad Larraín and Caroliña Bascuñan conducted a survey for UNICEF on child abuse. This survey, entitled Cuarto estudio de maltrato infantil (4th study on violence against children), was focused on children who, at the time of the survey, were attending the *octavo básico*.[5] Of 1,555 children surveyed, 14.7% had taken medication to improve their performance or behavior. Among the medications used, stimulants such as methylphenidate and other substances used to treat ADHD were mentioned (Larraín and Bascuñan 2012). According to the study, children are consuming medication not because it is necessary, but because their parents give it to them to improve their performance or behavior. The study does not indicate whether there is a matching medical diagnosis in these cases that justifies the use of medication. However, one could assume that the most probable scenario is that the estimate is not related to a medical condition since the figure is given under the wider description of one of the possible types of abuse to which children in Chile are being exposed. This was a national survey that was conducted with the use of a randomized probability sample and held to be representative of the Chilean context regarding the topic of child abuse.

In Chile, children's use of stimulant medication has been explored mainly by international agencies. In fact, it is due to their intervention that data regarding the topic have been produced. Sadly, the opinions of children have not been considered by Chilean experts exploring the topic. In addition, children have not been fully included in research and surveys conducted by experts in Chile. In the official national survey conducted by the Chilean Ministerio de Salud, the Encuesta Nacional de Salud (National Health Survey), only persons 17 years or older were considered as valid participants. A new version of this survey, which includes children, is being planned for launch in the future (Paula Margozzini, email message to the authors, March 8, 2014).[6]

It was only in 2013 that the first extensive epidemiologic study in relation to ADHD in Chile came to light. The research included a final sample of 1,558 children and adolescents from 4 different regions. The children ranged in age from 4 to 18 years. This is the largest study ever conducted in the national territory. The results showed that the total prevalence of ADHD in Chile was approximately 10%. In children 4 to 11 years of age, the prevalence among boys was 16.4% and the prevalence among girls was 14.6%. Among adolescents (12 to 18 years) the prevalence among boys was 2.1% and the prevalence among girls was 6.9%. Contrary to international diagnosis estimates, the 3:1 ratio of boys to girls was not shown (De la Barra et al. 2013). So far, there is no explanation for this finding. However, De la Barra and colleagues (2013) mention that sex differences in international diagnosis estimates are being challenged lately since they appear to be influenced by "referral bias and case identification problems." They also add that research conducted with specific populations reveals not only "a higher prevalence in women," but also a "more severe outcome in girls" (De la Barra et al. 2013: 5). Nevertheless, the explanation they provide is not specific for the Chilean context; this raises the need for further exploration of the topic in Chile.

As the authors of the aforementioned study reflect, the results presented are of great relevance and reveal that Chile has a higher prevalence of ADHD than the worldwide estimate shown in studies such as the one conducted by Polanczyk and colleagues (2007). The publication of the results of the study conducted by De la Barra and her colleagues (2013) makes us optimistic about many similar projects to come.

In a similar spirit, Margozzini's notification about future plans to develop a child-centered health survey fosters expectations of an eventual body of research that will aid in tackling the multiplicity of elements involved in dealing with ADHD in Chile. However, calls for research efforts considering the heterogeneity of elements involved in the composition of ADHD in Chile are not new. In 2000, the Ministerio de Planificacion y Cooperación published a document aimed at fostering and guiding both public and private initiatives targeting children and adolescents during the period from 2001 to 2010. In the document, the "hyperkinetic disorders" are one of many named as "key problems" for the Chilean state.

The emphasis by the government on "hyperkinetic disorders" has raised the suspicion of some researchers involved with child mental health. Some researchers (Abarzúa and González 2007) have argued that the prevalence of the disorder in Chile—which is normally higher than international figures—along with the strong emphasis used by the Ministerio de Salud to tackle and prevent hyperkinetic disorders as soon as possible, suggests that detection and treatment of the disorder are embedded in a high-level agenda to turn children into well-adapted, economically productive citizens. These researchers claim that the government's agenda does not necessarily pursue what is best for children in terms of mental health, but rather it is an attempt to gradually increase social control over a potentially disruptive population (Abarzúa and González 2007). Although we do not necessarily share this perspective, we find it useful in order to exemplify and understand the standpoint of some persons who challenge the diagnosis and use of Ritalin in the Chilean context.

Claims against the validity of the ADHD diagnosis, its high rates, and the use of stimulant medication appear to have become a sign of dissent that goes beyond the diagnosis itself, targeting the educational model implemented since Pinochet's dictatorship. This is reflected in the demands raised by students in the manifesto handed over to representatives of the Ministerio de Educación on May 4, 2012. This manifesto, entitled "Propuesta para la educación que queremos" ("Proposal for the education we want"), was delivered in the midst of student demonstrations that comprised the "Chilean Educational Conflict," which began in 2011 and has endured until the present day. The series of student-led protests aimed at changing the key elements of how education is being implemented and reflected on in Chile. Among the changes demanded by the Asamblea Coordinadora de Estudiantes Secundarios, or ACES, there is a call to cease the use of methylphenidate and the overdiagnosis of ADHD. This organization argues that the diagnosis rate reaches 40% in certain schools; this rate contradicts international evidence and underlines the possibility of an abuse of the diagnosis in Chile (ACES 2012).

These critiques, whether justified or not, put in the limelight one central concern that has been lurking since the beginning of our account. Can we really consider that the ADHD diagnosis operates and follows the same trajectories and rationale in Chile as it does in other parts of the world?

Conclusion

The trajectories of ADHD that we have traced in this chapter reveal the heterogeneous positions and relations that diverse actors play in framing this diagnosis in Chile. We have shown how particular institutional and political contexts—such as the Chilean educational system and its reforms—have influenced the ways in which social actors position themselves in relation to the diagnosis. We have also illustrated the increasingly widespread prescription and consumption of stimulant medication in Chile and the growing debates around these developments.

The so-called abuse of the diagnosis in Chile is an intriguing case study, which reveals how a psychiatric diagnosis that aims to be "global" is, at the same time, extremely contextual and local. As Santos (2001) has argued, in the conditions of the Western capitalist world system, there is no genuine globalization. We add that there can be no such thing as a pure or simple replication of a mental category or disorder from one place to the other. Globalization always entails a series of multiple processes and interactions, and therefore we see a struggle between the local becoming global, and the local as colonized and designated by the global.

When reflecting on ADHD in Chile, it is possible to witness how, by emphasizing the local determinants of the diagnosis, a new scenario comes into play. Educational policies and an extremely strong neoliberal economy appear to be at the base of a constant and sharp surveillance of children's actions and behaviors. This also entails the widespread use of methylphenidate, the easiest and quickest way to deal with the symptomatic manifestations of the disorder.

These interactions and determinations among different actors and scenarios become problematic, even contradictory at times. As we stressed above, there is relatively widespread agreement that stimulant medication is only one dimension of treatment and should be used on a short-term basis in conjunction with nonpharmacological interventions. However, this approach does not seem to be what is implemented in practice (EducarChile n.d.; Rojas 2010).

It is fair to say that the official approach sustained by the Chilean government has mostly failed to build an official program to tackle the real impact and extension of ADHD and its potential treatment. For now, all we can expect is for promises of future interventions and studies to become a reality, to enable the construction of a body of work that reveals a greater understanding of the realities of children and adolescents in Chile, while at the same time acknowledging the nuances involved in the local contexts and their social dynamics. It is crucial to develop approaches that are able to grasp these complexities. We expect that future approaches will be able to rescue the particular narratives and trajectories incurred by different actors—children, medical practitioners, educational experts, and policymakers, among others—involved in shaping the context around ADHD in Chile. After all, this is necessary in order to rescue the contextual aspects that are entailed in the particular Chilean characteristics of an apparently global category, such as ADHD.

NOTES

1. It is not clear in the reports collected by Jorge Rojas whether he is referring to Ritalin in a generic way to name methylphenidate—a usual practice in Chile—or if he is referring specifically to the medication synthesized by Ciba. Given the ambiguity of the word, we have chosen to use "methylphenidate" in our reflections. However, in this chapter we use the word "Ritalin" when the original sources consulted use that particular word, although we cannot be certain whether the consulted sources actually refer to one meaning or the other.

2. Child and adolescent psychiatry had a slow start in the Chilean context. Only in recent decades have various medical centers and medical faculties developed specific programs and started offering grants and the possibility of doing training in order to obtain that medical specialty. Before that, psychiatrists who were interested in child and adolescent mental health were mostly trained as neurologists (Heskia and Carvajal 2014).

3. *Psicopedagogo* is a professional trained particularly to deal with learning difficulties and impairments.

4. These rates and figures were obtained through the Ley de transparencia de la función pública y de acceso a la información de la administración del Estado, and given to us by the Ministerio de Salud. In order to access this information, a form must be filled out on the website of the Chilean Ministerio de Salud. In the form it must be clearly stated which data are being requested and the reason why the request is being made. The application is then transferred to the governmental institution that can provide the required information—in this case the Central de Abastecimiento del Sistema Nacional de Servicios de Salud, or CENEBAST, and the Ministerio de Salud. If approved, the Chilean Ley de transparencia de la función pública y de acceso a la información de la administración del Estado dictates that within a couple of weeks, the information must be delivered. In our case, it was sent in a PDF and Excel files via email to the lead researcher. What was received is not an official report, but various figures of medication consumption and ADHD prevalence divided according to age groups, gender, and geographical location.

5. *Octavo básico* is the final year of what is known in Chile as "basic education."

6. Paula Margozzini was the chief epidemiologist in charge of conducting the 2009–10 National Health Survey.

REFERENCES

Abarzúa, Marianella, and Marta González. 2007. "Salud mental infanto-juvenil como problemática pública." *Revista de Psicología* 16 (2): 79–95.

Aboitiz, Francisco, and Carolina Schröter. 2005. "Síndrome de déficit atencional: Antecedentes neurobiológicos y cognitivos para estudiar un modelo de endofenotipo." *Revista Chilena de Neuro-Psiquiatría* 43 (1): 11–16.

Aravena, Pedro, and Manuel Inostroza. 2015. "¿Salud pública o privada? Los factores más importantes al evaluar el sistema de salud en Chile." *Revista Médica de Chile* 143 (2): 244–51.

Araya, Olga. 1986. "Los niños y el psiquiatra." *Revista YA*, July 1, 13.

———. 1987a. "Enredos infantiles." *Revista YA*, March 17, 9.

———. 1987b. "El niño eléctrico." *Revista YA*, April 7, 7.

Asamblea Coordinadora de Estudiantes Secundarios (ACES). 2012. "ACES Chile; Propuesta para la educación que queremos." MovilizateChile. http://www.movilizatechile.cl/2012/05/aces-chile-propuesta-para-la-educacion-que-queremos/.

Barkley, Russell. 2005. *Attention-Deficit Hyperactivity Disorder: A Handbook for Diagnosis and Treatment.* 3rd ed. New York: Guilford.

Cabalin, Cristian. 2014. "The Conservative Response to the 2011 Chilean Student Movement: Neoliberal Education and Media." *Discourse: Studies in the Cultural Politics of Education* 35 (4): 485–98.

De la Barra, Flora, Benjamin Vicente, Sandra Saldivia, and Roberto Melipillan. 2013. "Epidemiology of ADHD in Chilean Children and Adolescents." *Attention Deficit and Hyperactivity Disorders* 5 (1): 1–8.

Devilat, Marcelo. 1993. "Editorial." *Boletín Sociedad de Psiquiatría y Neurología de la Infancia y Adolescencia* 4 (1): 4–5.

EducarChile. n.d. "Ritalín en la sala de clases." http://www.educarchile.cl/ech/pro/app/detalle?id=106430.

Elacqua, Gregory. 2012. "The Impact of School Choice and Public Policy on Segregation: Evidence from Chile." *International Journal of Education Development* 32 (3): 444–53.

Galvez, Karim. 1995a. "El déficit atencional Madura con y sin Ritalin." *Revista YA*, May 16, 6.

———. 1995b. "Mi vida es un drama total." *Revista YA*, July 4, 7.

Harvey, David. 2007. *A Brief History of Neoliberalism.* Oxford: Oxford University Press.

Heskia, Cristóbal, and César Carvajal. 2014. *Historias de Psiquiatras: Testimonios de psiquiatras chilenos.* Santiago: Universidad de los Andes.

International Narcotic Control Board (INCB). 2013. "Psychotropic Substances: Statistics for 2012. Assessments of Annual Medical and Scientific Requirements." United Nations. http://www.incb.org/documents/Psychotropics/technical-publications/2013/en/Tech_pub_2013.pdf.

Jaque, José Miguel, and Francisco Rodríguez. 2011. "Los 20 años de la generación Ritalín." *La Tercera*, June 4, sec. Tendencias.

Junta Nacional de Auxilio Escolar y Becas (JUNAEB). 2015. "Habilidades para la vida." http://www.junaeb.cl/habilidades-para-la-vida.

Lange, Klaus, Susanne Reichl, Katharina Lange, Lara Tucha, and Oliver Tucha. 2010. "The History of Attention Deficit Hyperactivity Disorder." *Attention Deficit Hyperactivity Disorder* 2 (4): 241–55.

Larraín, Soledad, and Carolina Bascuñan. 2012. *4to Estudio de maltrato infantil*. Santiago: UNICEF.

Lévi-Strauss, Claude. 1966. *The Savage Mind*. Chicago: University of Chicago Press.

Lincoln, Yvonna, and Norman Denzin. 2003. *Turning Points in Qualitative Research: Tying Knots in a Handkerchief*. Lanham, MD: AltaMira.

Marzouka, Nelly, and Ilse López. 1994. "Déficit atencional, hábitos televisivos y funcionamiento familiar." *Boletín Sociedad de Psiquiatría y Neurología de la Infancia y Adolescencia* 5 (3): 7–8.

Mayes, Rick, Catherine Bagwell, and Jennifer Erkulwater. 2009. *Medicating Children: ADHD and Pediatric Mental Health*. Cambridge, MA: Harvard University Press.

Ministerio de Educación. 2009. *Déficit Atencional: Guía para su comprensión y desarrollo de estrategias de apoyo, desde un enfoque inclusivo, en el nivel de educación básica*. http//www.mineduc.cl/usuarios/edu.especial/doc/201305151612430.Deficit_Atencional.pdf.

Ministerio de Salud. 2005. *Encuesta Mundial de Salud Escolar: Chile 2004 y 2005*. http://www.bvsde.paho.org/bvsdeescuelas/emse/chile/encuesta2005.pdf.

———. 2008. *Guía clínica atención integral de niñas/niños y adolescentes con trastorno hipercinético/trastorno de la atención (THA)*. http://www.hrrio.cl/documentos/GUIA%20CLINICA%20THA%2028%20agosto%2020081(final).doc

Montenegro, Hernán. 1983. "Disfunción cerebral y relación padres-hijos." *Revista YA*, November 1, 7.

Peña, Mónica, Patricio Rojas Navarro, and Sebastián Rojas Navarro. 2014. "¿Cómo diagnosticar un niño? Diagnóstico del Trastorno de Déficit Atencional con Hiperactividad desde una perspectiva discursiva crítica." *Atheneadigital: Revista de pensamiento e investigación social* 15 (1): 91–110.

Polanczyk, Guilherme, Maurício Silva de Lima, Bernardo Lessa Horta, Joseph Biederman, and Luis Augusto Rohde. 2007. "The Worldwide Prevalence of ADHD: A Systematic Review and Metaregression Analysis." *American Journal of Psychiatry* 164 (6): 942–48.

Rojas, Jorge. 2010. *Historia de la infancia en el Chile republicano: 1810–2010*. Santiago: OchoLibros.

Rojas, Juana, and Erna Imperatore. 1994. "Niños con déficit atencional: ¿verdaderamente agresivos? Enfoque de integración sensorial a través de la terapia familiar ocupacional." *Boletín Sociedad de Psiquiatría y Neurología de la Infancia y Adolescencia* 5 (3): 12.

Rojas Navarro, Sebastián, and Patricio Rojas. 2015. "The Making of Children Identities beyond Adult Given Classifications: Biomedical Diagnostic Categories and Processes of Resistance Performed by Chilean Children." In *Dialogue and Debate in the Making of Theoretical Psychology*, edited by James Cresswell, Andrés Haye, and Antonia Larraín, 321–29. Concord, ONT: Captus.

Ruiz, Alfredo. 1985. "Niños inquietos." *Revista YA*, June 25, 5.

Santos, Boaventura de Sousa. 2001. "Nuestra América: Reinventing a Subaltern Paradigm of Recognition and Redistribution." *Theory, Culture & Society* 18 (2–3): 185–217.

Sapelli, Claudio, and Cristián Aedo. 2001. "El sistema de vouchers en educación: una revisión de la teoría y evidencia empírica para Chile." *Estudios Públicos* 82: 35–82.

Schlager, German, and Ximena Keith. 1993. "XII Congreso de Psiquiatría y Neurología de la Infancia y Adolescencia." *Boletín Sociedad de Psiquiatría y Neurología de la Infancia y Adolescencia* 4 (2): 47.

Still, George. 1902. "Some Abnormal Psychical Conditions in Children: The Goulsto-nian Lectures." *The Lancet* 1: 1008–12.

Torres, Ana María. 2013. "Estudio de los proyectos de integración escolar de primer año de Educación Básica en establecimientos municipales y particulares subvencionados de la provincia de Valparaíso." *Perspectiva Educacional* 52 (1): 124–46.

Vicente, Benjamín, Sandra Saldivia, Flora de la Barra, Roberto Kohn, Ronaldo Pihan, Mario Valdivia, Pedro Rioseco, and Roberto Melipillan. 2012a. "Prevalence of Child and Adolescent Mental Disorders in Chile: A Community Epidemiological Study." *Journal of Child Psychology and Psychiatry, and Allied Disciplines* 53 (10): 1026–35.

Vicente, Benjamín, Sandra Saldivia, Flora de la Barra, Roberto Melipillan, Mario Valdivia, and Roberto Kohn. 2012b. "Salud mental infanto-juvenil en Chile y brechas de aten-ción sanitarias." *Revista Médica de Chile* 140 (4): 447–57.

Whitehead, Alfred North. 1968. *Modes of Thought.* New York: Touchstone.

16

The Development of Child Psychiatry and the Biomedicalization of ADHD in Taiwan

Fan-Tzu Tseng

A ttention deficit–hyperactivity disorder (ADHD) has been the most commonly diagnosed mental disorder of childhood and adolescence in Taiwan over the past decade. According to surveys based on community samples, the estimated prevalence of ADHD among children 7 to 15 years of age is between 6.3% and 12% (Huang 2008), which is higher than the estimated global average prevalence of 5% (Polanczyk et al. 2007). Compared with these estimates, the number of ADHD diagnoses in Taiwan's National Health Insurance (NHI) database of medical claims has been much lower. The most recent research using NHI data based on a random population sample of 378,881 patients 4 to 17 years of age found that the prevalence of the ADHD diagnosis between 2010 and 2011 was 2.3% (Chen et al. 2016). Another study, which recruited all newly diagnosed ADHD patients 18 years of age or younger from 2000 through 2011, revealed that the annual prevalence of ADHD increased 10.3 times (from 0.1% to 1.3%) throughout the duration of this study, and about 60% of the ADHD patients were prescribed medication to manage their condition (Wang et al. 2015). The same study also showed that the male-to-female ratio for ADHD was about 3.7 to 1 in Taiwan. Although more updated statistics are currently unavailable, ADHD diagnoses and the use of stimulant treatment among Taiwanese children and adolescents are believed to have continued to increase since 2011.[1]

The challenge lies in explaining the rising prevalence of ADHD and the increase in stimulant use to treat it. This condition is the archetype of the study of medicalization (Conrad 2006) in that deviant behaviors such as hyperactivity, impulsivity, and inattention are classified as medical conditions and therefore fall under medical jurisdiction. Related literature reveals that the engines driving the medicalization of ADHD include changing diagnostic criteria and diagnostic expansion, promotion by big pharma, campaigns led by parent associations, transformation of educational institutions and educational culture, and contemporary social and cultural changes (Degrandpre 1999; Lloyd and Norris 1999; Conrad and Potter 2000; Mayes, Bagwell, and Erkulwater 2008; Singh 2008; Bailey 2009; Vallée 2010; Edwards and Howlett 2013; Rafalovich 2013; Singh et al. 2013).

The case of Taiwan is seemingly similar to the classical medicalization thesis, and it emphasizes the imperialistic tendencies of the medical profession in which doctors monopolize power over the ADHD diagnosis and prescriptions. However, I argue that the medicalization of ADHD in Taiwan, as a latecomer to Western medicine, has a different trajectory from its original context. Taiwanese child and adolescent psychiatry was still struggling to establish itself as a specialty at the turn of the twenty-first century, by which point the biomedical framing of behaviors associated with ADHD and related medication treatment were already well established in American research and clinical practice. This context deeply shaped the local approach to ADHD in Taiwan, where the American medical model has guided medical education and health care since the Second World War (Liu 2012). Although the specialty of child psychiatry was yet to be established in the late twentieth century, long before the category of ADHD was introduced to Taiwan, knowledge and techniques of child psychiatry were already adopted by non-psychiatric professionals to address children's challenging behaviors in school contexts, especially the disciplinary problems related to acting out. However, the approach to child psychiatry at the time was very different from the current biomedical paradigm.

Considering this desynchrony, I conceptualize "child psychiatry" in Taiwan to be a "network" linking agents, objects, concepts, and techniques, as well as institutional and spatial arrangements, rather than a "profession" (Eyal 2013). This approach helps focus beyond child psychiatrists per se to follow "a history of tasks and problems" (Abbott 2014: 314) on the understanding and handling of the "problem child" in terms of knowledge and techniques of child psychiatry, which have been imparted to different actors outside the psychiatric profession.

During this process, the medicalization of ADHD in Taiwan has been co-produced with the stepwise formation of a child psychiatric network in local society.

The medicalization of deviant behavior in its original society usually includes five sequential and overlapping stages: defining a specific condition as deviant, related medical discovery, claims-making driven by medical and nonmedical interests, legitimation to secure medical turf, and institutionalization (Conrad and Schneider 1992). This theorization suggests an often fiercely disputed process, but, as the case of Taiwan will show, a latecomer usually learns the established medical knowledge and classification system directly from pioneering countries, which is justified as a step toward modernization and professionalization. The typically complex and contested history of a new medical category is left in the original society, whereas professional communities in the receiving society often take current knowledge for granted. Rather than competing with other claims-makers on the definitions and jurisdiction of deviant behavior, local actors in a latecomer country usually expend more efforts to put this medical category into clinical practice, given the shortage of health professionals and corresponding medical cognition regarding the problem at issue in the entire society.

This chapter attempts to elucidate how ADHD came to be extensively recognized, diagnosed, and treated in Taiwan. Considering the late development of child psychiatry as a professional specialty and the foreignness of the concepts of child mental disorders in Western psychiatry for local people, the clinical realization of ADHD as a medical problem was achieved by co-constructing a child psychiatric network consisting of related ideas, agents, instruments, activities, organizations, and institutions. Further, the network was not monolithic but reconfigured over time when its key components changed.

I draw on data from various sources to illustrate these points. The sources include the historical archives of the Department of Psychiatry and the Children's Mental Health Center at National Taiwan University Hospital, both of which were early builders that developed the Taiwanese child psychiatric network; the (auto)biographies of pioneering professionals; local newspaper articles on hyperactive children since the 1950s; relevant medical and educational academic research, popular literature, and government documents and regulations; brochures issued by relevant parental organizations; and discussions about ADHD in parenting forums such as *BabyHome* (www.babyhome.com.tw), the largest parenting website in Taiwan, and the "BabyMother" and "SP_Teacher" boards on PTT, the largest Chinese language-based bulletin board system. I also conducted fieldwork to gather data from 2013 to 2015. I participated as an audience member in ADHD health education activities held in medical institutions and as a speaker in various panel discussions on ADHD hosted by different organizations.

In the following sections, I contextualize the process of medicalizing ADHD in Taiwan into three historical periods: (1) the initiation of Taiwanese child psychiatric services and school-based mental health programs (1953–77); (2) the emergence and stabilization of the ADHD diagnosis as well as the expansion of the child psychiatric network (1978–97); and (3) the network reconfiguration and the biomedicalization of ADHD (1998–present). With the continuing reassembly of this child psychiatric network, the prevailing perspective on children's hyperactivity has changed from a "maladjustment" to a "biomedical condition," but the efforts to frame it as a medical problem and to expand the corresponding medical treatments remain unchanged and in full force.

The Initiation of Child Psychiatric Services and School-Based Mental Health Programs (1953–77)

After the Second World War, American aid to Taiwan became the major source of funds for recovery and reconstruction. From 1951 to 1965, the United States provided US$1.4 billion (Jacoby 1966) to help Taiwan achieve self-sustainable economic growth, thereby exerting considerable influence on a wide range of institutional establishments. Almost all of the domains of public service, including medical care and public health, benefited from this aid. With its strong economic power and political influence, the United States also presented new professional standards for the postwar Taiwanese generation of medical professionals. Since the 1950s, more than 85% of Taiwanese medical school graduates and young fellows have gone to the United States for further education (Liu 2012). The development of child psychiatry was not an exception to the influence of the United States.

The child psychiatric service in Taiwan was formed in 1951 when the Department of Psychiatry at National Taiwan University Hospital established the children's division, which was rebuilt as the Children's Mental Health Center (CMHC) in 1953 with support from the World Health Organization (WHO) and the Council on US Aid. The CMHC was formed to align with American child guidance clinics, which were popular in the 1940s and 1950s and provided treatments for so-called maladjusted children as an integral part of juvenile delinquency prevention programs (Jones 1999). Run by an interdisciplinary team composed of a psychiatrist, a clinical psychologist, and a social worker, the paradigm of diagnosis in the CMHC was one of dynamic psychiatry. This approach was dominant in the United States in the mid-1900s and was concerned with the biological, psychological, and social roots of mental maladjustment (Grob 2014).

The first child psychiatrist in Taiwan, Chen-Chin Hsu, obtained a two-year fellowship from the WHO to specialize in child psychiatry at the Jadge Baker Guidance Center in Boston and the Department of Psychiatry at Harvard University in the late 1950s. He was the only child psychiatrist in Taiwan until 1980, and he believed that the dynamic therapeutic approach emphasizing psychoanalysis and "talk therapy" was too laborious and time-consuming to be provided in a developing country like Taiwan, which lacked trained clinical experts (Hsu 1972). Moreover, traditional Chinese norms discourage open expression of personal emotions, especially strong and negative ones. According to the observations of the medical anthropologist and psychiatrist Arthur Kleinman (1980), experiences of illness and the perception of symptoms are culturally bounded, and Chinese culture, which is deficient in terms of a psychological orientation to illness, makes most Chinese patients incapable of describing their feelings and affect "in considerable detail and relat[ing] it to many different aspects of their lives," unlike middle-class Caucasian-American sufferers with similar conditions (Kleinman 1980: 141). Based on a similar understanding of Taiwanese society, Hsu introduced behavioral therapy in Taiwan and put it into practice. Thus, behavioral therapy replaced psychotherapy and became the main treatment provided at the CMHC. To objectively evaluate the traits of patients and the effectiveness of treatment, the CMHC also attempted to translate and localize various diagnostic scales over the following decade. These standardized tools included the Werry-Weiss-Peters Activity Scale (Werry 1968) and the Conners Comprehensive Behavior Rating Scales (Conners CBRS™; Conners 1968, 1970), both of which were later frequently used to assess hyperactive children in Taiwan.

However, as an outpatient clinic in a teaching hospital, the CMHC had a very limited number of patients given the lack of child psychiatric personnel and the severe stigma attached to psychosis in the culture at the time. Despite the agreement on mental illness as a medical condition among Taiwanese clinical experts, the stigma of "craziness" was exceedingly strong in Taiwanese society, which attributed responsibility to the family instead of to the individual because of the traditional idea of "karma" (retribution for sin), which suggested that the sufferer's parents or ancestors had done something immoral (Lin 1981). This family-oriented stigma undoubtedly prevented the majority of parents from taking their children to receive psychiatric services.

In addition to clinical work, improving community child mental health to prevent future disorders was also one of the main tasks of the CMHC from the outset. As the only professional agency in Taiwan focusing on the mental health of children, the CMHC first needed to address the problem of having only a "few clinical experts serving eight million children and adolescents" (Soong 2009: 1). The shortage of mental health care workers required psychiatric professionals to elicit the interest of schoolteachers in planning and implementing mental health programs.

This idea developed into an experimental mental health project launched in Taipei Municipal East-Gate Elementary School in 1960 to motivate and assist teachers in integrating mental health work into their daily teaching routine. In a comparison of teacher-reported "problem children" before and after a series of mental health seminars, the student population that teachers identified as "problem children" rose from 3.5% to 12%, and "acting-out disciplinary problems" remained as the greatest concern (Hsu and Lin 1969). The training provided in this experimental project equipped participating teachers with standardized scales to identify children's problems and basic behavioral therapy skills for managing such problems. Only the severe cases that required clinical treatment were referred to proper professional agencies. This experimental project led by child psychiatric experts eventually trained teacher-counselors, who could implement mental health work in a school-based counseling office. The East-Gate Elementary School then became a training center for teachers from other schools and served as a model for school mental health programs across the country. This development was the first step in the formation of a school-counseling profession in Taiwan.

According to the CMHC's archives, no exclusive diagnosis for hyperactive children existed until the late 1970s. The first official category of hyperkinesis—hyperkinetic reaction of childhood—was listed in the second edition of the *Diagnostic and Statistical Manual of Mental Disorders* (*DSM-II*), published by the American Psychiatric Association (APA) in 1968. However, at the time, the *DSM* system had minimal influence in both the United States and Taiwan. The most likely diagnosis for children who might have the symptomology of hyperkinesis was "minimal brain dysfunction" (MBD), which was generally considered to be one of the historical antecedents of the concept of ADHD (Barkley 2005). Notably, the first prescription of Ritalin in the CMHC was for a patient diagnosed with

MBD in 1977. Other patients were diagnosed with "behavioral problems" and "behavioral disorders" caused by conditions of the brain's nerve system. These children may now be deemed "ADHD" patients, given that ADHD is currently considered to be a neurodevelopmental disorder in the *DSM-5* (APA 2013).

In summary, the development of child psychiatry in Taiwan during the initial period focused on community child mental health and on dealing with the "problem child." The lack of human resources required the participation of schoolteachers in mental health programs. These teachers were taught the necessary knowledge, techniques, and screening tools to address behavioral problems. Although no exclusive diagnosis existed for hyperactive children in Taiwan, children with related symptomology were initially identified as maladjusted by teacher-counselors and then referred to clinical experts. These patients were subsumed under the terminologies of "minimal brain dysfunction," "behavioral problems," or "behavioral disorders" and were treated mainly by behavioral therapies.

Stabilization of the ADHD Diagnosis and the Expansion of the Child Psychiatric Network (1978–97)

In 1977, the WHO published the ninth edition of the *International Classification of Diseases (ICD-9)*, which included the first standard system of diagnosis and classification of mental disorders. This so-called common language medical coding system, which aimed to enable a consistent way of comparing and sharing health information across the specialties and sites of care, was proposed in 1965 by Tsung-Yi Lin, the first Taiwanese chief of the Department of Psychiatry at Taiwan University Hospital and an advisor to the WHO Mental Health Unit. In the following decade, Taiwan, representing the whole of China, was selected by the WHO as one of the nine "field research centers" to develop standardized procedures for the assessment of mental disorders (Wu 2012). Consequently, psychiatry in Taiwan moved toward standardization, and the Taiwanese minister of health then specified the implementation of *ICD-9* into clinical practice in 1978.

The category "hyperkinetic syndrome of childhood" in the *ICD* system immediately appeared in the medical records of the CMHC as the first official diagnosis specific to hyperactive children in Taiwan. This category accounted for approximately 12% of the number of new patients in the following decade, second only to mental retardation (Soong 1997a: 161). Significantly, Ritalin was imported systematically beginning in 1982 by Novartis Taiwan for the treatment of hyperkinetic syndrome of childhood, and the drug became a therapeutic choice alongside behavioral therapy. However, prescription practices in the CMHC remained conservative given the insufficiency of clinical trials for the safety of psychiatric medications in children. Records from new patients in 1980, 1985, and 1990 show that only 12.8% of patients in the CMHC received medications. Ritalin, as the only drug available in Taiwan for hyperkinetic syndrome, accounted for nearly 4% of all the treatments, but it still represented the most frequently used single medicine (Soong 1997b: 192).

Compared with the preceding emphasis on public health, the CMHC in this period ceased its organizational partnership with the WHO and local government, returning to the role of psychiatric clinic at a teaching hospital. In 1981, Wei-Tsuen Soong completed his child psychiatry specialty training program in Canada and engaged in the CMHC's work to develop a new clinical orientation. Benefiting from the stable increase in the number of patients in the CMHC, the research conducted in this period was based on large clinical samples rather than on case reports, as was common in previous decades. As mentioned above, hyperkinetic syndrome of childhood was a relatively new diagnosis and the second most common diagnosis; thus, a series of academic articles on this syndrome was published in the 1980s, including an overview of the condition, clinical characteristics, screening tests, and temperamental traits of children with hyperkinetic syndrome of childhood. Notably, all but one of these studies used the newly published *DSM-III* (APA 1980) as a reference because of its more concrete diagnostic criteria than the *ICD* system, reflecting the gradual adoption of the *DSM* system by Taiwanese psychiatrists. Since 1987, the *DSM-III-R* (APA 1987) rephrased the category of "attention-deficit disorder with or without hyperactivity" in the *DSM-III* to "attention deficit/hyperactivity disorder (ADHD)" which was immediately accepted in Taiwan and became the main, if not the only, designation addressing hyperactive children.

With the standardization of a diagnostic system and the development of clinical research, child psychiatry has since been incorporated into the existing psychiatric fellowship training and medical education in universities, with ADHD as an important area of focus. Although specialty training for child psychiatry was not formally established until the turn of the twenty-first century, an increasing number of psychiatrists were already interested in child mental disorders and organized a group based at the CMHC in the late 1980s. The affiliated members held seminars to exchange new knowledge and experiences regarding child mental disorders. This group was the precursor of the Taiwanese Society of Child and Adolescent Psychiatry.

Issues related to hyperactive children began to appear, aside from clinical and research domains, in popular medical and parenting magazines in the second half of the 1980s, as well as in books mainly written by psychiatrists. Given this new media of communicating with Taiwanese society, psychiatrists expected parents to be allies and provided them with basic knowledge on child mental disorders, techniques of behavioral therapy, and screening tools for early identification. As Hsu told parents, "Don't worry about undercutting the professional counselors if you know the ropes. This is exactly what we want. The better you do up front, the less we become burdened. Above all, it means that counseling practices will be spread widely and rooted deeply" (Hsu 1981: 309).

In the succeeding period, individual parents were not the only new allies who were expected to participate in this expanding child psychiatric network to address children's mental health. A new parental organization, the Association of Hyperactive Children, and burgeoning special education regulations were aligned to ensure the right to equitable education opportunities for hyperactive children. In the 1980s, Taiwan experienced a gradual political democratization that peaked when the 38-year martial law ended in 1987. This dramatic political reform coincided with the rapid upsurge of social movements, among which protests for disability rights were a powerful force (Chang 2007). Moreover, parents organized to advocate on behalf of their children for special education rights and social welfare services, which were limited in Taiwan at the time. During the confrontation between the stigma attached to disabilities and the fight for public resources, the medical profession was often an important resource for parents to justify the legitimacy of the condition in question.

In the mid-1990s, the discovery of new information regarding ADHD and the increase in the number of diagnoses during that time motivated a group of parents of children with ADHD to form the Association of Hyperactive Children (AHC). The objectives of this effort were to protest against disadvantaged school environments and to appeal for the justification of eligibility for special education of children with ADHD. Newspaper articles about students with ADHD often described fierce conflicts in the educational environment; teachers complained that such children frequently disrupted classes and aggravated other students, whereas parents of the students with ADHD claimed that their children were punished unjustly or even rejected by schools. On the one hand, the AHC's campaign initiated the definite reframing of ADHD from a condition of "badness" to a "sickness" (Conrad and Schneider 1992) with regard to the troublesome behavior of children in school environments, thereby highlighting the important role of psychiatrists in addressing this issue. On the other hand, the media emphasized "hyperactivity" and "impulsivity" as manifestations of ADHD and stressed that ADHD is a mental disorder that requires medical treatment and educational accommodations. In fact, the medical definition of ADHD included the aspect of "inattention." During this period, however, for both parents and schoolteachers in Taiwan, children's hyperactivity and impulsivity were the urgent issues that needed to be addressed.

Being diagnosed with ADHD does not automatically guarantee that a child will qualify to receive special education services. For example, in the United States, ADHD is listed under the Individuals with Disabilities Education Act (IDEA) eligibility category of "other health impaired." Children classified under this category may receive special education and related services if their conditions "adversely affect educational performance" (US Department of Education 2006: 46757). In addition, students with ADHD may qualify under "specific learning disabilities" or "severe emotional disturbance" (Kirk, Gallagher, and Coleman 2014: 224). Issued in Taiwan in 1988, the Evaluation Enforcement for Students with Disability and Giftedness listed ADHD under the category of "serious emotional disorders" (which, in 2002, was restated as "emotional and behavioral disabilities"). The article further noted that the evaluation of these disorders "may refer to the psychiatric diagnosis."

During this period, psychiatrists allied with the parental organization AHC and promoted the emerging field of special education. This growing network expanded the scope of the child psychiatry approach to include children's issues; however, specialty training for child psychiatry in Taiwan had not yet been formally started. Parents of children with ADHD organized themselves to fight for educational rights by actively adopting biological accounts of ADHD and drawing on the authority of psychiatrists. This close collaboration between the AHC and psychiatrists consolidated around a medical understanding of ADHD. Such an alliance had also been anticipated in behavioral therapy, which continued to be the main treatment for children with ADHD, although Ritalin had been an available treatment option since the early 1980s. Regardless of whether a child's hyperactivity or impulsivity was considered a daily behavioral problem, a type of mental disorder, or an indicator of the need for special education accommodations, psychiatrists have increasingly played an essential role in the management of ADHD. Thereafter, in view of this expanding network of child psychiatric expertise, the number of specialists became a weak "reverse salient" (Hughes 1987) that needed to be immediately addressed to accelerate the progress of the network.

Network Reconfiguration and Biomedicalization of ADHD (1998–Present)

In 1998, the Taiwanese Society of Child and Adolescent Psychiatry was established, and formal specialty training was subsequently launched. As a result, the number of certified child psychiatrists steadily increased in the following years. At present, child psychiatric services are provided in more than 100 medical institutions (Taiwanese Society of Child and Adolescent Psychiatry 2015). With ADHD becoming a more common diagnosis today, this condition remains a fundamental topic of research, teaching, and mass health education in the psychiatric profession.

Researchers have given considerable attention to the increasing prevalence of patients with ADHD. A series of studies used different scales in surveying specific local communities, and they estimated that the prevalence of ADHD ranged from 6.3% to 9.9% (Huang 2008). Considering that these scales are more biased toward hyperactivity than inattention because of the early understanding of hyperkinesis, Shur-Fen Gau, who was the first Taiwanese psychiatrist to specialize in ADHD, led a team to translate and publish the 26-item Swanson, Nolan, and Pelham scale, version IV (SNAP-IV) (Swanson et al. 2001), a *DSM-IV*-based ADHD rating scale that can be used in assessing and screening children with ADHD. With this new standardized instrument, Gau's team estimated that the prevalence of ADHD among Taiwanese children ranged from 7% to 12% (Liu et al. 2006). In the following years, this scale became the most widely used screening tool for ADHD in medical institutions, public health services, and special education settings. The Chinese version of the SNAP-IV scale is readily available on the Internet, and parents can obtain the tool and fill out the questions on their own to gauge whether their children may have symptoms of ADHD.

Although Ritalin was a regular medication for ADHD in Taiwan, pharmaceutical companies did not play a constructive role in this network with regard to ADHD until the extended-release Concerta was imported to Taiwan by Janssen-Cilag in 2003. The lack of interest on the part of Novartis Taiwan to actively promote Ritalin may be attributed to the NHI scheme in Taiwan, which is a single-payer compulsory social insurance program that centralizes the disbursement of health care funds through the NHI administration. The NHI provides a comprehensive package covering nearly all types of medical services and pre-scription drugs, and more than 99% of the population is enrolled in the NHI program, thereby boosting the administration's bargaining power with pharma-ceutical companies. For example, with regard to ADHD medications, the price of a minimum-dose Ritalin tablet has held at less than US$0.10 ever since the NHI was instituted in 1995 because the patents for regular Ritalin have already expired. However, when Concerta was first imported, the NHI set the price of a minimum-dose tablet to nearly US$2. Four years later, Lilly Taiwan introduced another ADHD medication called Strattera, which was priced at US$3 for a minimum-dose tablet. The differences in the prices set by the NHI administra-tion determine the profitability of these drugs for these pharmaceutical compa-nies, which in turn affect their willingness to conduct marketing campaigns to the medical community.

In addition to setting the prices of ADHD medications, the NHI administra-tion also determines the fee of other clinical therapies for mental disorders and has accordingly brought about an essential reconfiguration of treatment prac-tices for ADHD. The prices of psychotherapies vary depending on the treatment type and the provider's professional qualification. For instance, a 40-minute "inten-sive individual psychotherapy" session conducted only by psychiatrists costs between 1,203 and 1,718 points (approximately US$40–US$57), whereas a 60-minute "re-educative individual psychotherapy" session conducted by clini-cal psychologists costs between 344 and 515 points (approximately US$11–US$17). A 60-minute family therapy session provided by psychiatric social workers costs 515 points (approximately US$17). Given such low prices, providing these psycho-therapies and maintaining an interdisciplinary team that handles children's disorders would not be cost-effective for medical institutions and personnel. Ultimately, the NHI payment system compromised the incentive of child psychiatrists to commit to the biopsychosocial model while unintentionally en-couraging drug treatments for patients with ADHD.

With the approval of Concerta and Strattera for clinical use, Janssen-Cilag Taiwan and Lilly Taiwan have been expanding the child psychiatric network for ADHD treatment by providing active support for continuing medical education for psychiatrists. Janssen-Cilag Taiwan created a website dedicated to ADHD (www.adhd.club.tw), and its link is prominently displayed on the homepage of the Taiwanese Society of Child and Adolescent Psychiatry. A Google search for "ADHD" in Taiwan would yield the ADHD website as a recommended link, sec-ond only to the entry on "ADHD" from Wikipedia.

In addition to their engagement with the child psychiatric community, pharmaceutical companies have exerted considerable efforts to inform potential clients, mainly parents, while acceding to the Taiwanese government's prohibition on direct-to-consumer advertising for prescription medications by actively collaborating with the parental organization, which has been restructured as the Naivety ADHD Taiwan Association (NATA), to advocate for ADHD identification and treatment. Their collaborative efforts include conducting related speeches and joint workshops as well as sponsoring various brochures concerning ADHD issues for parents and teachers. These pamphlets typically contain the Chinese version of the SNAP-IV scale, and medication therapy is listed on top in the section on treatments. Aside from establishing rapport with parents who may recognize or suspect their children's condition, Janssen-Cilag Taiwan, in 2007, commissioned the prestigious mass medical magazine *Common Health* to publish a special issue that contained information on ADHD and had the issue delivered for free to 290,000 parents of first-year elementary school students nationwide. In that special issue, ADHD was depicted merely as a biological disease rather than a multifactorial disorder, and the extended-release medication was described as a "smart pill" and a "focus drug," with its effects emphasized as providing "improvement of academic achievement" by means of treating "inattention" (*Common Health* 2007: 49).

Based on my observation, the confidence of many Taiwanese child psychiatrists in ADHD medications is based on a series of Multimodal Treatment of ADHD (MTA) studies that were funded by the National Institute of Mental Health in the United States (MTA Cooperative Group 1999), although the influence of pharmaceutical companies is also undeniable. The MTA studies, which frequently appeared in mass health education materials on ADHD for Taiwanese psychiatrists, suggested that for core ADHD symptoms, medication management was superior to purely intensive behavioral treatment (MTA Cooperative Group 1999). The safety and adverse effects of these medications have already been assessed in follow-up studies (Swanson et al. 2007). This optimism toward medication is also reflected in the clinical practice of Taiwanese psychiatrists for patients with ADHD. At the CMHC, clinicians once tended to be more conservative in using stimulants in earlier years, but the medical records from 2002 to 2003 showed that approximately 36.5% of patients were diagnosed with ADHD, of which 55% were prescribed Ritalin (Gau et al. 2004). Another recent study based on the NHI database also revealed that the rate of nationwide medication use among patients with ADHD was about 60% (Wang et al. 2015). These statistics suggest that medications have become the main treatment approach for children with ADHD in clinical settings in Taiwan.

Schoolteachers are advised to directly refer students with suspected ADHD to child psychiatrists. A recent survey showed that approximately 97% of teachers have a positive opinion of drug therapy despite the medium to severe adverse effects reported among more than 60% of local children who receive medication (Meng and Hsieh 2012). Several reasons point to why most Taiwanese teachers readily accept ADHD diagnoses and medication therapies. On the one hand, teachers obtain knowledge about ADHD through various in-service training seminars. In general, school counseling offices organize seminars on topics related to ADHD, for which psychiatrists are the typical speakers. On the other hand, teachers often experience difficulty in managing students with ADHD, especially when they have to take care of more than 30 students in a class. As such, medication is a more convenient and effective means than other methods such as educational accommodations or modifications (Hsu and Chan 2008).

By contrast, parents are more ambivalent toward medication treatments. Nearly 38% of parents of children with ADHD rejected medications for their children; although 62% of parents accepted stimulants, 38.2% of them expressed concerns (Meng and Hsieh 2012). Based on my long-term observations from online parenting forums regarding ADHD, the primary concern of parents is the potential adverse effects of the medications, especially because negative information and stories about stimulant use are readily available online. Their hesitations were further heightened when, in 2011, a series of news reports uncovered that an after-school teacher illegally provided Ritalin to students who did not have ADHD to keep them quiet and focused. One reporter (Yan 2010) described Ritalin as "Kiddie Cocaine," and the interviewed government official revealed that methylphenidate, the main ingredient of Ritalin, is classified as a schedule III controlled drug in Taiwan,[2] and this schedule also includes the notorious Ketamine, which is often abused by local drug addicts, according to that official's additional remarks. This scandal stirred panic among parents of children with ADHD and even caused some of them to stop medicating their children.[3]

Furthermore, these concerns are aggravated by the doubts shared by many middle-class parents who find psychiatric diagnosis to be a seemingly subjective process. Some parents even question the validity of ADHD as a disorder on the basis of information that they find on foreign websites or their own childhood experiences. For example, Chia-Yan Lee, a family physician who refuses to attach the "ADHD" label to her son, openly described her own ADHD-like "bad deeds" during her childhood to question whether the prevailing excessive diagnosis of ADHD is a phenomenon "stemming from adults' impatience with restless children" (Hsiao 2013: 3). This distrust among parents with regard to ADHD and its diagnosis might account in part for the relatively low rate of diagnosis in the NHI database in Taiwan, at least until 2011.

During this period, the image of ADHD in Taiwanese mass media has shifted from "bad behavior" to "poor performance." At present, ADHD is portrayed as more of an academic issue rather than a disciplinary problem. This transformation is supported by the revision of the conceptualization of ADHD since the publication of the *DSM-IV* in 1994 (APA 1994). The latter version reformulated a subtype of ADHD for children with inattention but without hyperactivity or impulsivity. The Taiwanese Society of Child and Adolescent Psychiatry also holds an annual ADHD student academic contest sponsored by pharmaceutical companies that restricts entry eligibility to children receiving treatment. Although these contests and the response to mass media have contributed to destigmatizing children with ADHD and their parents to some extent, reported stories still consistently refer to ADHD as a pure neurological disorder and describe "miracles" attributed to medications.

Conclusion

This chapter traces the emergence, extension, and reconfiguration of the child psychiatric network to elucidate why and how ADHD can be identified and diagnosed more extensively and more comprehensively in Taiwan. The interwoven axes of the biomedicalization of ADHD in this country include the following: formation of the professional workforce for child psychiatry; transformation of the professional orientation from public health to the clinical setting; adoption of diagnostic categories; collaboration of related professionals and laypeople; construction and dissemination of evaluation tools for ADHD screening; emergence and use of medications; and campaigns of pharmaceutical companies and parental organizations.

The increase in the number of ADHD diagnoses is closely related to the development of child psychiatry in Taiwan. However, as a specialization with delayed development, the main goal of this profession appears to be focused on "catching-up." The routine practice appears to be directly invoking the latest knowledge and techniques from abroad. However, instead of the unreflective transplantation of psychiatric knowledge and techniques as well as the one-way imposition on auxiliary professionals, specialists in child psychiatry have persisted in considering local conditions and have constantly co-produced the "problem" and "task" with teachers and parents in relation to child behavior and learning. Accordingly, the network of expertise for governing the "problem child" continues to expand with the increase in the number of social sectors sharing the medical frame related to children's behaviors. However, physicians have always monopolized the power to diagnose and prescribe medications.

With the expansion of the child psychiatric network, the driving mechanism has gradually shifted from psychiatrists to the NHI and pharmaceutical companies in the past two decades. Since the second half of the 1990s, the NHI system has become an infrastructure that shapes nearly the entire medical practice. The seemingly impregnable position of psychiatrists in this network has begun to weaken with the formation of the NHI as a single-payment system restricting the clinical autonomy of physicians. The work of other medical professionals, including clinical psychologists and psychiatric social workers, has also been devaluated in terms of financial reimbursement for their services. As such, this payment system not only consolidates the inequality of status among different medical professionals but also reshapes the clinical practices of psychiatrists and reconfigures the treatment options for patients with ADHD. Although several child psychiatrists are still striving to provide more comprehensive care for children with ADHD under the unfavorable NHI reimbursement scheme, the reconfiguration of the network is gradually eroding the biopsychosocial model of understanding and treating children's mental disorders and is causing the disintegration of the multidisciplinary teamwork in holistic health care. Since influential pharmaceutical companies began intervening in this network in 2003, medication management for children with ADHD has gradually become a prevailing measure for controlling core symptoms. Thus far, the dominant conceptualization of children's hyperactivity and related behaviors has shifted from a maladjustment that might be caused by the interaction between innate dysfunctions and environmental factors to a disorder rooted in a biomedical condition.

This biomedicalization of ADHD is taken for granted by the majority of Taiwanese medical professionals. Given that Taiwan is a latecomer in the course of developing a modern medical infrastructure, the institutionalization of local child psychiatric and specialty training has lagged in terms of the biomedicalization of ADHD and other mental disorders that have occurred in many Western settings. The first goal of a latecomer profession is often to "catch up" by transplanting the latest developments from the pioneers, although there are still some disputes regarding how to diagnose and treat ADHD (e.g., Vallée 2011; Saul 2014) in several medically advanced countries such as the United States and France (e.g., Vallée 2011; Saul 2014). However, the lack of knowledge regarding the controversial history of ADHD appears to have resulted in the unreflective acceptance of simplistic biomedical explanations and treatments for this condition (Smith 2012). In addition, other related domains, such as special education, school counseling, and parental organizations have also been developed, if not underdeveloped, under the frame of child psychiatry, and they often align themselves with the psychiatric framing to lend scientific credibility to their claims. To some extent, their subordinate positions in this child psychiatric network prevent the emergence of alternative knowledge of ADHD.

In Taiwan, the prevailing view of ADHD is that it is a biological disorder, and in clinical practice, stimulant use is the most prevalent course of treatment. However, some parents and other professionals continue to resist biomedicalization in the child psychiatric network of ADHD. For example, doctors of traditional Chinese medicine have described a different etiology of ADHD and use herbal formulas and acupuncture for treatment (Yu, Huang, and Yen 2011). At the end of 2013, the family physician Chia-Yan Lee, as mentioned earlier, spoke out against the overdiagnosis and overmedication of hyperactive children on the basis of her personal experiences and clinical observation. Lee organized a series of campaigns intended to criticize how the medicalization of hyperactivity hinders the diversity of children's personalities and medicates powerless children solely to relieve parents' anxiety. Lee's earnest outcry has inspired many parents and educators who are ambivalent about stimulants while sending tremors throughout the child psychiatric community. However, the subsequent effects of this outcry on the dominant network and its biomedicalized approach to ADHD in Taiwan remain to be seen.

NOTES

1. Prevalence studies pertaining to adults with ADHD in Taiwan have concluded that the sample size of patients with ADHD who are 19 years of age or older among NHI enrollees before 2005 was too low to analyze significantly; the authors believed that underdiagnosis of adults might be due to lack of awareness of this disorder among the general population and even clinical practitioners (Huang et al. 2014). The first adult ADHD outpatient department in Taiwan was established in 2012, but in 2014, the cumulative number of patients remained less than 100. http://www.chimei.org.tw/main/cmh_de partment/59012/magazin/vol106/vol_106_38.html.

2. By definition, the schedule III substances have "potential for habitual use, dependence, abuse, and danger to the society" (Taiwan Food and Drug Administration 2011: 2).

3. See the discussion thread on the special education board in the PTT Bulletin Board System (in Chinese). https://www.ptt.cc/man/sp_teacher/D4E3/M.1263565974.A.A4F.html.

REFERENCES

Abbott, Andrew. 2014 (1988). *The System of Professions: An Essay on the Division of Expert Labor.* Chicago: University of Chicago Press.

American Psychiatric Association (APA). 1968. *Diagnostic and Statistical Manual of Mental Disorders (DSM-II).* 2nd ed. Washington, DC: American Psychiatric Association.

———. 1980. *Diagnostic and Statistical Manual of Mental Disorders (DSM-III).* 3rd ed. Washington, DC: American Psychiatric Association.

———. 1987. *Diagnostic and Statistical Manual of Mental Disorders (DSM-III-R).* 3rd ed., revised. Washington, DC: American Psychiatric Association.

———. 1994. *Diagnostic and Statistical Manual of Mental Disorders (DSM-IV).* 4th ed. Washington, DC: American Psychiatric Association.

———. 2013. *Diagnostic and Statistical Manual of Mental Disorders (DSM-5).* 5th ed. Washington, DC: American Psychiatric Association.

Bailey, Simon 2009. *Producing ADHD: An Ethnographic Study of Behavioural Discourses of Early Childhood.* PhD diss., University of Nottingham.

Barkley, Russell A. 2005. *Attention-Deficit Hyperactivity Disorder: A Handbook for Diagnosis and Treatment.* 3rd ed. New York: Guilford.

Chang, Heng-hao. 2007. "Social Change and the Disability Rights Movement in Taiwan: 1980–2002." *The Review of Disability Studies: An International Journal* 3 (1–2): 3–19.

Chen, Mu-Hong, Wen-Hsuan Lan, Ya-Mei Bai, Kai-Lin Huang, Tung-Ping Su, Shih-Jen Tsai, Cheng-Ta Li, Wei-Chen Lin, Wen-Han Chang, Tai-Long Pan, Tzeng-Ji Chen, and Ju-Wei Hsu. 2016. "Influence of Relative Age on Diagnosis and Treatment of Attention-Deficit Hyperactivity Disorder in Taiwanese Children." *Journal of Pediatrics* 172: 162–67.

Common Health. 2007. *A Parental Guidance for Promoting Health.* Taipei: *Common Health.* (In Chinese)

Conners, C. Keith. 1970. "Symptom Patterns in Hyperkinetic, Neurotic, and Normal Children." *Child Development* 41: 667–82.

———. 1968. "A Teacher Rating Scale for Use in Drug Studies with Children." *American Journal of Psychiatry* 126: 884–88.

Conrad, Peter. 2006. *Identifying Hyperactive Children: The Medicalization of Deviant Behavior.* Expanded ed. Burlington, VT: Ashgate.

Conrad, Peter, and Deborah Potter. 2000. "From Hyperactive Children to ADHD Adults: Observations on the Expansion of Medical Categories." *Social Problems* 47 (4): 559–82.

Conrad, Peter, and Joseph W. Schneider. 1992. *Deviance and Medicalization: From Badness to Sickness.* Expanded ed. Philadelphia: Temple University Press.

Degrandpre, Richard. 1999. *Ritalin Nation: Rapid-Fire Culture and the Transformation of Human Consciousness.* New York: W. W. Norton.

Edwards, Claire, and Etaoine Howlett. 2013. "Putting Knowledge to Trial: 'ADHD Parents' and the Evaluation of Alternative Therapeutic Regimes." *Social Science & Medicine* 81: 34–41.

Eyal, Gil. 2013. "For a Sociology of Expertise: The Social Origins of the Autism Epidemic." *American Journal of Sociology* 118 (4): 863–907.

Gau, Shur-Fen, Yen-Nan Chiu, Wen-Che Tsai, and Wei-Tsuen Soong. 2004. "Average Daily Dose of Methylphenidate for Children with Attention-Deficit Hyperactivity Disorder in a Medical Center." *Taiwanese Journal of Psychiatry* 18 (2): 136–41. (In Chinese)

Grob, Gerald N. 2014. *From Asylum to Community: Mental Health Policy in Modern America.* Princeton, NJ: Princeton University Press.

Hsiao, Alison. 2013. "ADHD Diagnoses May Be Harming Kids." *Taipei Times,* May 6.

Hsu, Chen-Chin. 1972. "Er Tong Jing Shen Yi Xue Er Shi Nian." In *Guo Li Tai Wan Da Xue Yi Xue Yuan Fu She Yi Yuan Shen Jing Jing Shen Ke Er Shi Wu Zhou Nian Ji Nian Kan,* edited by Hsien Rin, 30–50. Taipei: National Taiwan University Hospital. (In Chinese)

———. 1981. *He Chu Shi Er Jia: Yu Xue Sheng Sheng Huo You Guan De Xin Li Wei Sheng Wen Ti.* Taipei: Health World. (In Chinese)

Hsu, Chen-Chin, and Tsung-Yi Lin. 1969. "A Mental Health Program at the Elementary School Level in Taiwan: A Six-year Review of the East-Gate Project." In *Conference on Mental Health Research in Asia and the Pacific,* edited by William Caudill and Tsung-Yi Lin, 178–97. Honolulu, HI: East-West Center.

Hsu, Chiung-Chu, and Shih-Yi Chan. 2008. "A Survey Study on Aspects of Elementary School Teachers toward Students with Different Disabilities in Regular Classes." *Bulletin of Special Education and Rehabilitation* 19: 25–49. (In Chinese)

Huang, Charles Lung-Cheng, Chin-Chen Chu, Tain-Junn Cheng, and Shih-Feng Weng. 2014. "Epidemiology of Treated Attention-Deficit/Hyperactivity Disorder (ADHD) across the Lifespan in Taiwan: A Nationwide Population-Based Longitudinal Study." *PLoS ONE* 9 (4): e95014.

Huang, Huey-Ling. 2008. "Review of Attention Deficit Hyperactivity Disorder (ADHD) Research in Taiwan." *Research in Applied Psychology* 40: 197–219. (In Chinese)

Hughes, Thomas P. 1987. "The Evolution of Large Technological System." In *The Social Construction of Technological Systems: New Directions in the Sociology and History of Technology,* edited by Wiebe E. Biker, Thomas P. Hughes, and Trevor F. Pinch, 51–82. Cambridge, MA: MIT.

Jacoby, Neil H. 1966. *An Evaluation of U.S. Economic Aid to Free China, 1951–1965.* Washington, DC: Bureau for the Far East Agency for International Development.

Jones, Kathleen W. 1999. *Taming the Troublesome Child: American Families, Child Guidance, and the Limits of Psychiatric Authority.* Cambridge, MA: Harvard University Press.

Kirk, Samuel, James Gallagher, and Mary Ruth Coleman. 2014. *Educating Exceptional Children*. 14th ed. Belmont, CA: Cengage Learning.

Kleinman, Arthur. 1980. *Patients and Healers in the Context of Culture*. Berkeley: University of California Press.

Lin, Keh-Ming. 1981. "Traditional Chinese Medical Beliefs and Their Relevance for Mental Illness and Psychiatry." In *Normal and Abnormal Behavior in Chinese Culture*, edited by Arthur Kleinman and Hsung-Yi Lin, 95–114. Dordrecht: D. Reider.

Liu, Michael Shiyung. 2012. "From Japanese Colonial Medicine to American-Standard Medicine in Taiwan: A Case Study of the Transition in the Medical Profession and Practices in East Asia." In *Science, Public Health and the State in Modern Asia*, edited by Liping Bu, Darwin H. Stapleton, and Ka-che Yip, 161–76. New York: Routledge.

Liu, Yu-Chih, Shih-Kai Liu, Chi-Yung Shang, Chien-Ho Lin, Changling Tu, and Shur-Fen Gau. 2006. "Norm of the Chinese Version of the Swanson, Nolan and Pelham, Version IV Scale for ADHD." *Taiwanese Journal of Psychiatry* 20 (4): 290–304. (In Chinese)

Lloyd, Gwynedd, and Claire Norris. 1999. "Including ADHD?" *Disability & Society* 14 (4): 505–17.

Mayes, Rick, Catherine Bagwell, and Jennifer Erkulwater. 2008. "ADHD and the Rise in Stimulant Use Among Children." *Harvard Review of Psychiatry* 16 (3): 151–66.

Meng, Ying-Ru, and Chiung-Hui Hsieh. 2012. "The Study Related to Appearance Rates, Identification, Medical Care and Teaching Strategies for Students with Attention Deficit Hyperactivity Disorder in Elementary Schools." *Journal of Research in Special Education and Assistive Technology* 5: 1–36. (In Chinese)

MTA Cooperative Group. 1999. "A 14-Month Randomized Clinical Trial of Treatment Strategies for Attention-Deficit/Hyperactivity Disorder: The MTA Cooperative Group. Multimodal Treatment Study of Children with ADHD." *Archives of General Psychiatry* 56 (12): 1073–86.

Polanczyk, Guilherme, Maurício Silva de Lima, Bernardo Lessa Horta, Joseph Biederman, and Luis Augusto Rohde. 2007. "The Worldwide Prevalence of ADHD: A Systematic Review and Metaregression Analysis." *American Journal of Psychiatry* 164 (6): 942–48.

Rafalovich, Adam. 2013. "Attention Deficit-Hyperactivity Disorder as the Medicalization of Childhood: Challenges from and for Sociology." *Sociology Compass* 7 (5): 343–54.

Saul, Richard. 2014. *ADHD Does Not Exist*. New York: Harper.

Singh, Ilina. 2008. "ADHD, Culture and Education." *Early Child Development and Care* 178 (4): 347–61.

Singh, Ilina, Angela M. Filipe, Imre Bard, Meredith Bergey, and Lauren Baker. 2013. "Globalization and Cognitive Enhancement: Emerging Social and Ethical Challenges for ADHD Clinicians." *Currrent Psychiatry Reports* 15 (9): 385.

Smith, Mattew. 2012. *Hyperactive: The Controversial History of ADHD*. London: Reaktion.

Soong, Wei-Tsuen. 1997a. "Tai Da Er Tong Jing Shen Yi Xui Jin Er Shi Wu Nian De Fa Zhan." In *Wu Shi Zai Fu Chen: Tai Da Yi Yuan Jing Shen Bu Wu Shi Nian Ji Yao*, edited by Yue-Joe Lee, 155–78. Taipei: Department of Psychiatry at National Taiwan University Hospital. (In Chinese)

————. 1997b. "Tai Da Yi Yuan Er Tong Jing Shen Yi Xui Zhi Liao Mo Shi De Yan Bian." In *Wu Shi Zai Fu Chen: Tai Da Yi Yuan Jing Shen Bu Wu Shi Nian Ji Yao*, edited by Yue-Joe Lee, 179–201. Taipei: Department of Psychiatry at National Taiwan University Hospital. (In Chinese)

————. 2009. "Attention Deficit Hyperactivity Disorder (ADHD) and Autism Research in Taiwan." *Research in Applied Psychology* 41: 1–4. (In Chinese)

Swanson, James M., Glen R. Elliott, Laurence L. Greenhill, Timothy Wigal, L. Eugene Arnold, Benedetto Vitiello, Lily Hechtman, Jeffery N. Epstein, William E. Pelham, Howard B. Abikoff, Jeffrey H. Newcorn, Brooke S. G. Molina, Stephen P. Hinshaw, Karen C. Wells, Betsy Hoza, Peter S. Jensen, Robert D. Gibbons, Kwan Hur, Annamarie Stehli, Mark Davies, John S. March, C. Keith Conners, Mark Caron, and Nora D. Volkow. 2007. "Effects of Stimulant Medication on Growth Rates Across 3 Years in the MTA Follow-Up." *Journal of the American Academy of Child and Adolescent Psychiatry* 46 (8): 1015–27.

Swanson, James M., Helena C. Kraemer, Stephen P. Hinshaw, L. Eugene Arnold, C. Keith Conners, Howard B. Abikoff, Walter Clevenger, Mark Davies, Glen R. Elliott, Laurence L. Greenhill, Lily Hechtman, Betsy Hoza, Peter S. Jensen, John S. March, Jeffrey H. Newcorn, Elizabeth B. Owens, William E. Pelham, Ellen Schiller, Joanne B. Severe, Steve Simpson, Bbenedetto Vitiello, Karen Wells, Timothy Wigal, and Min Wu. 2001. "Clinical Relevance of the Primary Findings of the MTA: Success Rates Based on Severity of ADHD and ODD Symptoms at the End of Treatment." *Journal of the American Academy of Child and Adolescent Psychiatry* 40: 168–79.

Taiwan Food and Drug Administration. 2011. "Controlled Drug Act." http://www .taiwanservices.com.tw/org2/1/download_doDownload2/en_US/1106813.

Taiwanese Society of Child and Adolescent Psychiatry. 2015. "Doctors." http://www .tscap.org.tw/TW/Retail/ugC_Retail.asp.

US Department of Education. 2006. "34 CFR Parts 300 and 301. Assistance to States for the Education of Children With Disabilities and Preschool Grants for Children With Disabilities; Final Rule." http://idea.ed.gov/download/finalregulations.pdf.

Vallée, Manuel. 2010. "BioMedicalizing Mental Illness: The Case of Attention Deficit Disorder." In *Understanding Emerging Epidemics: Social and Political Approaches (Advances in Medical Sociology, Volume 11)*, edited by Ananya Mukherjea, 281–301. Bingley, UK: Emerald Group Publishing Limited.

————. 2011. "Resisting American Psychiatry: French Opposition to DSM-III, Biological Reductionism, and the Pharmaceutical Ethos." In *Sociology of Diagnosis*, vol. 12, Advances in Medical Sociology, edited by P. J. McGann and David J. Hutson, 85–110. Dallas: Emerald.

Wang, Liang-Jen, Sheng-Yu Lee, Shin-Sheng Yuan, Chun-Ju Yang, Kang-Chung Yang, Tung-Liang Lee, and Yu-Chiau Shyu. 2016. "Impact of Negative Media Publicity on Attention-Deficit/Hyperactivity Disorder Medication in Taiwan." *Pharmacoepidemiology & Drug Safety* 25: 45–53.

Werry, John S. 1968. "Developmental Hyperactivity." *Pediatric Clinics of North America* 15 (3): 581–99.

World Health Organization (WHO). 1977. *Mental Disorders: Glossary and Guide to Their Classification in Accordance with the Ninth Revision of the International Classification of Diseases.* Geneva: World Health Organization.

Wu, Harry Yi-Jui. 2012. "Jing Shen Yi Xue Zhen Duan Zhan Hou Fen Lei Ji Biao Zhun Hua De Li Shi." In *Nursing and the Society: The Transdisciplinary Dialogue & Innovation*, edited by Zxy-Yann Jane Lu, Hsien-Hsien Chiang, and Yi-Ping Lin, 249–82. Taipei: Socio. (In Chinese)

Yan, Yu-Long. 2010. "Ji Yi Shang Yin: Li Ta Neng Wei Tong Tai Du." *China Times*, January 12. (In Chinese)

Yu, Chao-Hui, Tzu-Ping Huang, and Hung-Rong Yen. 2011. "The Overview of Attention Deficit Hyperactivity Disorder in Chinese Medicine and Conventional Medicine and Its Evident Base Studies." *The Taipei Researches of Traditional Chinese Medical Journal* 14 (2): 79–93. (In Chinese)

17

Exploring the ADHD Diagnosis in Ghana

Between Disrespect and Lack of Institutionalization

Christian Bröer
Rachel Spronk
Victor Kraak

Taking ADHD to Ghana

This chapter explores the diagnosis and treatment of attention deficit–hyperactivity disorder (ADHD) in Ghana. The emergence of diagnosis and treatment in the Global South has been researched only partially. African countries remain particularly under-researched, with South Africa being the exception (Meyer and Sagvolden 2006; Snyman and Truter 2010; Seabi and Economou 2012). We know about the diverging prevalence of ADHD in different regions across the globe (Polanczyk et al. 2014). Much less is known about what ADHD means and how diagnosis and treatment are employed across different settings. We explore precisely this, from a biosocial perspective, attending to niche variation in ADHD in relation to contextual institutional differences (Singh 2012).

To our knowledge, this is the first study on the clinical use of the ADHD diagnosis and treatment in Ghana or any other sub-Saharan African country so far, apart from South Africa (e.g., Meyer and Sagvolden 2006; Snyman and Truter 2010). There are no prevalence statistics or clinical records concerning ADHD in Ghana. We therefore approached clinicians and policymakers and searched the media for references to ADHD. Since the ADHD diagnosis is only sparsely used in Ghana, we were able to survey almost the whole field. At present, there is some recognition of ADHD among children in mental health policy, limited provisions, and some calls for "upscaling" treatment. ADHD among adults and disparities among groups remain almost unknown. Researching Ghana therefore offers the opportunity to obtain an early introduction of the disease category.

We explore how the introduction of diagnosis and treatment is related to the following institutional contexts: mental health provisions, nongovernmental organizations (NGOs), educational facilities, and cultural understandings of intergenerational relations. The question of whether the introduction of the ADHD diagnosis and treatment addresses unmet needs or reflects social transformations is beyond the scope of this chapter. Even if medicalization is not at the center of the analysis, but rather the "glocalization" (Robertson 1995) of ADHD, this chapter points to some "vehicles of migration" (Conrad and Bergey 2014) of this medical diagnosis and its treatment.

Ghana has an estimated population of 25.4 million (World Bank Ghana 2014), 64% of whom live in rural communities. It is ranked as a "lower middle-income" country and has experienced a period of significant economic growth, boosted by oil and gas extraction. The gross domestic product per capita was $40.7 billion in 2012. Although many people live in poverty, a growing group in Ghana has access to modest financial resources. Not surprisingly, Ghana has a poorly developed mental health and educational sector. Even if psychiatric diagnoses seem to be on the rise, concerns about deviant behavior or— depending on one's perspective—mental health, are often couched within a spiritualistic explanatory model in Ghana (Doku et al. 2008; Read 2012; Read and Doku 2013).

Our exploration suggests that corporal punishment, traditional healing, and prayer seem to remain the first treatments for children who are brought to the attention of clinicians who diagnose and treat ADHD. This situation might change given the attempts of Ghanaian health professionals, policymakers, NGOs, pharmaceutical companies, and journalists to "raise awareness" about ADHD. And, even though the importance of school performance is an issue in Ghana almost as much as it is in the West, the difference lies in the fact that school performance more explicitly connotes family status and potential for income generation and upward social mobility, rather than academic accomplishment.

We find that "ADHD" is not a culturally established category, as it is, for example, in many countries in the West. However, there might be a niche in the making: disrespect for parents, teachers, and the elderly seems to be at stake when the ADHD diagnosis and medication are sought in Ghana.

Niches for ADHD Worldwide

Following up on Singh's (2012) comparison of the United States and the United Kingdom, this chapter asks whether ADHD in Ghana is used for child behavior in specific social situations and in combination with distinct cultural connotations. Our analysis seeks to avoid a strict nature-nurture divide (Singh 2002). This biosocial perspective situates diagnosis and treatment in institutional contexts and provides space for the ambiguities and politico-normative implications of diagnosis and medication. At the same time, the perspective is "biological" in the sense that a biological basis of ADHD is not ruled out; it is possible that one might find universal traits of ADHD, such as problems with self-control, and biology itself may be flexible and in need of translation through culture.

More specifically, we employ the concept of an "ecological niche" (Singh 2012), which "suggests that children's behavioral development must be seen as a fundamentally situated and relational process in which there is an on-going and mutual process of shaping and of transformation between child actors and their immediate and proximal social and physical spaces" (890). Such an approach will help elucidate how children's difficulty with self-control on the one hand, and the social environment on the other hand, interact to produce a distinctive phenotype as well as how children and parents understand the disease.

Singh's (2012) study describes different ecological niches that children inhabit and posits some mechanisms that may underlie the development of variations at the phenotypic level among children with the same diagnoses. For example, in the United States, a modal "performance niche" means that oftentimes children and families see ADHD as a disorder of academic performance and associate stimulant drug treatments with improvement in the classroom (Singh 2012: 895). Similarly, in the United Kingdom, a modal "conduct niche" means that "a child's difficulty with behavioral self-control finds its expression in, is shaped by, and gives shape to, a normative behavioural channel" (Singh 2012: 895). Niche variation is further illuminated in a small number of studies (Stolzer 2005; Mcintyre and Hennessy 2012; Bröer and Heerings 2013).

The current study is the first one to apply the niche model to a non-Western country. It explores when, where, and how ADHD diagnosis and treatment are employed among clinicians and NGOs, in policy, and in the media. We identify the institutional context and practices of diagnosis and treatment. Future research needs to address children to see which phenotypes might develop in Ghana.

Methods

Based in Cape Coast, Ghana, Kraak conducted the field research between November 2011 and March 2012, while Spronk was working on a different project concerning the emerging middle classes (Spronk, n.d.). The fieldwork was coordinated with Bröer through repeated online sessions.

The research design was exploratory and aimed at a broad survey of the field of ADHD diagnosis and treatment among clinicians and policymakers and in media reports in Ghana. Patients and relatives were not included in the present study, though they were referred to in the interviews. The findings from 2011–12 were checked and updated with desk research and through the ongoing contacts and fieldwork of Spronk in 2014.

At the start of the project, we had no idea about the scope of the ADHD diagnosis. We therefore started interviewing clinicians as a way to delineate the possibility of an ADHD niche. From there, we identified the specific context and practices in which a diagnosis comes about, the meanings attached to it, and the problems addressed in its application.

The contextual analysis included the institutions of mental health (including NGOs and hospitals) and partly those of education (particularly schools). Here, we assessed policy documents and interviewed policymakers and stakeholders. We gathered research literature, newspapers, and web sources, searching for explicit references to ADHD in Ghana. Most mental health treatment in Ghana is provided by inpatient and outpatient facilities in psychiatric hospitals (WHO 2007). We found that most clinicians involved in child mental health are also working in Accra, the capital of Ghana. We therefore focused on clinicians in Accra.

We approached all major mental health clinics, private clinics, and university departments to find clinicians using the ADHD diagnosis and asked for respondents to identify colleagues using the diagnosis. After several rounds, we were confident that we had spoken to almost all professionals using the ADHD diagnosis and treatment. We found hardly any professionals working on ADHD outside Accra. It is not uncommon that services are clustered in Accra, partly because people search for anonymity to avoid stigma (Dapaah 2012). One psychiatrist interviewed had worked in Kumasi, the second largest city of Ghana. He assessed children with special educational needs. We identified 10 relevant clinicians: 4 psychiatrists, 4 clinical psychologists, and 2 pediatricians, of whom we could interview 8 (see tab. 17.1). Interviews were held face to face (and one by phone) and lasted between 30 minutes and 1 hour. None of the respondents was

Table 17.1.   Overview of Clinicians in Our Study

Profession	Organization	Public or Private	Estimates of Number of Patients per Year
Psychiatrist	Accra Psychiatric Hospital	Public	60
Clinical psychologist	Korle-Bu Teaching Hospital, Department of Psychiatry	Public	12
Clinical psychologist	Korle-Bu Teaching Hospital, Department of Psychiatry	Public	4–5
Clinical psychologist	Ankaful Psychiatric Hospital	Public	Not provided
Pediatrician	Korle-Bu Teaching Hospital, Department of Child Health	Public	300–400
Psychiatrist	Smarthealth clinic and government clinic in Kumasi	Private	100
Developmental pediatrician	Child & Associates	Private	8
Psychiatrist	Peace Be Clinic	Private	8

able to provide more than an estimate of the number of cases. In addition to the clinicians, we interviewed two government officials.

We first called respondents to introduce ourselves; they received information about the study and were then finally interviewed. The interviews were held with a structured topic list, which we developed on the basis of initial conversations. The items included mental health policy, debates about ADHD and mental health, collaboration, the uptake of the diagnosis, clinical definitions, patient characteristics, and the professional background of the respondent. All interviews were recorded and transcribed verbatim with the respondents' consent.

We performed qualitative thematic content analysis (Mayring 2000; Hsieh and Shannon 2005) on the interviews and documents. Inductively, we established the local interpretation of ADHD-related concerns. Initially, interpretations were drawn up individually and then compared and discussed among team members. Deductively, we gathered information about the other items. Preliminary interpretations were repeatedly compared among members of our team.

Institutional Context

Below, we report the findings of our study, moving from the wider institutional context (education and health) to ADHD diagnosis and treatment more specifically.

EDUCATION

Ghana has more than 12,000 primary schools, more than 5,500 junior secondary schools, more than 500 senior secondary schools, more than 20 training
colleges, around 20 technical institutions, several diploma-awarding institutions,
and 5 universities. Most Ghanaians have, in theory, relatively easy access to good
education. In the past decade, Ghana's spending on education has increased
(Ghana Statistical Service 2013). School is mandatory from the age of 6 years until
at least 15 or 16 years. It comprises primary and secondary education.

According to official statistics, 85% of school-age children attended school in
2001, and by 2010, gross enrollment was reported to have reached 90% (Ministry of Education, Science, and Sports 2007). In 2011, primary school enrollment
was estimated at 107% due to the re-enrollment of over-aged children (World
Bank 2014). Primary school education in public schools is tuition-free, but the
financial contribution for books and school materials remains an obstacle to
school attendance. Social conditions in children's families are key contributing
factors to dropout, retention, and completion (Ananga 2011). Financial means
are a necessity for pursuing education in order to attain higher levels of formal
employment. There are therefore large differences in the rates of completion of
higher education among social classes.

As one of the interviewed professionals in this study stated, education is paramount in Ghana. This has been the case for a long period of time. One of the first
Ghanaian professors in psychology, Samuel Danquah, stated in 1987: "High
parental expectations are illustrated by the popular Ghanaian household saying,
'Seek first the kingdom of education and everything shall be added unto you.'"
Social capital is measured by educational achievement (Sackey 2005) and has
become an icon of social accomplishment. The pursuit of social mobility through
education can be found in lower and higher strata of society, and most Ghanaian
families invest a large part of their household budget in the education of (some
of) their children. Both girls and boys are equally represented, and school performance is slightly higher among girls (Ghana Statistical Service 2013). From
childhood on, engaging in this pursuit is an inescapable route, or expectation, of
growing up. The fear of not being able to generate an income, or of falling down
to less successful levels of society, hence of failing social expectations, is mentioned
as a driving force behind people's ambitions in one of our studies (Spronk, n.d.).
Not being successful is considered a disgrace and a personal failure of persever-
ance. Therefore, parents are very concerned about successful school results.

Mental Health in Ghana

As in most sub-Saharan countries, resources and facilities for mental health in Ghana are scarce (Asare 2010). The treatment gap is estimated to be 98% in sub-Saharan Africa and 98.8% in Ghana (WHO 2007). The Ghana Health Service estimated 6,316 inpatient cases and 26,559 outpatient cases in 2005. An estimated 2.8 million adults have a mental disorder according to World Health Organization (WHO) prevalence rates (WHO 2007). Inpatient facilities are offered by three psychiatric hospitals, some regional hospitals, and district hospitals, which are mainly based in the south of the country. Access to these institutions is free. The most common reasons for admission to a psychiatric hospital are schizophrenia, substance abuse, depression, and mania (Read 2012). The most common outpatient diagnoses are epilepsy, acute psychosis, substance abuse, and neurosis (Read 2012). Ghana has between 4 and 15 psychiatrists (WHO 2007; Asare 2010) and 4 psychologists working in the mental health field. Over the past decade, a few private institutions have been set up that offer outpatient services in Accra, often by professionals who also work in public service. We also believe that the numbers have increased since the turn of the century, with more and more students finishing their graduate education in psychology. No data are available on their numbers. Besides pressing financial limitations, the limited mental health sector has also been shaped by years of a lack of political commitment and the continuous emigration of highly skilled professionals (Connell et al. 2007).

The WHO has identified Ghana as one of the countries to receive intensified support by the Mental Health Gap Action Programme (mhGAP) to improve treatment for mental, neurological, and substance use disorders (http://www .who.int/mental_health/mhgap/en/). This is the result of the much broader initiative of the WHO Mental Health Programme, which seeks to improve access in low-income countries by scaling up mental health services and treatment, promoting human rights, stopping social exclusion, and developing mental health laws. Ghana is also participating in the Mental Health and Poverty Project (MHaPP), a Research Programme Consortium funded by the UK Department for International Development (DfID) for the benefit of developing countries. The purpose of the consortium is to provide new knowledge regarding "comprehensive multi-sectoral approaches to breaking the negative cycle of poverty and mental ill-health" (Mental Health and Poverty Project 2008; Kleintjes, Lund, and Flisher 2010; Faydi et al. 2011).

Mental health services for children are offered by some institutions such as the Accra Psychiatric Hospital and the Korle Bu Teaching Hospital, but children's facilities are not strictly separated from adult facilities. The implementation of the Mental Health Bill, passed in 2012 (Doku, Wusu-Takyi, and Awakame 2012), aims to separate children's facilities from adults', since there had previously been no national plan to support the implementation of provisions for children and adolescents. In rural parts of the country, there are several projects to set up community-based mental health services that also include children. In Accra, some privately based psychiatrists, clinical psychologists, and pediatricians offer outpatient psychiatric and psychological services for adults, families, and children—however, none specialize in ADHD. Respondents in this study report that families from all socioeconomic backgrounds patronize these facilities, and there is a clear trend among middle- and upper-class families to visit private clinics. There are no nationwide data available on the number of children who are treated for psychiatric problems.

ADHD Facilities for Children in Ghana

Considering the above, it is not surprising that there is no central body, government organization, or government policy focusing on ADHD. Nor is there any specialized center for the diagnosis and treatment of ADHD. Still, in 2010, the government included ADHD in the latest edition of the Standard Treatment Guidelines (http://ghndp.org/images/downloads/stg2010.pdf).

This document provides a description of ADHD as a disorder and its symptoms, together with treatment options for children only. Besides behavioral therapy, methylphenidate is recommended as the only pharmacological treatment option. It is also recommended that "children suspected to have ADHD should be referred to a child psychiatrist or pediatrician for full assessment and treatment" (160). This shows that there are efforts to formalize the diagnosis and treatment of ADHD by psychiatrists participating in the mental health workgroup of the Ghana Health Service.

Clinicians, Caseloads, and Treatment

The introduction of diagnosis and treatment of ADHD in Ghana was partly the result of the gradually growing number of clinicians who started diagnosing and treating children with ADHD symptoms, mainly in Accra and the rest of the coastal region. We found 10 clinicians who stated that they worked with children with ADHD symptoms. Eight of these clinicians were interviewed (see "Methods" for more details). The clinicians ranged in age from roughly 25 to 65 years and had begun their careers in the 1980s up to the present. With one exception, all of these professionals had spent at least part of their career in an educational institution in the West for graduate, doctorate, or postdoctorate education. Knowledge of ADHD was acquired during their studies either in the West or in Ghana.

All interviewed clinicians stated that they diagnosed children with ADHD at some point during their career, and more recently, in the institution where they were currently working. Clinicians typified ADHD-related behavior, for example, as "bouncing off the walls" (clinical psychologist, Ankaful Psychiatric Hospital). Respondents said they based their diagnoses on the *Diagnostic and Statistical Manual of Mental Disorders* of the American Psychiatric Association (APA) and on the *International Classification of Diseases* of the WHO. They described symptoms in interviews in the following ways:

- doesn't sit still
- fidgets a lot
- talks excessively
- gets up when they shouldn't
- restless/constantly in motion
- overactive/lots of energy
- throws things (at other children)
- destroys things/destructive
- doesn't follow instructions/not cooperative
- fights easily, quarrels, hits other children
- screams
- disruptive behavior/social disruption
- no friends/difficulty maintaining social relationships
- doesn't pay attention/inattention
- failure to progress academically
- impulsive
- distractible
- unable to complete tasks

All but one clinician established the diagnosis with unstructured observations and verbal reports. Clinicians mentioned diverse causes of ADHD: genetic factors, (neurochemical) disturbances in the brain, lower threshold for stimuli, trauma and perinatal factors, and mental retardation as both a cause and an effect. Mental retardation was said to mask ADHD. All respondents signaled extensive comorbidity. When describing children with ADHD, some clinicians pragmatically defined levels of severity of ADHD: "The children that do not severely have ADHD, they will slowly catch up (at school)" (clinical psychologist, Korle-Bu Teaching Hospital).

Quite a few clinicians implied that ADHD is underdiagnosed because schools and parents do not recognize the problematic behavior, or parents do not know where to get help. The reported number of children with ADHD whom clinicians see varies from between as few as two to up to several hundred per year. Most of the ADHD cases seem to be treated through the Accra Psychiatric Hospital and the Department of Child Health at Korle-Bu Teaching Hospital in Accra.

Following an ADHD diagnosis, psychiatrists and pediatricians offer the following pharmacological treatments: haloperidol, chlorpromazine, carbamazepine, imipramine, atomoxin, and methylphenidate. These differ from the Standard Treatment Guidelines, which only recommend methylphenidate. Scarcity of the medication is a problem; one government official stated: "I cannot assure you that once a product is listed [in the Essential Medication List] it is available in every facility. It should be, but it isn't" (policy official, Ministry of Health). One clinician has arrangements with pharmaceutical companies to import methylphenidate and sell it only under his prescription. We suspect that he, being a younger professional, is in conflict with senior colleagues who reject methylphenidate:

> I don't like it [methylphenidate]. Because it is an amphetamine, it is addictive . . .
> you should control drugs. You should be careful. (Psychiatrist, private clinic)

Medications that are provided by public services (Accra Psychiatric Hospital, Korle-Bu Teaching Hospital) are government-financed and cost little for patients. Ghana has a National Insurance Scheme that makes access to health care more available to larger groups in society. Haloperidol, chlorpromazine, carbamazepine, and imipramine are (partly) reimbursed under this scheme, but atomoxin and methylphenidate are not. The costs of atomoxin are estimated to be $200 a month, whereas methylphenidate is estimated to be $80 a month (compared to a per capita income of $1,770 per year; see World Bank GINI 2015). Although clinicians reported treatment compliance, the duration of treatment seems to depend on the costs of medication.

ADHD Advocacy

Based on the analysis of Ghanaian newspapers, television programs produced in Ghana, and news websites, there is limited public attention to ADHD. We found 14 newspaper and Internet-based articles for the period of 2008 to 2014 and 1 television item—lasting 10 minutes in a lifestyle program—in 2014. We did not find references to ADHD before 2008.

Half of the contributions introduce ADHD and are intended to "raise awareness." The others are more focused and concern the following factors: dietary advice, coping with an ADHD-diagnosed "husband" or "employee," ADHD and traffic accidents, and ADHD-related activities. ADHD is generally discussed in terms of a specific setting and limited focus, such as a failing spouse or employee. Since ADHD is mentioned so little, we cannot relate it to broader patterns, such as gender disparity. It was not possible to trace most of the authors of these articles, but one author was the globally operating mental health advocate Cory Couillard, who explicitly asked his readers to answer the question "do you have ADHD?" (http://vibeghana.com/2013/04/17/do-you-have-adhd/). NGOs and a pharmaceutical company also promote ADHD diagnosis and treatment. CareplusGhana is a UK-based patient organization that uses Janssen-Cilag's promotional video-footage (http://www.careplusghana.com/home/). Special Attention Project Ghana is an advocacy group for learning disabilities that also explicitly targets ADHD. The Ghanaian African Social Development Aid Foundation in 2010 collaborated with the Dutch National Committee for International Cooperation and Sustainable Development (NCDO) in a seminar on ADHD in Ghana (http://www.foundationasda.org/index.php?option=com_content&view =article&id=11&Itemid=13). As this site shows, the collaboration is initiated by Ghanaian expatriates in the Netherlands. A UK-based volunteer organization advertises special education projects and explicitly mentions ADHD care. These intermittent engagements show that since the turn of the century, ADHD has received more consideration, albeit sparsely.

Disease Etiology and Health-seeking Behavior in Ghana

In Ghana, an estimated 70% to 80% of people with mental health problems consult an herbalist, a traditional healer (Ae-Ngibise et al. 2010), or so-called Christian prayer camps (WHO 2007). There were an estimated 45,000 traditional healers in Ghana and a handful of practicing psychiatrists before the turn of the century (WHO 2007). The three existing psychiatric hospitals are understaffed and overcrowded, and patient living conditions are qualified as inhumane by mental health advocates (http://www.basicneeds.org/where-we-work /ghana/). Biomedical explanations of ill health stand next to or are combined with "traditional," "indigenous," or "ethno" medicine in Ghana (Twumasi 1979;

Tsey 1997). In Ghana, mental illnesses are generally believed to be the result of social pressure, life events and spiritual forces, curses, and charms (Lamensdorff, Ofori-Atta, and Linden 1995; Ofori-Atta, Read, and Lund 2010). Ae-Ngibise et al. (2010) describe how "juju, supernatural powers and evil spirits" are central in local etiology in their explanation of mental suffering (561).

Mental illnesses are feared in most communities in Ghana, and people suffering from mental illness are severely stigmatized (Kleintjes, Lund, and Flisher 2010). People have reported direct experiences of stigmatization, as well as the fear of stigma (Scambler 2009). Moreover, courtesy stigma (Goffman 2009), the extension of stigma to those close to the stigmatized person, is also a real threat (Quinn 2007; Sonuga-Barke et al. 2010). The stigmatization of mental illness can have a significant influence on one's willingness to disclose and seek help; on the quality of health care received; and on access to family, community, school, or work support for recovery. In a qualitative study involving persons who care for people with mental health problems, about half of the caregivers interviewed in Accra and Kumasi believed that mental illness could be explained by secular causes. In contrast, in the northern region, most caregivers explained mental illness in terms of spiritual or supernatural factors (Quinn 2007). Previously, Lamensdorff, Ofori-Atta, and Linden (1995) found that among schoolteachers, higher incomes and living in urban areas correlated with the view that mental health was caused by "internal" problems.

In our study, clinicians reported that parents often seek the help of traditional healers, herbalists, and faith healers before, during, or after ADHD treatment. Furthermore, corporal punishment is a common form of "treatment" at home and in school. Clinicians told us stories about children with ADHD in which spiritualistic beliefs were described:

> I even got someone from the UK. It was a girl, the father sent her away [back to Ghana], because the mother thought she was a witch and wanted to kill her. Now she is in university. Amazing, isn't it? (Pediatrician, Korle-Bu training hospital)

As far as we can infer from clinicians' reports and the sparse literature on mental health in Ghana, we have found that parents of unruly children might be pushed to see a clinician because the behavior of children can discredit the whole family. At the same time, seeking psychiatric help may also be associated with the fear of stigma. Therefore, clinicians repeatedly see parents who are seeking clinicians' advice outside their own community (this was also reported for other help-seeking behavior, such as seeking treatment for HIV/AIDS; see Dapaah 2012). Parents often complained of unruly children, which is indicative of the emergence of a particular niche.

INTERGENERATIONAL RELATIONS

Intergenerational relations in Ghana are based on explicit and pervasive notions of reciprocity (Twum-Danso 2009: 426). Whereas children depend on their parents to provide care for them as they grow up, parents are dependent on children later in life. Parents spare no efforts to support and educate their children—especially during adolescence—in order to raise their status and increase their ability to improve the welfare and resource base of the family. In return, parents expect their children to serve them: "The reciprocities between parents and their children are life-long ones and are backed not by legal requirements necessarily, but by moral and religious obligation. Society does not spare those parents and children who fail in their reciprocal obligations. The recalcitrant child or parent may be ridiculed or gossiped about by concerned others" (Awedoba cited in Twum-Danso 2009: 427). It is crucial for children to practice respect, to show their parents that they are grateful, as well as to assume responsibilities such as household chores, succeed in school, and secure an income. Paying respect and behaving respectfully are culturally treasured values in the gerontocratic culture in Ghana (Van der Geest 2004). Twum-Danso (2009: 420) outlines how "in Ghanaian culture children are trained from a very early age that they must respect and obey all elders, be humble towards adults, and take their advice."

Disrespect is a violation of social values, and disrespectful children are seen as failures on the part of their parents, which might lead to the stigmatization of the entire family. Not only are disrespectful children punished, they also risk incurring a curse. According to a child in Twum-Danso's study, "if you respect you will get a long life [because you are accepted], if you do not respect you will get a short life because someone will curse you" (Twum-Danso 2009: 420). Respect and obedience are considered duties of children, and failing to conform to these social values discredits children and may bring shame on their parents.

Clinical Practice

From our study, we can conclude that most children are referred to clinicians by their parents, often on the basis of school staff's advice. According to the clinicians with whom we spoke, parents' and teachers' primary concerns are class-room interactions and performance at school. ADHD seems to figure primarily in relations between "educators" and children, but reports of parents also include unruly behavior in public and at home. Although this seems similar to ADHD, as reported in schools in Western countries, a closer examination reveals differences. In the first quote, disruptive behavior in itself is deemed problematic, and school performance is considered secondary. A clinician outlines the reasons for referral:

> The reason why they come is, one, teachers advise parents to take them because of their disruptive behavior and, two, pre-school performance is declining. (Psychiatrist, public clinic)

Below, we will demonstrate that disruptive behavior at school is problematic because it signals disrespect toward elders; threatens family aspirations, status, and earning capacity; and reflects badly on parents as good educators and nurturers.

PAY ATTENTION TO YOUR TEACHER

The words "disruptive" and "social disruption" are used by informants repeatedly in relation to many aspects of classroom behavior that are associated with ADHD. As one clinician described a child:

> He was distractible and disruptive in the classroom . . . He was throwing things at children, he would engage in contact with children when he was not supposed to, and he was not paying attention to what the teacher was ordering him to do. (Developmental psychiatrist, private clinic)

Other clinicians stated:

> He had disruptive behavior, he could not sit down in the classroom, he was talking to others, he constantly had to be punished. (Pediatrician, public clinic)

> They are very restless, fidgeting, destructive and disrupting, paying little attention, they are not able to sit down, and the performance at school is poor. (Psychiatrist, public clinic)

Being disruptive means that the behavior is disturbing others, usually the child's classmates, and implies noncompliance with the teacher's orders and not paying attention to the teacher. Academic decline is mentioned, but not as a core concern.

"Performance" is a problem in addition to or as a consequence of "disruption." In two of the three citations, performance is not even mentioned. Instead, respondents expand on disruptive behavior.

Children suspected of having ADHD are repeatedly called "stubborn," which can be interpreted as not obeying the teacher's rules or instructions. In the statements below, ADHD is again related to not paying attention to the teacher because of stubbornness.

> He would not hear instantly when the teacher was talking to him, or he would pay some attention at what the teacher was ordering him to do, but after a short time he would be not doing it again. Stubborn. (Psychiatrist, Accra Psychiatric Hospital)

> Causing a lot of trouble and being stubborn. [Stubborn] means when children are "not hearing," they don't do this or that. They are not obeying instructions even after they have been repeatedly told things in the face of punishment. (Psychiatrist, private clinic)

In the descriptions of ADHD-related problems, the respondents emphasize the importance of obeying instructions and responding to punishment. Attention deficit is primarily a problem of not paying attention to elders, when children are "not hearing."

Children are labeled "disruptive" or "troublesome" when they violate norms about how to respect not only the teacher but also the older generations, as a pediatrician tells us when describing typical ADHD behavior:

> They can't sit down, they are all over the place, they talk excessively and interrupt others, that is what worries the relatives. Interrupting is rude here in Ghana, especially when it comes to the elderly. Children are typically not allowed to talk in front of elderly people. It is changing, but it is still here. Children here are not allowed to express their thoughts. Parents want their children then to be in check. So when a child cannot be controlled, it is like sticking up a sore thumb. They would be spanking the child, calling it troublesome. (Pediatrician, public clinic)

Here, ADHD-like behavior explicitly violates the belief that children have to keep quiet and "stand at attention" when in the presence of grownups. Moreover, disrespect might threaten the moral status of family members. ADHD-like behavior is associated with "badness" and can be disgraceful to parents. Being "bad" thus implies disrespect:

> [Parents] think that they have a bad boy, meaning that they will be abused, targeted and bullied, beaten by other children or their parents. These are the children who are called stubborn, obstinate. (Psychiatrist, public clinic)

Respect for the older generation is central to the gerontocratic culture of Ghanaian society. Elders should be greatly respected for their age and associated wisdom, and younger people are expected to listen and follow up on elders' advice. Not adhering to elders thus undermines generational reciprocity, which rests on the notion that respect expresses the generational contract.

DISRESPECT AND PUNISHMENT

When a child is considered stubborn or troublesome, what often follows is corporal punishment, at school and at home. Informants stated this when asked how teachers react to these behaviors:

> They cane them. Or they incarcerate them. Or they give them activities to do so they don't have to keep still. (Psychiatrist, private clinic)

Corporal punishment, or caning, is lawful in schools. It has a long history and is contested at the same time. On the one hand, certain severe forms of punishment are seen as outdated and unjust, while on the other hand, "a good beating with a well selected stick or belt still awaits the disobedient child" (Twum-Danso 2009: 421). In reaction to reports on abuse and injuring children through corporal punishment in the 1970s, the Ghana Education Service (GES) decided that caning should consist of a maximum of six strokes and be administered by a head teacher or person authorized by the head teacher. More recently, this partial ban has come under attack. For example, in 2007, Central Regional Minister Isaac Edumadze and the chairman of the School Management Committee in Antwiagyeikrom, Kwashie Boakye, reiterated that the partial banning of corporal punishment has contributed to a lack of discipline in schools and advocated for its full reintroduction (*Ghanaian Chronicle*, April 3, 2004). Similarly, in 2007, the chiefs and queen mothers of Mfantseman District called for the reintroduction of corporal punishment in schools (*Accra Daily Mail* 2007).[1] They viewed the ban on teachers' use of the cane in schools as responsible for a breakdown of discipline and identified public video shows, child labor, listening to music late at night, and broken homes as factors that inhibited good academic performance. In 2011, an opinion poll found that 94% of parents, 92% of students, and 64% of teachers favored the use of corporal punishment (Ghana News Agency 2011).

The debate about punishment bears upon ADHD and help-seeking behavior significantly. As one pediatrician stated:

> Discipline varies across schools or people . . . Quite a number of the new generation never have been caned. So we have two groups with different arguments: The ones that use harsh discipline for what they see as the disruptive behavior. They think they should beat children, that they should be disciplined for that [bad] behavior. But when they go through a barrier, when they see that even beating is not working, then they see there is something wrong and come for help. (Pediatrician, public clinic)

The emphasis on obedience and discipline legitimizes harsh punishment and (re) affirms the authoritative position of adults. At the same time, this practice seems to preclude psychiatric explanations and treatment.

School Failure

Although respect seems to be a major concern, clinicians also relate "academic decline" or "falling grades" to ADHD.

> We have stubborn children whose academic performance is declining, who would be described as brilliant but not doing well at school. And they would not sit still, be talking in class, making a mess, getting into quarrels, fights, losing books. (Psychiatrist, private clinic)

School performance is an issue of respect for teachers and parents, as we have seen. Failure easily leads to dropping out of or expulsion from school. As far as clinicians report on the issue, there might be two dimensions to school dropouts. First, they are the result of a general social failure, testifying to a child's intemperateness and possibly contributing to the marginalization of the child and even the family. Second, dropping out of school might be more closely tied to academic performance and upward social mobility or at least income generation. This is expressed, for example, in the following statement from a clinician:

> When children fail to perform, parents cannot cope with that. "It cannot be that my child cannot perform." They think that if their child is given this label,

that then they are potentially useless. They don't want to hear that. They don't know then what will come of them. (Pediatrician, private clinic)

The clinician refers to how parents may translate lack of performance into being "useless." Being "useless" is considered to be the inability to contribute financially to income and socially to status. It undermines the intergenerational contract. Among the upcoming middle class, the desire for mobility might even be more pronounced. Some clinicians suggested that low-income groups do not care about dropping out of school:

The low-income structures, they don't care. The children are expelled from school, they drop out of school and then they stay at home and that is it. With the middle and upper class, education is paramount. (Psychiatrist, private clinic)

From the perspective of the clinicians, disruptive and stubborn behavior might lead to a child dropping out of school when disciplining and caning fail. But the relationship between punishment and dropping out is more intricate; on the one hand, dropping out can be a reaction to punishment itself (e.g., Dunne and Ananga 2013); on the other hand, dropping out and failure are more than academic underperformance. They are also related to lack of obedience, lack of humility, and inability to endure discipline itself.

Respondents in our study indicate that some parents adopt strong negative attitudes to their unruly or mentally ill children, up to the point that children are abandoned in front of hospitals or psychiatric wards. According to some respondents in our study, a child who is not performing and being useless is a source of severe stigma for parents. In any case, the threat of a child dropping out is a major motivation for parents to seek help, first from traditional healers or priests and second from clinicians.

A Respect Niche

In this chapter, we analyzed ADHD in Ghana from an ecological perspective, which assesses the proximal and distant social context relevant to the phenotypical development of problematic behavior. Extending the line of research of Singh (2012), we identified relevant niches for ADHD within and across several countries in the Global West and South.

In Ghana, a handful of clinicians, mostly trained abroad, use the *DSM*-based ADHD diagnosis and treat this condition with haloperidol, chlorpromazine, carbamazepine, imipramine, atomoxin, or methylphenidate, depending on availability. More recently, advocacy groups—closely related to those in Western countries—and one pharmaceutical company have tried to raise "awareness." However, except for the inclusion of ADHD in governmental guidelines in 2010, there is hardly any standardized diagnosis or treatment. This lack of institutionalization coupled with scarce resources means that ADHD has yet to become a common diagnostic category. Still, clinicians do use the diagnosis for children who are referred to them by parents and teachers. Psychiatrists, clinical psychologists, and pediatricians are usually a last resort, after healers and priests have been consulted in vain.

From an ecological perspective, the lack of institutionalization means that other culturally available frames and mental health definitions and solutions come first. This shapes the understanding and identification of ADHD. Our exploratory research among clinicians suggests that in Ghana, ADHD is a problem of respect due to elders. Informed by cultural values where reciprocity and respect are key notions, unruly behavior at school is primarily an issue of disobeying teachers and not responding to disciplinary punishment.

This chapter points to a respect niche where "stubborn" children are diagnosed and treated with ADHD medication. Stubbornness and disobedience are generally described in Ghana as not listening and paying attention, speaking loudly in the presence of elders, being boisterous, and, in particular, not being humble. Stubbornness and disobedience are considered unacceptable behaviors because they are believed to result from a lack of respect.

Similar to observations in the West, schools are fertile grounds for medical diagnoses, and children's academic performance is a widely shared concern. But performance is itself a sign of respect and obedience. Underperformance, moreover, threatens family status and social aspirations. School failure and dropping out are not only tied to academic performance but also to the ability to abide by disciplinary measures. Problems of "attention" in relation to respect do not refer to tasks and learning (as studies in the United Kingdom and United States suggest), but to obedience and standing still at attention.

We find that the training of clinicians (often abroad), the import of pharmaceuticals, and the work of NGOs serve as vehicles for the migration of ADHD diagnosis and treatment to Ghana. Because of the lack of institutionalization and the stigma attached to a mental health diagnosis, it is unclear whether, in the long run, ADHD will serve as a way of dealing with problems of respect-related inattention and overactivity in Ghana. Nonetheless, these findings suggest that the global spread of ADHD to Ghana is not—as of yet—marked by hegemonic medicalization. In a trial-and-error way, clinicians and patients seem to piece together a local variant of ADHD around the central norm of respect.

NOTES

This chapter has been greatly improved thanks to the comments of the editor. An earlier version of this text greatly benefited from discussions with Ilina Singh. Christian Bröer has taken the initiative for this research and supervised the fieldwork carried out by Victor Kraak. Bröer took the lead in data analysis and writing, and at a later stage, Rachel Spronk has contributed to both. Language editing was provided by Gail Zuckerwise. The fieldwork on which this exploration is based has partly been made possible by a grant from the Dutch Council of Scientific Research and a grant from the program group Political Sociology of the University of Amsterdam.

1. The title of queen mother can relate to the rank of a paramount queen, a queen, or a sub-queen among certain ethnic groups. This woman is not necessarily the respective chief's mother. Her role in the system is to keep an eye on the social conditions.

REFERENCES

Accra Daily Mail. 2007. "Cane Them into Line," October 5. http://www.corpun.com /ghs00710.htm.

Ae-Ngibise, K., S. Cooper, E. Adiibokah, B. Akpalu, C. Lund, V. Doku, et al. 2010. "'Whether you like it or not people with mental problems are going to go to them': A Qualitative Exploration into the Widespread Use of Traditional and Faith Healers in the Provision of Mental Health Care in Ghana." *International Review of Psychiatry* 22 (6): 558–67.

Ananga, E. D. 2011. "Typology of School Dropout: The Dimensions and Dynamics of Dropout in Ghana." *International Journal of Educational Development* 31 (4): 374–81.

Asare, J. 2010. "Mental Health Profile of Ghana." *International Journal of Psychology* 7: 67–68.

Boakye, K. 2001. "Reintroducing Caning in Our Schools?" *Ghanaian Chronicle*, April 3, 1.

Bröer, C., and M. Heerings. 2013. "Neurobiology in Public and Private Discourse: The Case of Adults with ADHD." *Sociology of Health & Illness* 35 (1): 49–65.

Connell, J., P. Zurn, B. Stilwell, M. Awases, and J. Braichet. 2007. "Sub-saharan Africa: Beyond the Health Worker Migration Crisis?" *Social Science & Medicine* 64 (9): 1876–91.

Conrad, Peter, and Meredith R. Bergey. 2014. "The Impending Globalization of ADHD: Notes on the Expansion and Growth of a Medicalized Disorder." *Social Science & Medicine* 122: 31–43.

Dapaah, J. M. 2012. *HIV/AIDS Treatment in Two Ghanaian Hospitals: Experiences of Patients, Nurses and Doctors*. Leiden: African Studies Centre.

Doku, V., B. Akpalu, U. Read, A. Osei, K. Ae-Ngebise, D. Awenva, et al. 2008. "A Situational Analysis of Mental Health Policy Development and Implementation in Ghana." *Accra: Mental Health and Poverty Project.*

Doku, V., A. Wusu-Takyi, and J. Awakame. 2012. "Implementing the Mental Health Act in Ghana: Any Challenges Ahead?" *Ghana Medical Journal* 46 (4): 241.

Faydi, E., M. Funk, S. Kleintjes, A. Ofori-Atta, J. Ssbunnya, J. Mwanza, et al. 2011. "An Assessment of Mental Health Policy in Ghana, South Africa, Uganda and Zambia." *Health Research Policy and Systems/BioMed Central* 9. doi:10.1186/1478-4505-9-17.

Ghana Statistical Service. 2013. Population & Housing Census 2010, National Analytical report, Accra, Ghana.

Ghana News Agency. 2011. "94 Per Cent of Ghanaian Parents Endorse Corporal Punishment." August 18.

Goffman, E. 2009. *Stigma: Notes on the Management of Spoiled Identity.* New York: Simon & Schuster.

Hsieh, H. F., and S. E. Shannon. 2005. "Three Approaches to Qualitative Content Analysis." *Qualitative Health Research* 15 (9): 1277–88.

Kleintjes, S., C. Lund, and A. Flisher. 2010. "A Situational Analysis of Child and Adolescent Mental Health Services in Ghana, Uganda, South Africa and Zambia." *African Journal of Psychiatry* 13 (2).

Lamensdorff, A. M., A. Ofori-Atta, and W. Linden. 1995. "The Effect of Social Change on Causal Beliefs of Mental Disorders and Treatment Preferences in Ghana." *Social Science & Medicine* 40 (9): 1231–42.

Mayring, P. 2000. "Qualitative Content Analysis." *Forum: Qualitative Social Research* 1 (2).

Mcintyre, R., and E. Hennessy. 2010. "'He's just enthusiastic. Is that such a bad thing?' Experiences of Parents of Children with Attention Deficit Hyperactivity Disorder." *Emotional & Behavioural Difficulties* 17 (1): 65–82.

Mental Health and Poverty Project. 2008. *Breaking the Vicious Cycle of Mental Ill-Health and Poverty.* Policy Brief 11, University of Cape Town.

Meyer, A., and T. Sagvolden. 2006. "Fine Motor Skills in South African Children with Symptoms of ADHD: Influence of Subtype, Gender, Age, and Hand Dominance." *Behavioral and Brain Functions* 2: 33.

Ministry of Education, Science, and Sports. 2007. *Preliminary Education Sector Performance Report.* Accra: Ministry of Education.

Ofori-Atta, A., U. Read, and C. Lund. 2010. "A Situation Analysis of Mental Health Services and Legislation in Ghana: Challenges for Transformation." *African Journal of Psychiatry* 13 (2).

Polanczyk, G. V., E. G. Willcutt, G. A. Salum, C. Kieling, and L. A. Rohde. 2014. "ADHD Prevalence Estimates across Three Decades: An Updated Systematic Review and Meta-regression Analysis." *International Journal of Epidemiology* 43 (2): 434–42.

Quinn, N. 2007. "Beliefs and Community Responses to Mental Illness in Ghana: The Experiences of Family Carers." *International Journal of Social Psychiatry* 53 (2): 175–88.

Read, U. 2012. "'I want the one that will heal me completely so it won't come back again': The Limits of Antipsychotic Medication in Rural Ghana." *Transcultural Psychiatry* 49 (3–4): 438–60.

Read, U. M., and V. Doku. 2013. "Mental Health Research in Ghana: A Literature Review." *Ghana Medical Journal* 46 (2): 29–38.

Robertson, R. 1995. "Glocalization: Time-Space and Homogeneity-Heterogeneity." *Global Modernities*, 25–44.

Sackey, H. A. 2005. "Poverty in Ghana from an Assets-Based Perspective: An Application of Probit Technique." *African Development Review* 17 (1): 41–69.

Scambler, G. 2009. "Health-Related Stigma." *Sociology of Health & Illness* 31 (3): 441–55.

Seabi, J., and N. Economou. 2012. "Understanding the Distracted and the Disinhibited: Experiences of Adolescents Diagnosed with ADHD within the South African Context." *Contemporary Trends in ADHD Research*: 165–82.

Singh, Ilina. 2002. "Biology in Context: Social and Cultural Perspectives on ADHD." *Children and Society* 16 (5): 360–67.

———. 2012. "A Disorder of Anger and Aggression: Children's Perspectives on Attention Deficit/Hyperactivity Disorder in the UK." *Social Science & Medicine* 73 (6): 889–96.

Snyman, S., and I. Truter. 2010. "Complementary and Alternative Medicine for Attention Deficit/Hyperactivity Disorder: An Eastern Cape Study." Scientific Letter. *South African Family Practice* 52 (2): 161–62.

Sonuga-Barke, E. J., J. R. Wiersema, Jacob J. van der Meere, and H. Roeyers. 2010. "Context-Dependent Dynamic Processes in Attention Deficit/Hyperactivity Disorder: Differentiating Common and Unique Effects of State Regulation Deficits and Delay Aversion." *Neuropsychology Review* 20 (1): 86–102.

Spronk, R. n.d. "LIONS of Ghana: Aspiration and Praxis in the Formation of the Middle Classes." Unpublished manuscript.

Stolzer, J. 2005. "ADHD in America: A Bioecological Analysis." *Ethical Human Psychology and Psychiatry* 7 (1): 65–75.

Tsey, K. 1997. "Traditional Medicine in Contemporary Ghana: A Public Policy Analysis." *Social Science & Medicine* 45 (7): 1065–74.

Twumasi, P. A. 1979. "A Social History of the Ghanaian Pluralistic Medical System." *Social Science & Medicine Part B: Medical Anthropology* 13 (4): 349–56.

Twum-Danso, Afua. 2009. "Reciprocity, Respect and Responsibility: The 3Rs Underlying Parent-Child Relationships in Ghana and the Implications for Children's Rights." *International Journal of Children's Rights* 17 (3): 415–32.

Van der Geest, S. 2004. "Grandparents and Grandchildren in Kwahu, Ghana: The Performance of Respect." *Africa* 74 (1): 47–61.

World Health Organization (WHO). 2007. *Ghana, a Very Progressive Mental Health Law.* Geneva: World Health Organization, Department of Mental Health and Substance Abuse.

World Bank Ghana. 2014. http://data.worldbank.org/country/ghana.

World Bank GINI. 2015. http://data.worldbank.org/indicator/NY.GNP.PCAP.CD/countries /GH-XN?display=graph%20as.

18

Reflections on ADHD in a Global Context

Peter Conrad
Ilina Singh

This chapter is a reflection on some of the findings presented and issues raised in the depictions of ADHD in the 16 countries presented in this book. As noted in the introduction, this volume is not meant to be a comprehensive depiction or comparative study per se, but rather a series of chapters presenting the state of ADHD in a global context. The goal of this final chapter is to highlight some patterns and idiosyncratic situations in the chapters, but we stop short of drawing conclusions. In working on this book, we have been struck powerfully by the paucity of a research-based understanding of the social dimensions, contributors, and drivers of ADHD in a global context. Our present phase of knowledge production requires more questions and more investigations, ahead of conclusions. Indeed, we hope that the many unresolved problematics arising across the chapters in this volume will inspire further international social science studies of ADHD.

Critics and advocates alike recognize that in the past three decades there has been a widespread medicalization of children's behavior, learning, and attention problems. By medicalization, we mean the process by which nonmedical problems become defined and treated as medical problems that often require medical treatment (Conrad 1992, 2007). Medicalization describes a sociological process (like industrialization and secularization). This process is not necessarily a problem, although critics have often used the term that way. ADHD is a classic case of medicalization (Conrad 1975) that has its roots in the United States, although the diagnosis and treatment of ADHD are becoming increasingly common in Europe, South America, and Asia. The chapter on the United States gives a brief history of the medicalization of ADHD and the growing prevalence of the condition among both children and adults in that country. Some might argue with the specific chronology, but, like many psychiatric disorders, the diagnosis we know as "ADHD" developed iteratively, in response to a changing constellation of behaviors, alongside shifting etiological models, and in direct partnership with psychopharmaceutical treatments (Singh 2002). More recently, researchers have suggested that the spread of the ADHD diagnosis reflects the globalization (Conrad and Bergey 2014; Hinshaw and Scheffler 2014) of a medicalized category. The 16 chapters in this volume provide evidence of the continued medicalization of certain behaviors of children (and increasingly of adults) in a range of countries. This suggests that globalization may be an important lens for understanding the spread and migration of the diagnosis.

Many signs point to a globalization of ADHD, if we understand "globalization" as an increase in global awareness of ADHD among parents and practitioners, a probable increase in the diagnosis of ADHD globally, and increasing global consumption of the most well-known ADHD drug treatment (methylphenidate and amphetamine-based medications). Even just a decade ago, ADHD was thought to be an "American disorder"; today, a widely cited estimate suggests that 5% of children in the world meet the criteria for ADHD diagnosis (Polanczyk et al. 2007). More recently, after examining 179 prevalence studies, Rae Thomas and her colleagues (2015) have estimated that the pooled global prevalence of ADHD is 7.2%.

The assumption underlying such prevalence figures is that ADHD is a global category. Indeed, one response to the global prevalence estimate has been to argue that it demonstrates definitively that ADHD is not a cultural phenomenon (Moffitt and Melchior 2007). However, as several scholars have pointed out, the fact that a global prevalence estimate can be generated statistically does not make this assumption true (Parens and Johnston 2011; Singh et al. 2013). By definition, such epidemiological estimates leave out as much as they include, in the sense that comparative statistics can only be generated from studies that meet a priori criteria, including, most important, consistency in the diagnostic methods used to estimate prevalence. As the epidemiologists themselves note in these papers, this methodological constraint means that many papers must be omitted from the meta-analysis. Polanczyk et al. (2007) have proposed that the solution to this problem is greater global standardization of diagnostic methods. But this proposal side-steps the fraught questions that exist around the validity of the ADHD diagnosis, or, following Ian Hacking (1999), its status as a "natural kind." Hacking's "natural kind" concept refers to a group of things that share a set of properties or capacities with a common structure and ontology. We think this book demonstrates that ADHD is most appropriately conceived as another kind of sociological object—a biosocial assemblage (Deleuze and Guattari 1988), composed of fluid, heterogeneous elements that have a relation to each other but do not have a fixed ontology. Envisioning ADHD as an assemblage acknowledges the contribution of a range of social, natural, and technological factors to the cluster of symptoms, signs, and markers associated with ADHD. It is the job of social science to identify these factors and to describe their relations across particular contexts, thereby continually reshaping and enlarging our understanding of what ADHD is.

Another question raised by the emerging globalization of ADHD is whether the global prevalence estimates of ADHD represent an increase in the number of children who meet criteria for the ADHD diagnosis around the world. In other words, is there a sudden "epidemic" of ADHD in children globally, or is something else going on? In the United States, the prevalence of ADHD is considered to be between 11% and 15%, depending on whose numbers one believes (Schwarz 2016). A recent meta-analysis (Polanczyk et al. 2014) concludes that the actual number of children (globally) who could potentially meet the standard criteria of the fourth edition of the *Diagnostic and Statistical Manual of Mental Disorders* (*DSM-IV*) is not increasing. What is changing, according to this analysis, is the number of practitioners who are adopting *DSM-IV* (and now the similar *DSM-5*) criteria for ADHD, which establishes a lower threshold for diagnosis than other guidelines (see the discussion on the *International Classification of Diseases* [*ICD*] below). Therefore, what looks like rapid escalation in ADHD cases around the world may be driven by external factors such as a change in the diagnostic threshold. Some observers argue that this increase in ADHD diagnosis around the world is not a bad thing—that it reflects better identification and treatment of children's needs. More research is needed to understand whether lowering the diagnostic threshold also results in more misdiagnosis of ADHD or in problematic medicalization of children's behavior (Schwarz 2016).

Another measure of the globalization of ADHD is the consumption of ADHD drugs, specifically methylphenidate, which is tracked globally by the UN International Narcotics Control Board (INCB). INCB data clearly indicate that the use of methylphenidate is no longer just an American phenomenon; in the past decade, the proportion of US consumption has fallen from 85% of the world's stock to 66% (http://www.incb.org/pdf/annual-report/2007/en/annual-report-2007.pdf). Analysis of Organisation for Economic Co-operation and Development (OECD) data and INCB data on consumption of ADHD drugs over the past decade has shown that increases in Northern European countries have far outpaced increases in historically high-consuming countries such as the United States and Canada (Scheffler et al. 2007). In fact, at least one review suggests that consumption of methylphenidate in the United States has stabilized over the past decade (Zuvekas and Vitiello 2012). This stabilization may be in part due to the introduction and promotion of longer-lasting medications such as Adderall.

Notwithstanding the increasing global consumption of methylphenidate, the chapters in this book indicate that there are national differences in how ADHD is treated post-diagnosis. Some countries (e.g., the United States, Canada, Australia, Germany, and Chile) adopt what can be called a "medications first" response, whereas others (e.g., France, the United Kingdom, Brazil, and Japan) use a "psychosocial first" approach, with medications used less frequently or reserved for severe cases. In the United States, approximately 9% of children may be medicated, whereas in France, for example, fewer than 0.5% may receive stimulant medications (Wedge 2012). In France, ADHD is considered to be a medical condition with predominantly psychological and social roots; the treatment of choice is some kind of psychotherapeutic or family intervention. Relatively few children receive medications as part of a medical intervention. In another example, in Portugal, ADHD is treated largely in the context of what might be called a "psycho-pedagogic" alternative, emphasizing psychosocial intervention as a primary response.

As all the chapters in this book demonstrate, and most clearly in the chapter on New Zealand, the choice of treatments for ADHD, and indeed, the ADHD diagnosis itself, are mediated by national health care systems. The nature of health care coverage for ADHD diagnosis and treatment within a country has significant effects on access to services and treatments. Some health care systems, such as that in the United Kingdom, take an evidence-based, cost-effectiveness approach to diagnostic practice and treatment. This approach tends to limit the types of practitioners who can conduct an evaluation of ADHD and the number and types of treatments that can be offered to a diagnosed patient. In Germany, for instance, stimulants may be prescribed only by specialists. The stark differences between the number of ADHD drugs available to patients in the United States (more than a dozen) and the number available to patients who receive care in the British National Health Service (four) is indicative of the ways in which national health care systems can drive or inhibit the use of ADHD drug treatments.

Of course, it is not necessarily the case that if more kinds of ADHD drugs are available to patients, more patients will therefore seek a diagnosis and medication. However, it is likely that with more competition for the ADHD market, pharmaceutical companies will try harder to convince practitioners to prescribe their drugs. Pharmaceutical detailing (targeted engagements with physicians) has been shown to influence physician-prescribing practices (Soumerai and Avorn 1990).

The types of nonmedical services provided to families of children with ADHD also vary across countries. In the United States, Australia, and Canada, for example, children diagnosed with ADHD can in certain circumstances apply for educational accommodations under national disability policies. France is in the process of reframing ADHD as a cognitive disability, and in Portugal ADHD may fall into a learning-disability category for special education and treatment purposes. Cuts in public spending and austerity measures in some European countries have had a negative impact on the availability of nonmedical services for ADHD children, leading to agitation by advocacy groups and physicians. National policies on provision of educational services for children with ADHD may be helpful to schools as well as to families and children. The chapter in this volume on Chile, for example, clearly lays out the resource benefits to schools associated with the ADHD diagnosis. Although some critics have suggested that children who receive ADHD medications benefit teachers (in the form of a more manageable classroom), this chapter illustrates that national policies on ADHD can have positive resource implications at the school level as well as at the classroom level.

The availability of services for children with ADHD under a national disability policy may have the effect of driving up diagnosis-seeking among families hoping to obtain more support for a difficult child or for a child who is struggling in school (Mayes, Bagwell, and Erkulwater 2009). Such an effect will depend on cultural views of disability and mental disorders. In countries such as Japan, Taiwan, and Ghana, the inclusion of ADHD under a disability umbrella would, at this point in time, more likely have the effect of decreasing help-seeking, given the stigma associated with disability and mental disorders.

Notwithstanding these cultural factors, we might still predict that in countries with generous resource provision to children with ADHD in schools, there might be some implicit or explicit encouragement to have children diagnosed. We might further predict that such a dynamic would be more likely in highly competitive schools, where children's achievement is a reputational concern. We do see some indication of this dynamic in parts of the United States, where, in highly affluent areas with competitive schools, prescription of ADHD drugs increases at certain times of the academic year when children are likely to be taking exams (King, Jennings, and Fletcher 2014). But among the lessons of this book is the following: we should not indulge in generalizations about the dynamics behind ADHD diagnosis and treatments across global contexts. For example, we do not see the affluent suburban dynamics of the United States in the Japanese context, which is known for its highly competitive schooling in the middle and upper classes. Rather, there is a low prevalence of ADHD diagnosis and low rates of consumption of ADHD drug treatments in Japan. This may be due to the lack of agreement over ADHD at a national policy and health care level, or it may be due to cultural attitudes toward psychotropic drugs; and these factors may themselves be a function of continued stigma associated with mental illness in Japan.

ADHD Advocacy and Diagnostic Migration: Sources and Contributors

The extent to which national education and health policies provide additional services to children may be, in part, a function of the power of ADHD advocacy in the country. We make a distinction between advocacy and migration because we see them as linked activities with potentially different outcomes, to the extent that advocacy activities may or may not enable and support migration of ADHD diagnosis and treatments across international territories. Moreover, this kind of migration may or may not be an explicit or intended goal of ADHD advocacy, whereas activities to promote diagnostic migration will generally involve some level of ADHD advocacy work.

As depicted in this volume, advocacy entails a range of activities, including parent and patient support activities, knowledge production and dissemination, education, and research. Advocacy campaigns frequently involve parents, patients, physicians, and the pharmaceutical industry; moreover, smaller constellations of these stakeholders may engage in distinctive advocacy activities.

Almost all our authors note the work of advocacy groups, except in contexts such as Ghana, Taiwan, and Japan, where stigma, lack of knowledge about ADHD, or both may still make it difficult for such groups to have a public presence. Advocacy groups exist in various forms, with local chapters forming bigger groups (e.g., Centre for ADHD Awareness Canada [CADDAC], Children and Adults with Attention Deficit Hyperactivity Disorder [CHADD] in the United States, and HyperSupers in France); these groups allow parents to access real support groups run by lay members. The chapters in this volume detail the advocacy work of such groups as the HyperSupers in France, ADHD Deutschland in Germany, and the UK Adult ADHD Network (UKAAN) and Attention Deficit Disorder Information and Support Service (ADDISS) in the United Kingdom. The authors of the chapters on Brazil, France, and Portugal note the role that physicians have played in ADHD advocacy, and the connections among pharmaceutical companies, advocacy, and research science emerge in many chapters, including those from Brazil, the United Kingdom, and the United States.

We must also note that advocacy in relation to ADHD does not refer only to advocacy for ADHD diagnosis and treatments. It is also possible that groups organize against ADHD, with some groups seeking to limit the proliferation of ADHD diagnosis and treatment in a country. In many of the countries described in this volume, parent and practitioner groups have organized against ADHD in the name of various agendas for the protection of children. These groups contest the claims about diagnosis and treatment and highlight what they see as the potential dangers of mass diagnosis. In most cases, the key issue is the use of stimulant drugs, with "for" and "against" groups arising to challenge each other's positions. Mobilization for and against ADHD creates a complex situation in which parent groups with shared claims about the child's best interests have opposing agendas in relation to the use of medication. Too often, this contestation quickly becomes ideological and polemical, in which form it frequently ignores the need to provide a balanced argument for what is in the best interests of the child.

ADHD Advocacy and ADHD Migration

Research that takes the form of "citizen science" campaigns (e.g., Edwards et al. 2014) is perhaps the most novel and structurally interesting kind of ADHD advocacy because successful citizen science forges an impactful relationship between parent-patient advocacy and scientific knowledge production. This combination is a powerful way to enable ADHD migration. The strongest example in this volume describes how the French advocacy group HyperSupers conducted the first survey on the epidemiology of ADHD in France in collaboration with the US scientist Stephen Faraone, one of the world's leading ADHD researchers. As a consequence, ADHD came to be viewed by some as a bona fide child mental health concern, even though disputes continue over its etiology and appropriate management and treatment.

A more prosaic, but nonetheless powerful way to enable ADHD migration is in the form of training of local researchers in the biological approach that dominates in the *DSM*. In Brazil, leading ADHD researchers were trained and continue strong collaborations with psychiatrists from the United States, the United Kingdom, and Europe, with the consequence that Brazilian researchers lead the world in a global epidemiological research on ADHD. These researchers do not necessarily engage in ADHD advocacy per se; however, their work has undoubtedly encouraged some degree of Brazilian support of ADHD diagnosis and treatments. Similar influences of training in biological psychiatry and the *DSM* approach on ADHD migration are evident throughout the chapters in this volume.

THE INTERNET AS A CONTRIBUTOR TO ADHD ADVOCACY AND MIGRATION

Although the authors of this volume do not often explicitly refer to the role of the Internet in ADHD advocacy, it is clear that the Internet is a major vehicle for parent-patient advocacy, with online ADHD support groups found in countries across Europe and South America (Conrad and Bergey 2014). There are literally hundreds of online groups, many of which are connected to well-established organizations such as the American-based CHADD or the UK-based ADDISS. Many online sites promote information about the diagnosis or treatment of ADHD and encourage identification and diagnosis, sometimes using checklists for screening or self-diagnosis. Some online groups and websites may be financed by pharmaceutical companies, but others are independent. The more sophisticated websites are aimed at educational or medical professionals, and some outline calls for policy changes (e.g., seeking to shape national guidelines regarding treatment). Because there are no international boundaries on information found on the Internet, we have to assume that online advocacy around ADHD is a powerful driver for global ADHD knowledge production and dissemination and potentially also for the migration of the diagnosis.

BIG PHARMA AS A CONTRIBUTOR TO ADHD ADVOCACY AND MIGRATION

It has become fairly standard to point to the pharmaceutical industry's long-standing role in the growth of ADHD as a diagnosis and in the prescription of stimulant medications. Whether it is promoting ADHD and its treatment to physicians or to the public (e.g., direct-to-consumer advertisements in the United States and New Zealand), pharmaceutical companies work hard to expand their markets. Not only does pharmaceutical promotion contribute to expanding markets globally, but it also works to promote a medical approach to treatment in new internal markets, such as adult ADHD. In this regard, the chapters on Taiwan and the United Kingdom illustrate the pharmaceutical industry's role in continuing medical education. However, what the chapters in this volume also make abundantly clear is that big pharma is rarely if ever an independent actor in ADHD advocacy. In particular, if pharmaceutical industry activities are to go beyond advocacy to achieve migration of diagnosis and treatments, big pharma needs national support at the policy level as well as local institutional partners, in order to facilitate research and regulatory pathways that ultimately lead to penetration of new markets. But it is also evident that market research companies have documented the potential "growth of ADHD markets" in many countries, virtually ensuring an increased global expansion of ADHD diagnoses and treatment (see Conrad and Bergey 2014: 36).

North American Psychiatry and *DSM* Criteria as Contributors to ADHD Migration

The psychiatric profession in the United States has increasingly become dominated by biological psychiatry (Carlat 2010). As the chapter in this volume on the US context illustrates, treatment of ADHD with psychoactive medications both predates the rise of biological psychiatry and serves as an exemplar of the biomedical approach to psychiatric problems. One mechanism by which *DSM*-based diagnostic practice may spread is through physicians receiving training abroad in countries that use the *DSM* diagnostic criteria (e.g., the United States, Canada, and Australia). Having been exposed to the diagnosis and psychoactive treatment of ADHD in these contexts, they may return to their countries of origin bringing such perspectives and practices along with them, as the chapter on Taiwan notes.

As chapters in this volume suggest, psychoanalytic approaches are still strong in some countries (e.g., France, Italy, and Argentina). The lingering importance of psychoanalysis motivates a robust resistance to strict alignment with *DSM* diagnostic criteria for ADHD and to adoption of biological and pharmaceutical approaches to ADHD. These cases, however, are in the minority, and one wonders whether, with the next generation of psychiatrists, biological psychiatry will come to prevail in these regions as well.

For the past few decades, there have been two major systems for diagnosing mental health conditions. In much of Europe until the past decade, a related diagnosis was based on the *ICD-9* and was called "hyperkinetic syndrome." In the United States, Canada, and Australia, the dominant diagnosis of ADHD was based on the American Psychiatric Association's (APA) *DSM*—particularly the *DSM-IV*. Although these diagnoses had much in common (both focused on children with "inattention, impulsivity, and overactivity"), the *ICD-9* had a much stricter set of criteria for diagnosis. Thus, when the *DSM-IV* criteria are adopted in countries that previously used the *ICD*, the threshold for diagnosing certain behavioral characteristics is broadened. The reasons for this change seem to include a desire for standardization of diagnoses, the influence of US psychiatry, and the fact that most of the published research uses the *DSM-IV* (and now the *DSM-5*).

LOCAL CONTRIBUTORS TO ADHD MIGRATION

In addition to the contributors to ADHD advocacy and migration at the macro-level, the chapters in this volume also reveal more local contributors to the migration of ADHD diagnosis and treatment. Relatively idiosyncratic links and relationships play a major role in this migration. For example, when methylphenidate was unavailable in Ireland, Irish families crossed into the United Kingdom for prescriptions, prompting physicians there to engage with Irish physicians around the need to provide ADHD drug treatments in Ireland. Similarly, links between an Argentinian hospital and a Chilean hospital might have facilitated the introduction of methylphenidate in Chile. The authors of the chapter on Ghana note the ways in which a small number of Ghanaian psychiatrists work to achieve an effective balance between local beliefs about appropriate management and treatment of problem child behavior and the approaches of biological psychiatry. Similarly, in Portugal, an interdisciplinary group of professionals works to balance a historical emphasis on "psycho-education" with neuropsychology and with developmental and dimensional approaches to the diagnosis. Such fine-grained accounts of local routes of ADHD migration enable a rich understanding of the dynamics surrounding ADHD globalization, when combined with an understanding of the power of macro-level drivers such as the Internet, the pharmaceutical industry, and the globalizing influence of US psychiatry (Conrad and Bergey 2014).

Selected Observations for Further Examination

As we reflect on the 16 countries described in this volume, we note four particular cross-cutting dimensions of globalization: age, gender, stigma, and inequalities.

THE AGE SPECTRUM

When ADHD was first described in the 1970s, it was suggested that children between the ages of 6 and 13 years could be diagnosed. The disorder was placed in the childhood disorders section of the *DSM-III*, with the view that the majority of children would eventually outgrow the disorder (APA 1980). A new or extended category—adult ADHD—began to emerge in the 1990s in the United States (Conrad and Potter 2000). This category describes adults who have attention and performance problems. As opposed to persons with classic childhood ADHD, those with adult ADHD were not diagnosed in childhood and were most often self-referred in their adult years. This suggests that ADHD has come to be considered a lifespan disorder for which lifetime treatment may be the expectation. Some researchers suggest that roughly 4 million people have adult ADHD in the United States alone (Hinshaw and Scheffler 2014). Many countries beyond the United States still either do not use the definition or do not diagnose and treat adult ADHD. But similar to ADHD in children, adult ADHD as a diagnosis is beginning to be more common and has started to migrate to other countries as well. For example, in less than a decade, the number of adult ADHD clinics in the United Kingdom has grown from less than 5 nationwide to approximately 30 (http://aadduk .org/help-support/specialists-support-and-coaches/).

At the same time, attention is turning to early identification of ADHD. In the United States, the age at which childhood ADHD can be screened and diagnosed has recently been reduced to 4 years (AAP 2011), and an increasing number of preschool-age children are being treated with stimulant drugs (Visser et al. 2015). An emerging research paradigm is investigating treatment of ADHD at the preclinical or prodromal stage in preschool-age children (DuPaul and Kern 2011; Graf and Singh 2015). Thus, ADHD is increasingly described as a set of specific challenges for which different kinds of interventions could be deemed appropriate over the life course.

GENDER BALANCE

In the early days of diagnosing hyperkinetic or hyperactive syndrome (1970s), the gender ratio of boys to girls was typically 10:1. By the late 1980s, the focus changed from hyperactivity to inattention. This led to an increasing number of diagnoses of inattention problems in girls, and the gender ratio narrowed (Rucklidge 2010). In countries in which the authors noted the gender ratio (e.g., Ireland), the ratio of boys to girls is now consistently 3:1 or 4:1. A notable exception, however, is Chile. In this book, the chapter on Chile reports the gender ratio to be roughly 1:3. Overall, it is unclear why the gender ratio is shifting to include more girls; likely drivers are an increased focus on inattention as a discrete symptom of ADHD (without hyperactivity) and an accompanying emphasis on the cognitive symptoms of ADHD rather than on the behavioral symptoms. We expect that biological research into ADHD alongside sociocultural dynamics will influence the gender epidemiology of ADHD such that the disorder will no longer be considered a "disorder of boyhood" (Pollack 1999) in the future.

Stigma

In some countries, it appears that an ADHD diagnosis carries with it a certain amount of stigma that may affect the willingness of doctors to identify, diagnose, and treat ADHD as a disorder. We find this most strongly in Japan and Taiwan, but it is also present in countries that retain a strong psychoanalytic tradition, such as Argentina and France. Societal stigma around ADHD is present in just about all the countries in this book, although European countries are undergoing a change in attitudes toward ADHD. In Germany, as medicalization of ADHD increased, the stigma of an ADHD diagnosis was reduced. In Ireland, ADHD was at first unrecognized. It later became a contested condition, and now it is an accepted disorder. Acceptance does not mean that families are willing to be open and transparent about a child's diagnosis, however. In many countries, parents report feeling stigmatized for pursuing an ADHD diagnosis and treatment for their children. There appears to be a pattern of stigmatization in which a wave of acceptance of the diagnosis is followed by critical media reports of increasing diagnoses, which is followed by societal critique of the diagnosis. This critique does not necessarily mean that parents will choose not to pursue diagnosis for a child, but it may encourage parents to keep a child's diagnosis secret from persons other than key caregivers.

Such dynamics of critique and secrecy inevitably have an impact on a child and may result in self-stigmatization (Singh 2011). We suggest that these dynamics around societal, family, and self-stigma across different settings are important to understand sociologically because they are likely to influence the acceptability of ADHD diagnosis and treatment and the child's experience of ADHD diagnosis and associated behaviors. A productive goal of such studies would be to better understand how to encourage a child's resilience against the harmful effects of stigma, particularly because these are likely to exacerbate difficulties that a child is already experiencing.

Inequalities

The chapters in this book raise other issues about the acceptance of ADHD and its treatment in various countries. These include the role of social class in diagnosis and treatment, as well as the influence of neoliberal regimes and austerity measures, particularly in countries that are just transitioning to acceptance of ADHD diagnosis and treatments. From the evidence available, it is impossible to reach any general conclusions about the relative impacts of social class, cultural values, and national health care policies on rates of ADHD diagnosis and use of diverse treatments across countries. Many countries do not collect data that provide information on the ethnic and racial makeup of people diagnosed with ADHD or treated with stimulant drugs, so we cannot know at this point if some of the disparities found across American settings generalize to other countries. It is also difficult to tell to what degree, if any, advocacy groups and critical or resistance groups are effective in identifying or reducing unequal access to ADHD diagnosis and treatment, on the one hand, or oppressive uses of ADHD diagnosis and treatment, on the other. While compulsory schooling seems to be a major contextual factor related to the emergence of ADHD in society (Hinshaw and Scheffler 2014), the role of schools and teachers in access to diagnosis and treatment and in rates of diagnosis and treatment remains unclear in many countries discussed in this book.

One of our major conclusions of this book is that there is a globalization of the medicalized ADHD diagnosis and treatment, but this process is manifested in sometimes markedly different ways in various countries. At the same time, there is little doubt that diagnosis and treatment of ADHD are becoming worldwide phenomena and can be expected to continue to grow, albeit with different social manifestations and outcomes. These processes make up the grist of the social science mill and are worthy of further systematic research and investigation.

REFERENCES

American Academy of Pediatrics (AAP). 2011. "AAP Expands Ages for Diagnosis and Treatment of ADHD in Children." www.aap.org/en-us/about-the-aap/aap-press-room/pages/AAP-Expands-Ages-for-Diagnosis-and-Treatment-of-ADHD-in-Children.aspx.

American Psychiatric Association (APA). 1980. *Diagnostic and Statistical Manual of Mental Disorders (DSM-III)*. 3rd ed. Washington, DC: American Psychiatric Association.

Carlat, Daniel. 2010. *Unhinged: The Trouble with Psychiatry; A Doctor's Revelations about a Profession in Crisis*. New York: Simon & Schuster.

Conrad, Peter. 1975. "The Discovery of Hyperkinesis: Notes on the Medicalization of Deviant Behavior." *Social Problems* 23 (1): 12–21.

———. 1992. "Medicalization and Social Control." *Annual Review of Sociology* 18: 209–32.

———. 2007. *The Medicalization of Society: On the Transformation of Human Conditions into Treatable Disorders.* Baltimore: Johns Hopkins University Press.

Conrad, Peter, and Meredith R. Bergey. 2014. "The Impending Globalization of ADHD: Notes on the Expansion and Growth of a Medicalized Disorder." *Social Science & Medicine* 122: 31–43.

Conrad, Peter, and Deborah Potter. 2000. "From Hyperactive Children to ADHD Adults: Observations on the Expansion of Medical Categories." *Social Problems* 47 (4): 559–82.

Deleuze, Gilles, and Félix Guattari. 1988. *A Thousand Plateaus: Capitaliam and Schizophrenia.* Translated by Brian Massumi. London: Continuum.

DePaul, George J., and Lee Kern. 2011. *Young Children with ADHD: Early Identification and Intervention.* Washington, DC: American Psychological Association.

Edwards, Claire, Etaoine Howlett, Madeleine Akrich, and Vololona Rabeharisoa. 2014. "Attention Deficit Hyperactivity Disorder in France and Ireland: Parents' Groups' Scientific and Political Framing of an Unsettled Condition." *BioSocieties* 9: 153–72.

Graf, William D., and Ilina Singh. 2015. "Can Guidelines Help Reduce the Medicalization of Early Childhood?" *Journal of Pediatrics* 166 (6): 1344–46.

Hacking, Ian. 1999. *The Social Construction of What?* Cambridge, MA: Harvard University Press.

Hinshaw, Stephen P., and Richard M. Scheffler. 2014. *The ADHD Explosion: Myths, Medication, Money, and Today's Push for Performance.* New York: Oxford University Press.

King, Marissa D., Jennifer Jennings, and Jason M. Fletcher. 2014. "Medical Adaptation to Academic Pressure: Schooling, Stimulant Use, and Socioeconomic Status." *American Sociological Review* 79 (6): 1039–66.

Mayes, Rick, Catherine Bagwell, and Jennifer L. Erkulwater. 2009. *Medicating Children: ADHD and Pediatric Mental Health.* Cambridge, MA: Harvard University Press.

Moffitt, Terrie E., and Maria Melchior. 2007. "Why Does the Worldwide Prevalence of Childhood Attention Deficit Hyperactivity Disorder Matter?" *American Journal of Psychiatry* 146 (6): 856–58.

Parens, Erik, and Josephine Johnston. 2011. "Troubled Children: Diagnosing, Treating, and Attending to Context: A Hastings Center Special Report." *Hastings Center Report* 41 (2): S1–S32.

Polanczyk, Guilherme V., Maurício Silva de Lima, Bernardo Lessa Horta, Joseph Biederman, and Luis Augusto Rohde. 2007. "The Worldwide Prevalence of ADHD: A Systematic Review and Metaregression Analysis." *American Journal of Psychiatry* 164 (6): 942–98.

Polanczyk, Guilherme V., Erick G. Willcutt, Giovanni A. Salum, Christian Kieling, and Luis A. Rohde. 2014. "ADHD Prevalence Estimates across Three Decades: An Updated Systematic Review and Meta-regression Analysis." *International Journal of Epidemiology* 43 (2): 434–42.

Pollack, William. 1999. *Real Boys: Rescuing Our Sons from the Myths of Boyhood*. New York: Holt.

Rucklidge, Julia J. 2010. "Gender Differences in Attention-Deficit/Hyperactivity Disorder." *Psychiatric Clinics of North America* 33 (2): 357–73.

Scheffler, Richard M., Stephen P. Hinshaw, Sepideh Modrek, and Peter Levine. 2007. "The Global Market for ADHD Medications." *Health Affairs* 26 (2): 450–57.

Schwarz, Alan. 2016. *ADHD Nation: Children, Doctors, Big Pharma, and the Making of an American Epidemic*. New York: Scribner.

Singh, Ilina. 2002. "Biology in Context: Social and Cultural Perspectives on ADHD." *Children and Society* 16: 360–67.

———. 2011. "A Disorder of Anger and Aggression: Children's Perspectives on Attention Deficit/Hyperactivity Disorder in the UK." *Social Science & Medicine* 73 (6): 889–96.

Singh, Ilina, Angela M. Filipe, Imre Bard, Meredith Bergey, and Lauren Baker. 2013. "Globalization and Cognitive Enhancement: Emerging Social and Ethical Challenges for ADHD Clinicians." *Current Psychiatry Reports* 15 (9): 385–95.

Soumerai, Stephen B., and Jerry Avorn. 1990. "Principles of Educational Outreach ('Academic Detailing') to Improve Clinical Decision Making." *JAMA* 263 (4): 549–56.

Thomas, Rae, Sharon Sanders, Jenny Doust, Elaine Beller, and Paul Glasziou. 2015. "Prevalence of Attention-Deficit/Hyperactivity Disorder: A Systematic Review and Meta-analysis." *Pediatrics* 135 (4): e994–e1001.

Visser, Susanna N., Rebecca H. Bitsko, Melissa L. Danielson, Reem M. Ghandour, Stephen J. Blumberg, Laura A. Schieve, Joseph R. Holbrook, Mark L. Wolraich, and Steven P. Cuffe. 2015. "Treatment of Attention Deficit/Hyperactivity Disorder among Children with Special Health Care Needs." *Journal of Pediatrics* 166 (6): 1423–30.

Wedge, Marilyn. 2012. "Why French Kids Don't Have ADHD." https://www.psychologytoday.com/blog/suffer-the-children/201203/why-french-kids-dont-have-adhd.

Zuvekas, Samuel H., and Bernedetto Vitiello. 2012. "Stimulant Medication Use among U.S. Children: A Twelve-Year Perspective." *American Journal of Psychiatry* 169 (2): 160–66.

Index

Page numbers in *italics* indicate figures and tables.

Abbott, 195
ADD. *See* attention deficit disorder
Adderall, 15, 102, 266, 299, 379. *See also* psychostimulants
Adderall XR, 39
ADD Midwest (Ireland), 143, 145, 153
ADHD. *See* attention deficit–hyperactivity disorder
ADHD Coaches Organization, 17, 21
ADHD coaching, 17, 21, 25
ADHD Europe, 155–56, 233
Administración Nacional de Medicamentos, Alimentos y Tecnología Médica (Argentina), 163, 174–75
adult ADHD, 13–14, 82, 248, 262, 270, 280, 386; awareness of, 48, 154, 280; coaching and, 25; nonreporting of, 39; practices related to, 87; prevalence rates for, 20. *See also individual nation listings*
advocacy groups, 17, 20–22, 55, 123, 233, 380–82. *See also individual nation listings*
Aedo, Cristián, 318
Ae-Ngibise, K., 365
AFT Pharmaceuticals, 303
Agence Nationale de la Sécurité des Medicaments (France), 239, 240, 249
Agência Nacional de Vigilância Sanitária (Brazil), 187, 190–92
Agenzia Italiana del Farmaco, 210, 212, 216
American Academy of Pediatrics, 24, 129
American Psychiatric Association, 1–2, 9. See also *Diagnostic and Statistical Manual of Disorders*
Americans with Disabilities Act, 13
amphetamines, 10–11, 265. *See also* Adderall; methylphenidate; psychostimulants
Anderson, Jessie, 292, 293

antidepressants, 170–72
anxiolytics, 170
Argentina, 4; ADHD definition in, 179; ADHD diagnosis in, 166, 167–68, 176, 178; ADHD's emergence in, 162; ADHD treatment in, 169–76; analysis in, of ADHD, 162–63, 167; *DSM*'s preeminence in, 179; health care in, 164–65, 169; *ICD-10* in, 179; medicalization in, 164–65; methylphenidate in, 163, 166, 169–76, 180–81; neoliberalism in, 167; opposition in, to psychotropic medication, 175–76; pharmaceutical industry in, 167, 176–79, 181; psychoanalysis in, 165–66; social security sector in, 165; socio-economics in, and ADHD, 169–70
Arizaga, M. Cecilia, 175
Associação Brasileira de Psiquiatria, 199–200, 201
Associação Brasileira de Saúde Mental, 199, 200
Associação Brasileira do Deficit de Atenção, 194–95, 199
Associazione Italiana Famiglie ADHD, 209, 210, 211, 216, 222, 225
Astra-Zeneca, 195
atomoxetine, 171, 173, 174, 176, 265–66, 294. *See also* psychostimulants
attachment theory, 144
attention deficit disorder, 1–2, 12, 80
attention deficit–hyperactivity disorder: acceptance of, 48; adult, 1 (*see also* adult ADHD); advocacy groups and, 6, 17, 14, 380–82; aggression and, 276; age spectrum for, 386; alternative approaches to, 24–25, 35; behaviors related to, 2, 6, 10, 108; blame and, 219–22, 224–25; Brazilian category for, 121; care models for, 124–27; challenges to,

attention deficit–hyperactivity disorder (*cont.*)
6, 22–23, 65–66, 113–15, 322, 345–46, 382;
children's experiences of, 107–8, 272; citizen
science and, 382; comorbidity and, 49,
100, 103, 168, 246–47, 248, 273, 362–63;
confusion about, based on diagnostic
translations, 121–22; as constructed social
object, 224–25; context for, 2, 302, 327,
380–81; definition of, 246; depression and,
276; developmental disorders and, 274, 275;
diagnosis of, 1–2, 17–19, 24, 87, 87–89, 290,
378 (*see also individual nation listings*);
diagnostic migration and, 381–85; diagnostic
threshold for, 378; diet and, 22; as disability,
13–16, 48–49, 61–62, 170, 341, 380–81;
drugs for, 9, 15–17, 19–20, 379–80 (*see also*
Adderall; atomoxetine; methylphenidate;
psychostimulants); as dynamic process, 119;
early identification of, 386; ecological niche
for, 356; educational accommodations for,
380; establishment of, 10–13, 377; etiology
of, 11, 79, 80; factors in, 216; false positives
and, 302; family physicians and, 41; future
for, 23–26; gender and, 17, 19, 37–40, 83–84,
91, 149, 188, 248, 262, 273, 292, 325, 359,
386–87; globalization of, 3, 25–26, 377–79;
"glocalization" of, 355; holistic approach to,
42, 44; vs. hyperkinetic disorder, 2–3;
identity and, 155; international responses to,
3–6; Internet groups for, 383–84; label of,
69; as lifespan disorder, 1, 12–14, 129, 219,
386 (*see also* adult ADHD); management of,
21, 24–25; marketing and, 16–17, 26 (*see also*
pharmaceutical industry); media coverage
of, 114–15; medicalization of, 64, 78, 81, 85,
256, 333–35, 347–48; migration of, 382–85;
mild, 69; as multifaceted problem, 130–31;
multidisciplinary approach to, 82, 193 (*see
also* multimodal treatment); national health
care systems and, 379–80 (*see also individual
nation listings*); as natural kind, 378; as
neurodevelopmental disorder, 81, 278, 338;
niche model for, 356–57; noninstitutional-
ization of, 372–73; nonmedical services for,
44–46, 380; nosography of, 210; overdiagnosis of, 22, 23, 24, 83; parents and, 101, 150
(*see also* parents); patient types, 89;
persistence rates of, 84; pharmaceuticalization of, 290; positive attributes of, 155;
predecessors to, 10–12; prevalence of, 2, 6,
9, 17–19, 24, 56, 91, 98–100, 377, 378;
prodromal, 116; professional groups and, 6;
psychoanalytic approaches to, 384; school
entry age and, 38; scientific publications on,
worldwide, 237; Scientologists and, 22–23;
social control and, 85; as social phenomenon, 7, 70, 254, 276, 277; socioeconomics
and, 6, 169–70; stigmatization and, 107–8,
380, 387 (*see also* stigmatization); subtypes
of, 14, 55, 82, 273; suburban dynamics and,
381; symptoms of, 2, 238, 275 (*see also*
attention deficit–hyperactivity disorder:
diagnosis of); three-dimensional image of,
97–98; traditional Chinese medicine and,
348; treatment of, 2, 6, 24–25, 124, 155, 379
(*see also individual nation listings*); types of,
214; underdiagnosis of, 146, 169; unifying
theory for, 122; as unsettled condition,
240–49; validity of, 23; vocabulary for,
158n4; worldwide diagnoses of, 1, 37, 292, 378
Attention Deficit Disorder Association (US),
17, 21
Attention Deficit Disorder Information and
Support Service (UK), 6, 382
Attention Deficit Hyperactivity Disorder
Rating Scale, 272, 273, 279
Australia, 4, 61–63; ADHD diagnosis in,
58–60; ADHD guidelines in, 56–58, 66–67;
ADHD prevalence in, 56, 187; ADHD's
acceptance in, 55; ADHD's emergence in,
54–58; ADHD treatment in, 57–60, 67–68;
antimedication views in, 64–66; educational system in, 58, 60, 61–63; health care
system in, 58, 61–63; identity development
in; medication usage in, 26, 54–56, 294,
295; national identity in, 68; perceptions in,
of society's medicalization, 64; pharmaceutical industry in, 57, 70; public debate in,
about ADHD, 64–66; student support policy
in, 61–63; support groups in, 70; US
influence in, 54
autism spectrum disorder, 63, 262–63, 274,
275–76
Autism Spectrum Screening Questionnaire, 273
A-Zee of ADHD (Hadd Ireland), 151
Azevêdo, Paulo, 188

Bachelet, Michelle, 319
Bagwell, Catherine, 16
Banaschewski, Tobias, 233
Banzato, Claudio, 201–2
Barkley, Russell A., 23, 47, 86, 122, 285, 312–13

Barthe, Yannick, 241
Basaglia, Franco, 197
Bascuñan, Caroliña, 324
Baylé, Franck, 233
behavior, 334, 367–69: ADHD-related, 2, 6,
    10, 108; brain damage and, 11; expectations
    for, 261–62, 264–65, 313–18; genetics and,
    225; management of, 216–17, 284; as moral
    failing, 78–79
behavioral therapy, 336
Belgium, medication usage in, 26
Benasayag, León, 167
Berbatis, Constantine, 292
Bergey, Meredith, 178, 181, 292
biological psychiatry, 384
biomedicalization, 164–65
biopower, 164
biosocial communities, 91
biosociality, 93n13, 164
biotechnology, 90, 164
Birleson Depression Self-Rating Scale for
    Children, 273
blame, discourses of, 218, 219–22, 224–25
Boakye, Kwashie, 369
Boletín de la Sociedad de Psiquiatría y Neu-
    rología de la Infancia y Adolescencia (Bulletin
    of the Society of Psychiatry and Neurology of
    Childhood and Adolescence; Chile), 311–12, 316
Bonati, Maurizio, 213
Bowlby, John, 144
Bradley, Charles, 10–11
Bradley Home (RI), 10–11
Bradshaw, Maria, 156
brain damage, behavior and, 11
brain malfunction, moral control and, 79
Branson, Richard, 155
Brazil, 4, 26, 187, 197, 201; ADHD activism in,
    193; ADHD diagnosis in, 186; ADHD policy
    in, 199; ADHD prevalence in, 187–89, 192;
    ADHD treatment in, 186, 192, 193; ADHD's
    emergence in, 189–90; ADHD's medicaliza-
    tion in, 198, 200; Constitution of, 196–97;
    local researchers trained in, 383; medication
    control in, 190–92; mental health care in,
    196–98; methylphenidate production in,
    190; methylphenidate regulation in,
    198–200; methylphenidate use in, 190–93,
    196; patient support groups in, 193–95;
    pharmaceutical industry in, 194–96
Breggin, Peter, 23, 36
Bristol-Myers-Squibb, 194–95

Bröer, C., 357
Bronfenbrenner, Urie, 107
Brown, Thomas E., 154
bullying, 106–7, 108
Bulsara, Max, 292
Busfield, Joan, 290, 291–92, 297–98, 299
Buss-Perry Aggression Questionnaire, 273

Cabalin, Cristian, 312
Cabral Barros, J. Augusto, 176
Caiani, Manuela, 156
Callon, Michel, 241
Cameron, David, 106
Canada, 4; accommodations in, for ADHD, 46;
    ADHD assessment in, 41; ADHD clinical
    guidelines in, 40, 42–46, 49–50; ADHD
    diagnosis in, 37–43, 45; ADHD treatment
    in, 37–46; ADHD's legitimation in, 48–49;
    adult ADHD in, 39, 48; advocacy groups in,
    34, 40, 42, 43, 46–49; CHADD in, 35;
    educational system in, and ADHD, 44–46;
    medication usage in, 26, 37, 56, 239, 294;
    suspicion in, about ADHD, 34–37; US
    influence in, 34–37, 43
Canadian ADHD Resource Alliance, 40,
    42–46, 47
Caponi, Sandra, 171
Carbajal, Mariana, 175
Carey, David, 144
Carlini, Elisaldo A., 192
Cassels, Alan, 176, 178
Centre for ADHD Awareness Canada, 43,
    47–48, 381
Céspedes, Amanda, 323
CHADD. *See* Children and Adults with
    Attention-Deficit / Hyperactivity Disorder
CHADD-Canada, 47
Childers, Nessa, 156
child guidance clinics, 335–36
childhood: medicalization of, 131, 186, 200;
    pathologization of, 162, 163, 180; risk and,
    218–19, 224
child psychiatry, 144, 148, 152, 316; network
    approach to, 333–47
Children and Adolescent Mental Health
    Services, 138, 147, 148–49
Children and Adults with Attention-
    Deficit / Hyperactivity Disorder (US), 6, 14,
    17, 21, 35, 46–47, 48, 178, 382
Children's Mental Health Center (Taiwan),
    335–39, 344

Chile, 4, 318; ADHD denounced in, 322; ADHD guidelines in, 310–11, 320; ADHD management in, 320–21; ADHD prevalence in, 315–18, 320, 321–22, 325; ADHD's emergence in, 312–13, 316–18; ADHD studies in, 310–11, 321–27; ADHD treatments in, 323; childhood behavior in, attitudes toward, 313–18; child psychiatry in, 316; educational model in, for ADHD, 326; educational system in, 318–21, 323; hyperkinetic disorders in, 325–26; methylphenidate use in, 313, 314–18, 322–24; public health system in, 321–22; Ritalin generation in, 315, 317
China, medication usage in, 26
Christian prayer camps, 364
Church of Scientology, 22–23, 113–14
Ciba, 313
citizen science, 382
Classification française de troubles mentaux de l'enfant et de l'adolescent, 179
clínica ampliada (amplified clinic), 198
Close Up (Argentina), 177
coaching, 21, 25
cognitive behavioral therapy, 82, 129, 210, 216, 284
cognitive enhancement, 87–89
Cohen, David, 291
Colombia, ADHD prevalence in, 187
combined type (ADHD subtype), 14
Common Health (Taiwan), 344
Concerta, 15, 19, 110, 126, 195, 266, 294, 342, 343. See also methylphenidate
conduct disorder, 103
conduct niche, 356
Conners tests, 129, 272, 316, 336
Conrad, Peter, 64, 70, 85, 164, 176, 178, 181, 292
contextualization, 87–88
Corboz, Robert, 80
Coridys (France), 250
Cornoldi, Cesare, 215
corporal punishment, 365, 369–70
Couillard, Cory, 364
Council on US Aid, 335
courtesy stigma, 365
Cruise, Tom, 22

Danquah, Samuel, 359
Darling, Rosalyn Benjamin, 223–24
Davies, Julie, 224

Decreto 170 (Chile), 312, 318–20
De la Barra, Flora, 325
Della Porta, Donatella, 156
democratic psychiatry movement, 197
Denhoff, Eric, 11
Der Struwwelpeter (Hoffmann), 10
developmental coordination disorder, 273–76
developmental disabilities, 278
developmental disorders: ADHD and, 274, 275; symptoms of, 273
deviant behavior, medicalization of, 334
dexamfetamine, 99, 102
Dexedrine, 294
diagnosis, as social act, 217
Diagnostic Interview for ADHD in Adults (Kooij and Franken), 129
diagnostic masking, 168
Diagnostic and Statistical Manual of Disorders (American Psychiatric Association), 1, 9, 99–100, 200, 214, 362, 384; DSM-II, 12, 337; DSM-III, 1–2, 12, 17, 80, 121, 179, 245, 293, 339; III-R, 2, 12, 81, 168, 292–93, 313, 339; DSM-IV, 3, 12, 14, 26, 43, 57, 80–81, 82, 167, 186, 188, 245–46, 290, 293, 320, 342, 346, 385; DSM-IV-R, 210; DSM-IV-TR, 278; DSM-5, 3, 24, 26, 37, 43, 55–56, 60, 81, 180, 278, 337; adoption of, increasing, 378; in Canada, 35; diagnostic criteria of, 3; opposition to, 162; translation of, 121–22
diagnostic substitution, 63
Didoni, Anna, 215
direct-to-consumer advertising, 16, 111, 177–79
disability, 13–14. See also attention deficit–hyperactivity disorder: as disability
disability tax credits, 48–49
disease, manufacturers of, 303
disease regime, 140
Donzelot, Jacques, 170
Duchess of Cambridge, 106
Dueñas, Gabriela, 167
Dugas, Michel, 235, 238, 248, 255–56
Duke of Cambridge, 106
Dumit, Joe, 138
DuPaul, George, 297

ecological model, 107
ecological niche, 356
Edumadze, Isaac, 369
Ehrenberg, Alain, 171
Eli Lilly, 110, 112, 194, 195
El Mercurio (Chile), 312

Elvanse, 110, 111
environmental coordination, 266
epidemiology, gaps in, 377–78
epistemic community, 242–45
Erkulwater, Jennifer, 16
Europe, ADHD advocacy in, 155–56. *See also individual nation listings*
evidence-based activism, 140, 143

family interventions, 129
family status, ADHD diagnosis and, 18
Farah, Martha J., 24
Faraone, Silvia, 175
Faraone, Stephen V., 248–49, 382
Farmoz, 126
Fayyad, John, 84
Feingold, Ben, 22
Fergusson, David, 293
"Fidgety Philip" (Hoffmann), 10, 77–78
Fitzgerald, Michael, 144, 156
Fórum sobre Medicalização da Educação e da Sociedade (Brazil), 193, 200–201
Foucault, Michel, 140, 164, 177
France, 3, 4, 234, 379; ADHD assessment in, 253–54; ADHD debate in, 233–35, 236, 254, 256–57; ADHD diagnosis in, 251–54; ADHD prevalence in, 247–49; ADHD reports in, 239–54; ADHD screening in, 251–52; ADHD's emergence in, 233–39, 255; ADHD treatment in, 234, 249–54; adult ADHD in, 248; advocacy organizations in, 240; educational support in, 250–51; epistemic community in, 242–45; health system in, 249–50; labels in, for ADHD, 245–46; methylphenidate use in, 238–39, 249; prescribing conditions in, 300; working groups in, 255
Frazzetto, Giovanni, 217
Freier, Antonio, 188
Fuchs, Flavio D., 188
Fukuyama, Francis, 90

Galanakis, Emmanouil, 26
Galvez, Karim, 317
Gau, Shur-Fen, 342
geography, ADHD diagnosis and, 19
Georgieff, Nicolas, 254
Germany, 4, 26; ADHD contested in, 77; ADHD defined as disease in, 91; ADHD guidelines in, 81–82; ADHD persistence in, 84; ADHD prevalence in, 83–84; ADHD's

emergence in, 78–81, 235; ADHD's medicalization in, 81; ADHD treatment in, 82, 84; adult ADHD in, 82; advocacy groups, 86; concern in, over methylphenidate, 90; health care system in, 83, 379; methylphenidate use in, 81, 86, 127; moral system in, 78–79; neuro-enhancement in, 91–92; prescription regulation in, 82–83; reactions in, to ADHD, 85–86; self-help groups in, 85
Gétin (Gétin-Vergnaud), Christine, 233, 248, 250, 252
Ghana, 4; ADHD advocacy in, 363–64; ADHD diagnosis in, 357–58, 361–63, 367–69; ADHD guidelines in, 361; ADHD in, ecological perspective on, 371–72; ADHD introduced in, 354–55; ADHD noninstitutionalized in, 372–73; ADHD treatment in, 355, 361–63, 365–66, 369–70; children in, ADHD facilities for, 361; corporal punishment in, 365, 369–70; disrespect in, 366–69; disruptive behavior in, 367–69; educational system in, 359; financial resources in, 355; gerontocratic culture in, 366–69; health care system in, 364–65; intergenerational relations in, 366, 369, 371; mental health in, approach to, 355, 357–58, 360–66; methylphenidate in, 361, 363; National Insurance Scheme in, 363; respect niche in, 372; school performance in, 355, 370–71; social capital in, 359; stigmatization in, 365–66; traditional healing in, 364–65
Giù le mani dai bambini (Italy), 209, 210, 211
GlaxoSmithKline, 194
globalization, 3, 25–26, 327, 377–79, 388
Global South, ADHD in, 354
Göllnitz, Gerhard, 80
Golse, Bernard, 238, 246, 248
Gomes, R., 192
Goodman, Robert D. Neves dos Santos, 188
Griesinger, Wilhelm, 78
Guardiola, Ana, 188

Haas, Peter M., 242
Habilidades para la Vida (Skills for Life; Chile), 321
Hacking, Ian, 378
HADD Cork (Hyperactive Attention Deficit Disorders Cork; Ireland), 142
HADD Ireland, 144, 154, 155
Hamamatsu School Cohort (Japan), 272–76

"Hans Guck-in-die-Luft" ("Johnny Head-in-Air; Hoffmann"), 77–78
Harman, Jeffrey S., 20
hattatsu shogai, 262–63, 264, 278
Haut Comité de la Santé Publique (France), 239, 245
Haute Autorité de la Santé (France), 240, 242
Hawthorne, Daniel, 292
health activism, 140
Hess, David J., 149
Hinshaw, Stephen P., 26
HKD. See hyperkinetic disorder
Hoagwood, Kimberly, 20
Hoffmann, Heinrich, 10, 77
Horton-Salway, Mary, 220
Horwood, John, 293
Hsu, Chen-Chin, 336, 340
Humphreys, Tony, 144–45, 148
hyperactive syndrome, 11
hyperactivity, 2, 12, 119, 120; adulthood, 13; American phenomenon, 291; gendered aspect of, 121–22; knowledge of, in Australia, 55; as medical condition, 122–23; prioritizing, 121
hyperkinesis, 11, 337
hyperkinetic disorder, 2–3, 55, 79–81, 82, 99–100, 325–26
hyperkinetic impulse disorder, 11
hyperkinetic reaction (syndrome) of childhood, 12, 338, 339
HyperSupers (France), 6, 233, 235–38, 240, 249–50, 250, 252–53, 255–56, 382

ICD. See International Classification of Diseases
Iceland, medication usage in, 26, 56, 239, 288, 294
IDEA. See Individuals with Disabilities Education Act
impulsivity, 2, 10–12, 81, 82, 120–21, 216, 275–76, 341
IMS Health, 26
inattention, 2, 10–12, 17, 24, 79, 121, 169, 193, 220, 262, 273–76, 341, 372
INCB. See International Narcotics Control Board
Individuals with Disabilities Education Act (US), 13–14, 341
Institut National de la Santé et de la Recherche Médicale (INSERM; France), 240, 241, 242, 245–48, 251–52, 255–56

International Classification of Diseases (WHO), 2, 26, 35, 362, 378; ICD-9, 81, 338, 385; ICD-10, 55, 67, 80–81, 82, 91, 99–100, 179, 186, 214, 245
International Monetary Fund, 152, 165
International Narcotics Control Board, 16, 26, 175, 190, 191, 288, 292, 294, 322, 378–79
Ireland, 3, 4, 140–41; ADHD as psychiatric disorder in, 148–49; ADHD diagnosis in, 150; ADHD in educational realm, 149; ADHD organizations in, 153–56; ADHD prevalence in, 146, 148–49; ADHD's emergence in, 138–39, 141–48; ADHD support groups in, 138; ADHD therapies in, 150; ADHD treatment in, 151, 153–54; ADHD underdiagnosed in, 146; adult ADHD in, 154; child psychiatry in, 144, 148, 152; demand in, for mental health services, 152; disability legislation in, 141; health activism in, 140, 153–56; health care system in, 141, 150–51, 152, 154, 157; knowledge dissemination in, 140; methylphenidate use in, 147, 150–51; parental blame in, 144; public opinion in, on ADHD, 149–50, 155; specialist ADHD centers in, 146; special needs assistance in, 141; support groups in, 141, 142
Iriart, Celia, 176
Irish National Council of ADHD Support Groups, 140, 142, 143–44, 146, 154–55
Israel, medication usage in, 26, 288, 294, 295
Istituto Superiore di Sanità (Italy), 212, 215, 216
Itaborahy, Claudia, 196
Italy, 3, 4; ADHD diagnosis in, 211–14, 218, 226; ADHD legislation and public policy in, 211–14; ADHD narratives in, 217–25; ADHD prevalence in, 214–16; ADHD regional reference centers in, 212–13, 216, 217; ADHD's emergence in, 208–11, 219; ADHD treatment in, 211–14, 216–17, 226; adult ADHD in, 215, 217; advocacy groups in, 209; national ADHD register in, 212–13, 215–16; psychostimulant use in, 210–14

Janin, Beatriz, 167
Janssen-Cilag, 17, 110, 194, 195, 364
Janssen-Cilag Taiwan, 342, 343, 344
Japan, 4, 283; ADHD assessment in, 272; ADHD classifications in, 262; ADHD diagnosis guidelines in, 279–80; ADHD

prevalence in, 262, 270–74; ADHD-related legislation in, 276–78; ADHD's emergence in, 263–65, 272; ADHD's medicalization in, 261, 262–63; ADHD stigma in, 261–65, 270; ADHD treatment in, 266, 279–80, 281–82; adult ADHD in, 262, 270, 280; autism spectrum disorder and ADHD in, 262–63; childhood behavioral expectations in, 261–62, 264–65; chronic conditions in, cultural understanding of, 280–83; conformity in, 284; disability rights in, 267; environmental coordination in, 266; health care delivery in, 261; medical culture in, 266; medications in, 265–67; negative attitudes in, toward pharmacotherapy, 261, 265–67, 280; nonstimulant drug therapy in, 261; psychosocial ADHD treatment in, 280–83; schooling in, for disabled students, 278–79
Jaque, José Miguel, 315–17
Jornal Brasileiro de Psiquiatria, 195–96

Keenan, Sinéad, 217
Kelleher, Kelly J., 20
Kendall, Tim, 101–2
Kildea, Sarah, 224
Killelea, Deirdre, 143–44
Kirk, Stuart, 290
Klawiter, Maren, 140, 142, 153
Kleinman, Arthur, 336
Konofal, Eric, 248–49
Kraak, Victor, 357
Kramer, Franz, 2, 10, 79–80
Kramer-Pollnow syndrome, 10

Lakoff, Andrew, 177, 224
Lamensdorff, A. M., 365
Lang, Jack, 251
Lange, Michael, 84
Larraín, Soledad, 324
Lascoumes, Pierre, 241
Latour, Bruno, 139
Laufer, Maurice, 11
lay experts, 223–24
Le Carnet Psy, 245–46
Lecendreux, Michel, 248–49
Lee, Chia-Yan, 345–46, 348
Lempp, Reinhart, 80
Lévi-Strauss, Claude, 311
Ley Nacional de Salud Mental 26.657 (Argentina), 162–63, 178, 179–80, 181n1
L'hyperactivité chez l'enfant (Dugas), 235

Lilly Taiwan, 343
Lin, Tsung-Yi, 338
Linden, W., 365
lisdexamfetamine, 99
Lynskey, Michael, 293

Malacrida, Claudia, 40
managed care, 15, 164
Maniowicz, Deborah, 175
Margozzini, Paula, 325
Maschietto, Dino, 215
Mattos, Paulo, 192
Mayes, Rick, 16, 312–13
MBD. *See* minimal brain dysfunction
McCabe, Sean Esteban, 23–24
McGee, Rob, 292–93
McKinlay, John, 303
McNicholas, Fiona, 146, 156
medicalization, 64, 69–71, 85, 164, 256, 262–63, 333–34, 376–77; bottom-up, 91; of children, 125; defined, 164; of deviant behavior, 334; dynamics of, 89, 91; methylphenidate and, 238–39; self-governed, 86–87; stages of, 334
medical-pharmacological model, 124, 126–27
Medicating Kids (PBS), 23
medications-first approach, 379
mental control, 165
mental disorders: vs. medical diseases, 202; standardized assessment of, 338–39
mental health, diagnostic systems for, 384–85. See also *Diagnostic and Statistical Manual of Disorders*; *International Classification of Diseases*
methylphenidate (Ritalin), 2, 15, 81, 266; consumption of, 288, 289, 290, 292, 378–79 (*see also individual nation listings*); criticism of, 22, 36; efficacy of, 301; modifications in, 171–72; need for, 85; overuse of, 290; regulation of, 85; research on, 322–23; warnings about, 174, 176, 301; world production of, 190. *See also* psychostimulants
mindfulness, 155
minimal brain damage, 11, 80
minimal brain dysfunction, 1, 11–12, 80, 120, 337–38
Ministère de la Santé (France), 234, 239–40, 250, 252
Ministère de l'Education (France), 234, 240, 250
Ministerio de Educación (Chile), 310, 321

Ministerio de Salud (Chile), 310, 321, 324, 326
minority groups, ADHD diagnosis and, 18
Montenegro, Hernán, 314
Morgan, Paul J., 18
Motora, Yuzero, 262
Moyano Walker, José M., 167
Moynihan, Ray, 176, 178
Moysés, Maria Aparecida, 193, 200
multimodal treatment, 213–14, 216, 217
Multimodal Treatment Study of ADHD
    (NIMH; US), 295, 301, 304
Mylan, 126

Nakamura, Kazuhiko, 270
National Health Insurance (Taiwan), 332,
    342–43, 347
National Health and Medical Research
    Council (Australia), 57, 66
National Health Service (UK), 98, 110
National Institute for Clinical and Care
    Excellence (UK), 99–103, 110
National Survey of Children's Health, 17, 18
natural kind, 378
neoliberalism, 167, 177
Netherlands, ADHD in, 3, 26, 235
Neumärker, Klaus-Jürgen, 79–80
neuro-enhancing, 90–92
neurofeedback, 82, 129
New Zealand, 4; ADHD Clinical Practice
    Guidelines, 293; ADHD prevalence in,
    292–93; ADHD treatment in, 295; adult
    ADHD in, 295–97; cost of living in,
    299–300; health care system in, 294,
    297–303, 379; prescribing conditions in,
    300; psychostimulant use in, 290–91,
    294–303; regulatory agencies in, 300–301
Nomura, Kenji, 270
nonstimulant drug therapy, 261
Norway, medication usage in, 26
Novartis, 17, 123, 194, 195, 303
Novartis Taiwan, 337–39, 342

Ofori-Atta, A., 365
Ohnishi, Masafumi, 270
Ohnuki-Tierney, Emiko, 280
Oliver, Jamie, 155
Ortega, Francisco, 196
Ouakil, Diane Purper, 233

Panei, Pietro, 213
parental entrepreneurs, 223–24

parents: associations of, 154, 209, 222–25;
    attitudes of, 108–9; blame and, 144, 221,
    224; involvement of, 105–6, 340; training
    of, 101, 129, 216–17, 284–85
Parsons, Talcott, 88, 92n1
pathologization, 209
performance niche, 356
PHARMAC (New Zealand), 298–300
pharmaceutical detailing, 380
pharmaceutical industry, 16–17, 26; ADHD
    advocacy and, 70, 110, 156, 383–84; ADHD
    education and, 110–11; ADHD migration
    and, 383–84; benefits for, of subsidized
    medication, 303; marketing by, 36–37, 70,
    110–12, 176–77, 193, 343–44, 380; research
    linked to, 66, 195–96; worldwide sales of,
    288–90
pharmaceuticalization, 288–92
Philalithis, Anastas, 26
physician-oriented marketing, 177–79
Pillen für den Störenfried (Pills for the Trouble-
    maker; Voss), 85
Pinochet, Augusto, 318
Polanczyk, Guilherme V., 26, 192, 325, 378
Pollnow, Hans, 2, 10
Pondé, Milena Pereira, 188
Ponnow, Hans, 79–80
Portugal, 3, 4, 126–27; ADHD contested in,
    123–24; ADHD diagnosis in, 128–29; ADHD
    prevalence in, 127–28; ADHD's emergence
    in, 118–19, 122–24; ADHD studies in, 128;
    ADHD treatment in, 124–29; advocacy
    groups in, 123; challenges in, for future of
    ADHD, 130–32; child mental health in, 120;
    pharmacological model in, 127; psychiatric
    practice in, 120; psycho-pedagogic
    treatment in, 379; psychostimulants
    licensed in, 126; public health in, 131–32;
    special education in, 125–26
poverty, ADHD and, 104, 105
prodromal ADHD, 116
psychiatric biomarker discovery, 100
psychoanalysis, 165–67
psycho-behavioral therapy, 216
Psychological Society of Ireland, 148
psychopedagogic model, 124–26
psychosocial-first approach, 379
psychosocial maladaptation, 273, 275–76
psychosocial treatment, 280–83
psychostimulants, 2; adverse effects of, 345;
    early use of, 10–11; globalization of, 293–94;

US use of, 9. *See also* Adderall; Concerta;
methylphenidate; Strattera
psychotherapy, methylphenidate and, 196
psychotropic drugs, 22

Quality Standard on ADHD (NICE; UK), 101,
102–3

Rabinow, Paul, 164
Re, Anna Maria, 215
Rebelo, José, 121
reciprocity, 366, 369, 371
Report on Attention Deficit Disorder in Ireland
(Joint Committee on Health and Children),
145–47
Revista YA, 312, 313–14, 317–18
Ritalin. *See* methylphenidate
Ritalina LA, 126
Ritalin-SR, 294, 298, 300
Rodríguez, Francisco, 315–17
Rohde, Luis Augusto, 192
Rojas, Jorge, 313, 328n1, 323
Rose, Nikolas, 170
Rosenberg, Charles, 123
Rothenberger, Aribert, 233
Rotta, Newra T., 188
Rubifen, 126, 294
Rubifen-SR, 294, 298, 300
Ruiz, Alfredo, 315
Russell, Ginny, 104

Sandoz, 126
Santos, Boaventura de Sousa, 119, 327
Sapelli, Claudio, 318
Sarkozy, Nicolas, 251
Saul, Richard, 322
Scheffler, Richard M., 26
Schlander, Michael, 83
School Education Act (Japan), 276–78
Schubert, Ingrid, 81
Schwarz, Alan, 114
Schwarz, Oliver, 83
Schwerdtfeger, Walter, 82
Scientology. *See* Church of Scientology
self, contextualization of, 87–88
Self-Concept Scales, 129
self-help, 85, 165
self-legitimation, discourse of, 218, 222–24
self-stigmatization, 387
Sept, Carla, 233–34
Sepúlveda, Juan, 314

Shire Labs, 17, 110, 111, 156, 194, 303
Shorter, Edward, 171
Singh, Ilina, 189, 217, 248, 356, 371
Skounti, Maria, 26
Smith, M. Elizabeth, 24
social control, 64, 78, 85
social factors, ADHD and, 103–5
social movements, 142, 193–94
Società Italiana di neuropsichiatria
dell'infanzia e dell'adolescenza, 211, 214, 215
socioeconomic status, ADHD treatment and,
67–68
sociomedical disorders, 90
Solomons, Gerald, 11
Soong, Wei-Tsuen, 339
South Africa, ADHD in, 354
Spain, 127, 187, 235, 295
specific language impairment, 250–51
Spronk, Rachel, 357
Stevens, Jack, 20
Stevens, Rozanne, 155
Stiglitz, Gustavo, 167
stigmatization, 261–65, 336–37, 365–66,
380, 387
Still, George Frederic, 2, 10, 79, 313
stimulants, 15–17, 19–20, 22, 56, 59–60;
cognitive enhancement and, 87–89;
German regulation of, 82–83; information
about, 111; used for cognitive enhancement,
23–24. *See also* Adderall; methylphenidate;
psychostimulants
Strattera, 39, 99, 110, 265–66, 294, 299, 300,
343
Strümpell, Ludwig, 79
Sunderland, Bruce, 292
support groups, 46–49, 70, 110, 141, 142, 156,
193–95, 383–84
Sweden, medication usage in, 26, 295
Switzerland, psychostimulant use in, 288, 294,
295
Szasz, Thomas, 23

Taipei Municipal East-Gate Elementary
School, 337
Taiwan, 4; ADHD management in, 341–42;
ADHD prevalence in, 332–33, 342; ADHD's
medicalization in, 333–35, 347–48; ADHD's
reconceptualization in, 346; ADHD's
validity questioned in, 345–46; ADHD
treatment in, 343–45; adopting the DSM
system, 339; American medical model in, 333;

Taiwan (*cont.*)
 behavioral therapy introduced to, 336; child
  psychiatry in, 333–47; democratization
  of, 340; direct-to-consumer advertising
  prohibited in, 344; National Health
  Insurance in, 342–43, 347; pharmaceutical
  companies in, 342–44, 347; psychostimulants in, 338–39, 342–45; reframing ADHD,
  340–41; school counseling profession in,
  337; special education in, 341; stigmatization in, of "craziness," 336–37
Taiwanese Society of Child and Adolescent
  Psychiatry, 340, 342, 346
Tanaka, Yasuo, 283
Taylor, Eric, 114, 233
TDAH (trouble déficit de l'attention/
  hyperactivité), 246, 255
*Terremotos y Soñadores (Earthquakes and
  Dreamers)*, 167
Teruyama, Junko, 262–63
THADA (trouble hyperactivité avec déficit de
  l'attention), 248–49
Thomas, Rae, 26, 377
Timimi, Sami, 113, 114
toxic childhood, rhetoric of, 220
traditional Chinese medicine, ADHD and, 348
transcendental meditation, 165
Trott, Götz Erik, 83
Twum-Danso, Afua, 366

Uchiyama, Satoshi, 270
UN Convention on the Rights of the Child,
  162, 163, 180, 181n1
UNICEF, 324
United Kingdom, 3, 4, 97; ADHD advocacy in,
  109–12; ADHD best practices in, 102–3;
  ADHD diagnosis in, 98–100, 102–3, 108–9;
  ADHD guidelines in, 8; ADHD prevalence
  in, 98–100, 109, 187; ADHD's emergence in,
  235; ADHD treatment in, 42, 100; bullying
  in, 106; conduct disorder in, 103; emotional
  reticence in, 108–9; health care system in,
  99–102, 297–98, 379–80; licensed drug
  treatments in, 99–102; national values of,
  98; parental attitudes in, 108–9; pharmaceutical industry in, 110–12; poverty in, and

ADHD, 104, 105; pre-licensing restrictions
  in, 111, 112; response in, to ADHD, 98,
  107–8; schooling in, and ADHD, 104–9;
  Scientology in, 113–14; social factors in, and
  ADHD, 103–9
United States, 2, 3, 4; ADHD as disability in,
  341; ADHD diagnosis in, 17–19; ADHD
  established in, 10–13; ADHD medication in,
  379–80; ADHD prevalence in, 17–19, 293,
  378; ADHD's emergence in, 235; ADHD's
  future in, 23–26; ADHD treatment in,
  19–20, 42, 290, 293–94; adult ADHD in,
  295–97; advocacy groups in, 20–22;
  biological psychiatry and, 384; challenges
  in, to ADHD, 22–23; child guidance clinics
  in, 335–36; international influence in,
  34–37, 43, 54, 335; market in, for ADHD
  drugs, 16; medication use in, 56, 239, 266,
  293–94; prescribing conditions in, 295, 300;
  socioeconomic status in, and ADHD
  treatment, 68; US Food and Drug Administration, 15, 16; US Supreme Court, 15–16
Uruguay, ADHD in, 166

Vallée, Manuel, 256, 292
Visacovsky, Sergio E., 166
Vision for Change, A (government of Ireland), 148
VOICES (Voices on Identity Childhood, Ethics
  and Stimulants: Children Join the Debate)
  study (UK), 107, 109, 111
Vyvanse, 15, 39, 99, 110

Web, Elspeth, 103–4
Werry, John, 292, 293
WHO. *See* World Health Organization
Working Group for Guidelines on the
  Diagnosis and Treatment of ADHD (Japan),
  279, 280, *281–82*
World Health Organization, 2, 26, 324, 335,
  336, 338, 339, 360
Wright, John, 224

"Zappelphillipp" (Fidgety Philip; Hoffmann),
  10, 77–78
Zola, Irving, 90
Zorzanelli, Rafaela, 201–2